Otolaryngology Study Guide

Nikolaos Tsetsos • Marios Stavrakas
Konstantinos Garefis
Editors

Otolaryngology Study Guide

A Case-Based Approach

Springer

Editors
Nikolaos Tsetsos
ENT Head and Neck Surgery Department
424 General Military Hospital
Thessaloniki, Greece

Konstantinos Garefis
2nd Academic ORL, Head and Neck Surgery Department
Aristotle University of Thessaloniki, Papageorgiou Hospital
Thessaloniki, Greece

Marios Stavrakas
ENT Head and Neck Surgery Department
University Hospitals Plymouth NHS Trust
Plymouth, UK

ISBN 978-3-031-77373-0 ISBN 978-3-031-77374-7 (eBook)
https://doi.org/10.1007/978-3-031-77374-7

This Springer imprint is published by the registered company Springer Nature Switzerland AG
The registered company address is: Gewerbestrasse 11, 6330 Cham, Switzerland

To my wife, Katerina

To my children, Filippos and Alexandros

Nikolaos Tsetsos

To my parents, Dimitrios and Amalia

Marios Stavrakas

To my parents, for giving me life

To my wife and children, who show me how to enjoy life

To my teachers, for their inspiring support in otolaryngology-head and neck surgery life

To my patients, who seek a better quality of life

Konstantinos Garefis

Preface

Ούκ ἔνι ἰατρικήν εἰδέναι, ὅστις μή οἶδεν ὅ τι ἐστίν ἄνθρωπος.
Ἱπποκράτης (c. 460 BC–377 BC)

Hippocrates, who lived thousands of years before our time, espoused radical views on the holistic approach to medicine, divorcing it from religious considerations. This quotation underscores the importance of profound understanding and highlights the significance of comprehending not only medical matters but also the human condition.

These values of deep knowledge and self-development are embraced in this endeavor, which seeks to offer a comprehensive study guide. This guide serves not only as a tool for revision but also as a companion in everyday practice and the management of ENT cases.

Each chapter is structured around a common ENT scenario and adheres to a standardized format, featuring carefully chosen multiple-choice questions and comprehensive answers. These are grounded in the latest evidence and guidelines. We aspire for the "Otolaryngology Study Guide: A Case-Based Approach" to evolve into a valuable resource for ENT surgeons, trainees, medical students, and allied healthcare professionals.

Thessaloniki, Greece — Nikolaos Tsetsos

Plymouth, UK — Marios Stavrakas

Thessaloniki, Greece — Konstantinos Garefis

Contents

Part III Rhinology

Contributors

Despoina Beka ENT Head and Neck Surgery Department, General Hospital of Athens "Laiko", Athens, Greece

Harry Carter ENT Head and Neck Surgery Department, Morriston Hospital, Swansea, UK

Angelos Chatziavramidis 2nd Academic ORL, Head and Neck Surgery Department, Aristotle University of Thessaloniki, Papageorgiou Hospital, Thessaloniki, Greece

Manuela Cresswell Derriford Hospital, University Hospitals Plymouth NHS Trust, Plymouth, UK

Dimitrios Daskalakis ENT Head and Neck Surgery Department, 424 General Military Hospital, Thessaloniki, Greece

Christodoulos Dimakis ENT Head and Neck Surgery Department, Athens Naval Hospital, Athens, Greece

Polychronia Eftychidou 1st Department of Dermatology and Venereology, School of Medicine, Aristotle University, Thessaloniki, Greece

Kidus Eshete University Hospitals Plymouth NHS Trust, Plymouth, UK

Evropi Forozidou ENT Head and Neck Surgery Department, "G. Papanikolaou" General Hospital, Thessaloniki, Greece

Maria Garefi Department of Paediatrics, Faculty of Medicine, School of Health Sciences, University of Thessaly, Larissa, Greece

Konstantinos Garefis 2nd Academic ORL, Head and Neck Surgery Department, Aristotle University of Thessaloniki, Papageorgiou Hospital, Thessaloniki, Greece

Konstantinos Geronatsios ENT Head and Neck Surgery Department, 424 General Military Hospital, Thessaloniki, Greece

John Goudakos ENT Head and Neck Surgery Department, 424 General Military Hospital, Thessaloniki, Greece

John Guy University Hospitals of Leicester NHS Trust, Leicester, UK

Fotini Ieridou University Hospitals Plymouth NHS Trust, Plymouth, UK

Vaios Kaminiotis Harefield Hospital, Guy's and St Thomas' NHS Foundation Trust, London, UK

Yazan Kanaan University Hospitals Plymouth NHS Trust, Plymouth, UK

Paraskevi Karamitsou ENT Head and Neck Surgery Department, "G. Papanikolaou" General Hospital of Thessaloniki, Thessaloniki, Greece

Adamantios Kilmpasanis Private Practice, Thessaloniki, Greece

Iordanis Konstantinidis 2nd Academic ORL, Head and Neck Surgery Department, Aristotle University of Thessaloniki, Papageorgiou Hospital, Thessaloniki, Greece

Konstantinos Markou 2nd Academic ORL, Head and Neck Surgery Department, Aristotle University of Thessaloniki, Papageorgiou Hospital, Thessaloniki, Greece

Vasilios Nikolaidis 2nd Academic ORL, Head and Neck Surgery Department, Aristotle University of Thessaloniki, Papageorgiou Hospital, Thessaloniki, Greece

Alexandros Poutoglidis ENT Department, Lister Hospital, East and North Hertfordshire NHS Trust, Stevenage, UK

Peter Rea University Hospitals of Leicester NHS Trust, Leicester, UK

Eleni I. Sakellari Faculty of Health Sciences, Aristotle University of Thessaloniki, AHEPA University Hospital, Thessaloniki, Greece

Nikolaos I. Sakellaris Department of Otolaryngology, "G. Gennimatas" General Hospital of Athens, Athens, Greece

Elena Sotiriou 1st Department of Dermatology and Venereology, School of Medicine, Aristotle University, Thessaloniki, Greece

Marios Stavrakas ENT Head and Neck Surgery Department, University Hospitals Plymouth NHS Trust, Plymouth, UK

Aikaterini Tsentemeidou 1st Department of Dermatology and Venereology, School of Medicine, Aristotle University, Thessaloniki, Greece

Nikolaos Tsetsos ENT Head and Neck Surgery Department, 424 General Military Hospital, Thessaloniki, Greece

Ram Vaidhyanath University Hospitals of Leicester NHS Trust, Leicester, UK

Zoi Zachou 1st ORL, Head and Neck Surgery Department, National & Kapodistrian University of Athens, Hippocration Hospital, Athens, Greece

Part I

General ENT/Emergencies

1 Epistaxis

Harry Carter

Abstract

Epistaxis is a common, potentially life-threatening condition which arises from damaged blood vessels within the nasal cavity. The common causes include: trauma, hypertension, bleeding diatheses, allergies, dry environment, anticoagulants and intranasal drugs. There is a bimodal peak in childhood and older adulthood. Epistaxis is often classified into 'anterior' and 'posterior', although there is no definitive border between these two. Anterior epistaxis commonly originates from Kiesselbach's plexus (Little's area), which denotes the confluence of arteries on the anterior nasal septum. Posterior epistaxis is much less common due to better protection from trauma, heat and dryness than the anterior nasal cavity. Therefore, these bleeds are more commonly associated with underlying pathology such as hypertension, anticoagulation or bleeding disorders. Epistaxis is always managed with first-aid principles initially: by pinching the cartilaginous nose and sitting forward. If these measures fail, a treatment ladder should be followed: nasal cautery, packing and examination under anaesthesia. In severe, irretractable cases, embolisation, sphenopalatine artery ligation or carotid tie-off may all be considered but carry significant risks.

Case Presentation

A 71-year-old woman presents by ambulance to the emergency department with right-sided epistaxis which has been ongoing for 2 h. The bleeding was preceded by two smaller bleeds which stopped spontaneously. Despite constant nasal pressure, the bleeding persists and is mostly flowing into her oropharynx. She admits to swallowing some blood. She is known to have hypertension and paroxysmal atrial fibrillation. Her medication includes Apixaban and Ramipril. Her pulse is 120 beats per minute and irregular. Her blood pressure is 102/58 mmHg. Her haemoglobin on venous blood gas is 94.

Figure 1.1 shows the basic toolkit for epistaxis management.

H. Carter (✉)
ENT Head and Neck Surgery Department,
Morriston Hospital, Swansea, UK

N. Tsetsos et al. (eds.), *Otolaryngology Study Guide*, https://doi.org/10.1007/978-3-031-77374-7_1

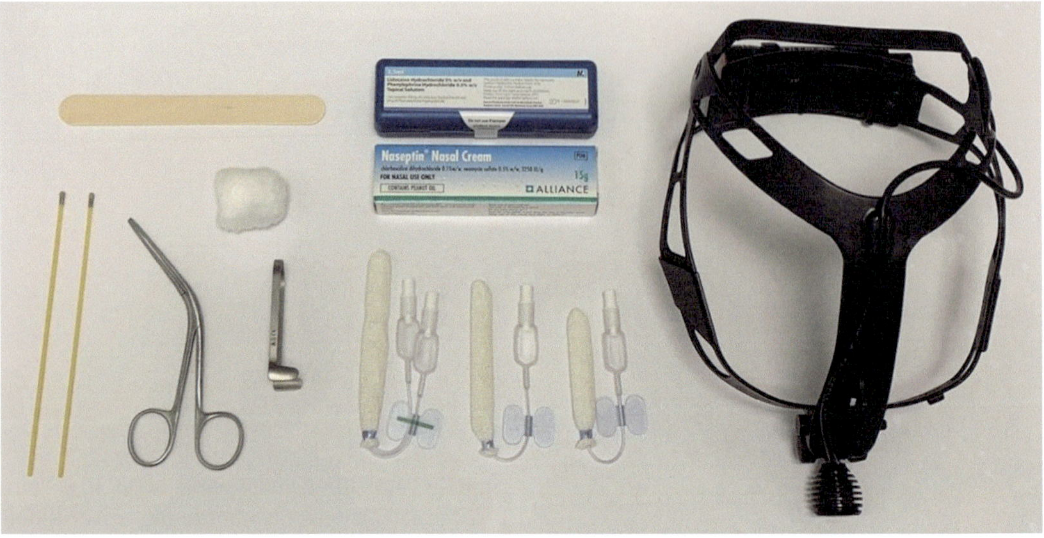

Fig. 1.1 The basic toolkit for epistaxis management. (Image rights belong to Mr. Harry Carter)

Questions

1. When you arrive, the emergency physicians have already placed bilateral anterior nasal packs. However, bleeding continues through the packs and into the oropharynx. You remove the packs but see no areas to cauterise on anterior rhinoscopy. What is your next step?
   A. Peri-arrest call
   B. Insert a posterior, double balloon pack
   C. Insert a Foley catheter and inflate the balloon in the posterior nasal space
   D. Book for emergency examination under anaesthesia
   E. Re-pack the nose with absorbable packing
2. Despite maximal ward-based packing, the epistaxis has not resolved and continues to flow into the oropharynx. You call haematology for advice on medical therapies which may improve the epistaxis. Which agent is likely to be suggested as first-line treatment?
   A. Vitamin K
   B. Idarucizumab
   C. Tranexamic acid
   D. Andexanet alpha
   E. Prothrombin complex concentrate
3. You book the patient in the emergency theatre for an examination under anaesthesia. In theatre, the view is obscured by heavy blood flow. You decide to re-pack the nose. What do you use?
   A. Rapid Rhino
   B. Nasopore
   C. Floseal
   D. Bismuth iodoform paraffin paste (BIPP) gauze
   E. Keracel
4. The intraoperative packing has slowed the bleeding but it is still collecting in the oropharynx. The patient's haemoglobin reached 58, and blood is being actively replaced by the anaesthetist. You decide to perform sphenopalatine artery (SPA) ligation. Which artery does not originate from the external carotid artery?
   A. Anterior ethmoidal artery
   B. SPA
   C. Greater palatine artery
   D. Superior labial artery
   E. Facial artery
5. Another patient is assaulted and sustains blunt trauma to the face. There is obvious deformity of the nose and brisk, pulsating epistaxis. Which artery is likely the source?

A. Greater palatine artery
B. Sphenopalatine artery
C. Anterior ethmoidal artery
D. Maxillary artery
E. Superior labial artery

Answers

1. **B**

The first step in epistaxis management is always first-aid measures, with constant pressure applied to the anterior third of the nose for 15 min [1]. If this fails, medical attention should be sought in the emergency department [2]. Anterior rhinoscopy should be performed with a nasal speculum and headlight, with suction to remove blood clots [3]. In adults, chemical cautery with silver nitrate sticks should be attempted if there is a clear bleeding vessel, following administration of adrenaline and local anaesthetic [4]. If cautery fails or a bleeding vessel cannot be seen, nasal packing should be considered next [2]. In the case above, a brisk posterior bleed is likely and therefore the easiest and safest option is to insert a single posterior, double balloon pack [5]. Although bilateral packing is common, it is very uncomfortable for patients and there is little evidence to support its efficacy [6]. Absorbable packing is less appropriate for arterial bleeding as it only exerts low pressure on the bleeding vessels [5]. A posterior Foley catheter is an advanced technique which carries a risk of irreversible pressure necrosis of the alar rim [7].

2. **C**

Tranexamic acid is a synthetic lysine analogue that binds plasminogen, inhibiting plasmin formation and preventing fibrinolysis (clot breakdown). Although often associated with improving trauma outcomes [8], tranexamic acid is used widely and is recommended by the National Institute for Health and Care Excellence (NICE) in the United Kingdom as an adjunctive medical therapy to be used in severe epistaxis [2]. However, evidence for its efficacy in epistaxis is limited [9]. Vitamin K could be given in the context of a patient with epistaxis taking warfarin, with a raised International Normalized Ratio (INR) [10]. New reversal agents have been created for Direct Oral Anticoagulants (DOAC); these include 'Idarucizumab' for Dabigatran [11] and 'Andexanet alpha' for Rivaroxaban and Apixaban [12]. Prothrombin complex concentrate may also be used in haemorrhage with advice from haematology [13].

3. **D**

BIPP is sterile ribbon gauze, impregnated in bismuth subnitrate, iodoform and paraffin. It acts to apply pressure, causing haemostasis, and provides moisture and antisepsis to the nasal cavity [14]. It is more commonly inserted under general anaesthetic as the packing process takes time and is uncomfortable. Loops of gauze are advanced into the nostril with Tilley's forceps and pushed superiorly into the roof of the nasal cavity, compressing the pack. This approach is sometimes used alongside a posterior Foley catheter to compress the choana [15]. A posterior Rapid Rhino is a quick and safe alternative but not if this measure has previously failed. Haemostatic agents such as Floseal may be used as an adjunct but are most effective when applied directly in anterior epistaxis [16]. Keracel is a wound dressing and should not be used in epistaxis.

4. **A**

The anterior ethmoidal artery is a branch of the distal ophthalmic artery, which originates from the internal carotid artery. All other arteries supplying the nasal cavity originate from the external carotid artery [17]. SPA ligation is considered for severe, persistent posterior epistaxis. In refractory cases where SPA ligation fails, external carotid tie-off or angiographic embolisation may be indicated [13, 18, 19].

5. **C**

The anterior ethmoidal artery is vulnerable to damage in nasal trauma; however, associated epistaxis usually stops with first-aid measures [20]. Intractable bleeding from the anterior ethmoidal artery may require formal ligation, which may be achieved in an open or endoscopic approach [18].

References

1. Nosebleed causes & treatments. NHS inform. [cited 2022 Aug 1]. https://www.nhsinform.scot/illnesses-and-conditions/ears-nose-and-throat/nosebleed.
2. Epistaxis (nosebleeds). Health topics A to Z. CKS | NICE. [cited 2022 Aug 8]. https://cks.nice.org.uk/topics/epistaxis-nosebleeds/.
3. Diamond L. Managing epistaxis. J Am Acad Physician Assist. 2014;27(11):35–9. https://pubmed.ncbi.nlm.nih.gov/25303882/.
4. Beck R, Sorge M, Schneider A, Dietz A. Current approaches to epistaxis treatment in primary and secondary care. Dtsch Arztebl Int. 2018;115(1–2):12–22. https://doi.org/10.3238/arztebl.2018.0012.
5. Flint P, Haughey B, Lund V, Robbins K, Thomas JR, Lesperance M, et al. Cummings otolaryngology: head and neck surgery. 7th ed. Elsevier; 2020.
6. Hettige R, Mackeith S, Falzon A, Draper M. A study to determine the benefits of bilateral versus unilateral nasal packing with Rapid Rhino® packs. Eur Arch Otorhinolaryngology. 2014;271(3):519–23. https://pubmed.ncbi.nlm.nih.gov/23765062/.
7. Leadon M, Hohman MH. Posterior epistaxis nasal pack. In: StatPearls. StatPearls Publishing; 2022. https://www.ncbi.nlm.nih.gov/books/NBK576436/.
8. Roberts I, Shakur H, Coats T, Hunt B, Balogun E, Barnetson L, et al. The CRASH-2 trial: a randomised controlled trial and economic evaluation of the effects of tranexamic acid on death, vascular occlusive events and transfusion requirement in bleeding trauma patients. Health Technol Assess (Rockv). 2013;17(10):1–80. https://pubmed.ncbi.nlm.nih.gov/23477634/.
9. Reed MR, Woolley LT. Uses of tranexamic acid. Contin Educ Anaesth Crit Care Pain. 2015;15(1):32–7. https://linkinghub.elsevier.com/retrieve/pii/S1743181617300185.
10. Scenario: Warfarin. Management. Anticoagulation—oral. CKS. NICE. [cited 2022 Aug 8]. https://cks.nice.org.uk/topics/anticoagulation-oral/management/warfarin/.
11. Garrett AD. Idarucizumab for dabigatran reversal, Drug topics, vol. 159. Advanstar Communications Inc.; 2015.
12. Andexanet alfa for reversing anticoagulation from apixaban or rivaroxaban. NICE. 2021 [cited 2022 Aug 8]. https://www.nice.org.uk/guidance/ta697.
13. Tunkel DE, Anne S, Payne SC, Ishman SL, Rosenfeld RM, Abramson PJ, et al. Clinical practice guideline: nosebleed (epistaxis). Otolaryngol Head Neck Surg (United States). 2020;162(1_Suppl):S1–38. https://pubmed.ncbi.nlm.nih.gov/31910111/.
14. Randhawa GK, Graham R, Matharu KS. Bismuth iodoform paraffin paste: history and uses. Br J Oral Maxillofac Surg. 2019;57(10):e53–4. http://www.bjoms.com/article/S0266435619305480/fulltext.
15. Amen F, Pace-Balzan A. Technical tutorial: How to pack a nose with bismuth iodoform paraffin paste gauze safely and effectively. Emerg Med J. 2009;26(1):52. https://emj.bmj.com/content/26/1/52.
16. Wakelam OC, Dimitriadis PA, Stephens J. The use of FloSeal haemostatic sealant in the management of epistaxis: a prospective clinical study and literature review. Ann R Coll Surg Engl. 2017;99(1):28–30. https://pmc.ncbi.nlm.nih.gov/articles/PMC5392783/.
17. Sobiesk JL, Munakomi S. Anatomy, head and neck, nasal cavity. In: StatPearls. StatPearls Publishing. http://www.ncbi.nlm.nih.gov/pubmed/31334952.
18. Saraceni Neto P, Mendes Acatauassu Nunes L, Carlos Gregório L, Rodrigo de Paula S, Macoto Kosugi E. Surgical treatment of severe epistaxis: an eleven-year experience. Braz J Otorhinolaryngol. 2013;79(1):59–64.
19. Waldron J, Stafford N. Ligation of the external carotid artery for severe epistaxis. J Otolaryngol. 1992;21:249. https://pubmed.ncbi.nlm.nih.gov/1527828/.
20. Jones NS, Woolford TJ. Endoscopic ligation of anterior ethmoidal artery in treatment of epistaxis. J Laryngol Otol. 2000;114(11):858–60. https://pubmed.ncbi.nlm.nih.gov/11144836/.

Post-tonsillectomy Bleeding 2

Maria Garefi and Konstantinos Garefis

Abstract

Tonsillectomy is a prevalent surgical procedure in otolaryngology and is recommended mainly for recurrent throat infections and obstructive sleep-disordered breathing. Post-tonsillectomy bleeding (PTB) represents the most frequent and significant complication after tonsillectomy, manifesting in approximately 5% of all cases, and it can lead to death. It is classified as primary or secondary bleeding. Primary bleeding can occur within 24 h, whereas secondary can occur at any time after the first 24 h. Primary PTB is typically attributed to insufficient hemostasis during the operation, while secondary is linked to the separation of the crust from the tonsillar bed, disregarding dietary instructions and wound separation. The risk factors of the PTB are age, reason for tonsillectomy, surgical approach, and the proficiency of the surgeon. Children with minor bleeding episodes should be closely monitored for possible development in severe bleeding. Severe PTB cases need surgical hemostasis, possible intubation, and management of hemodynamic instability.

Case Presentation

A 9-year-old boy weighing 26 kg presented to the emergency department with bleeding from his mouth. According to his history, he underwent a tonsillectomy 6 days ago due to recurrent episodes of tonsillitis. The child exhibited warm extremities, capillary refill time <2 s, a heart rate of 150 beats per minute, 96% oxygen saturation, a Glasgow scale of 15/15, and blood pressure of 108/65 mmHg. After 10 min, the bleeding stopped. His laboratory evaluation included hematocrit of 38% and hemoglobin level of 12.5 g/dL. During the mouth examination, a blood clot was found in the inferior pole of the right tonsillar fossa (Fig. 2.1).

Questions

1. Which of the following statements are true about PTB? (more than one correct answer possible)
   A. The highest occurrence of bleeding typically happens from 9 to 15 days post-surgery
   B. Primary bleeding is potentially more life-threatening than secondary bleeding

M. Garefi
Department of Paediatrics, Faculty of Medicine, School of Health Sciences, University of Thessaly, Larissa, Greece

K. Garefis (✉)
2nd Academic ORL, Head and Neck Surgery Department, Aristotle University of Thessaloniki, Papageorgiou Hospital, Thessaloniki, Greece

N. Tsetsos et al. (eds.), *Otolaryngology Study Guide*, https://doi.org/10.1007/978-3-031-77374-7_2

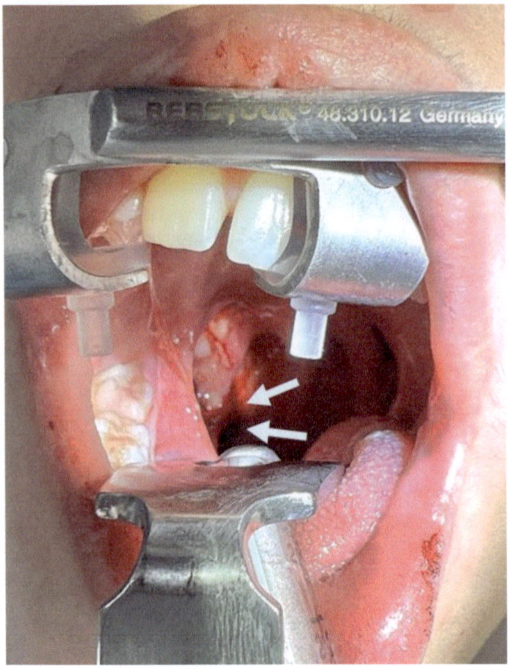

Fig. 2.1 Arrows showing the blood clot in the inferior pole of the right tonsillar fossa

C. A minor bleeding is usually preceded by a light one
D. The incidence of secondary bleeding is between 0.1% and 4.8%
E. Approximately 30% of all minor bleeding progress to severe

2. Which factors are commonly linked to PTB? (more than one correct answer possible)
   A. Patient's age
   B. Chronic–cryptic tonsillitis
   C. Von Willebrand disease
   D. Peri-operative antibiotics
   E. All of the above
3. Up to what volume of blood is the patient likely to have lost?
   A. 300 mL
   B. 273 mL
   C. 50 mL
   D. 176 mL
   E. 430 mL
4. Which is the first step for the patient's treatment? (more than one correct answer possible)
   A. Administration of intravenous 520 mL isotonic crystalloid fluids
   B. Placement of two peripheral venous lines
   C. Antibiotics
   D. Blood transfusion with one unit of red blood cells
   E. Suturing of the tonsillar pillars with local anesthesia
5. After conservative management, an active bleeding episode is occurring 6 h later. Which intervention could be employed for the definitive treatment of the new episode? (more than one correct answer possible)
   A. Electrocautery of bleeding vessels
   B. Suture ligation
   C. Direct pressure with an adrenaline-soaked swab
   D. Packing of the tonsillar fossa with gauze
   E. Carotid artery ligation

Answers

1. **B, C, D**

   Secondary PTB is more frequent than primary PTB, and the incidence is between 0.1% and 4.8%. On the contrary, the incidence of primary PTB is between 0.2% and 2.2% [1]. Primary PTB is typically viewed as more dangerous for the patient due to the potential risk of aspiration or laryngospasm and the concealed ingestion of blood, leading to a subsequent compromise in blood circulation [2]. Most instances of PTB occur within the period ranging from the fifth to the tenth days following the surgery [3]. A total of 41% of minor PTB incidents have been demonstrated to be preceded by a light bleeding event, and 10.2% of all instances of minor bleeding progress to severe bleeding [4]. Patients frequently describe minor PTB that has ceased by the time they arrive at the emergency department.
2. **A, B, C**

   It is essential for healthcare providers to assess risk factors preoperatively to mitigate the risk of PTB. Age is the most extensively recorded risk factor with older patients being at a higher risk. This may stem from a prolonged history of chronic tonsillitis in older patients and could be associated with reduced adherence to postoperative liquid diet and rest instructions [1, 3, 5, 6]. The

Table 2.1 Classification of hypovolemic shock

	Class I	Class II	Class III	Class IV
Blood loss (% blood volume)	<15%	15–30%	30–40%	>40%
Heart rate	Mild tachycardia	Tachycardia	Hypotension	Hypotension
Systolic blood pressure	No change	No change	Reduced	Very low
Respiratory rate	Normal	Tachypnea	Tachypnea	Severe tachypnea
Urine output	Normal	Normal	Reduced	Minimal
Extremities	Normal	Pale	Pale	Cold
Capillary refill time	Normal	Prolonged	Prolonged	Prolonged
Mental status	Alert	Anxiety	Confused	Lethargy

indication of chronic–cryptic tonsillitis as the reason for tonsillectomy also correlates with an increased risk of PTB [7]. PTB has also been linked with various coagulopathies, most frequently both treated and undiagnosed Von Willebrand disease [1, 8, 9]. According to US national guidelines, the incidence of PTB typically remains unaffected by the administration of perioperative antibiotics [6, 10].

3. **B**

   It is important to identify the type of hemorrhagic hypovolemic shock the patient is in before starting to calculate up to what volume of blood is likely to have lost. The patient has tachycardia with 150 beats per minute (normal value of heart rate 60–110 mmHg for his age) with normal blood pressure (normal value of systolic pressure 90 + 2 × age) and no other signs and symptoms of severe hypovolemic shock [11]. According to the classification of hypovolemic shock, the patient is in hemorrhagic hypovolemic shock type I with volume loss up to 15% of total blood volume (Table 2.1) [12].

   The child's blood volume and the permissible blood losses must be calculated based on his age (Table 2.2) [11].

   The circulating volume of a child 9 years old is approximately 70 mL/kg [11, 13].

   15% of 1820 mL = 273 mL. Therefore, he has lost up to 273 mL of blood.

4. **A, B**

   The initial evaluation should concentrate on identifying any active bleeding and assessing the patient's hemodynamic status. Fluids are administered during the initial treatment phase to replenish volume and ensure sufficient blood supply to vital organs. Initially, the placement of two peripheral venous lines and administration of isotonic crystalloid solutions is recommended, regardless of the type of shock, in a single dose of 20 mL/kg = 520 mL intravenously or intraosseously [14]. A patient in hypovolemic shock type I, who is hemodynamically stable and with normal level of hematocrit and hemoglobin for his age, does not require transfusion [15]. The administration of antibiotics after tonsillectomy is a contentious topic. They are usually used for prophylaxis rather than for the treatment of post-tonsillectomy bacteremia [16]. However, there is no additional advantage in using antibiotics following tonsillectomy to reduce the risk of PTB [16–18].

Table 2.2 Estimated circulating blood volume corresponding to the age

Child age	Volemia (mL/kg)
Preterm newborn	90
Term newborn–3 months	80–90
3 months–2 years old	78–80
>2 years old	70

5. **A, B**

   In patients without active bleeding, conservative treatment is the first step in proper patient management. In-hospital monitoring is crucial for patient safety, as bleeding can be life-threatening. In cases of active bleeding that does not cease or in the occurrence of a new severe episode, surgical intervention is necessary. Cauterization, with local or general anesthesia, and/or suture ligation can effectively stop ongoing blood loss. If bleeding persists and the patient's life is in danger, carotid artery ligation may be considered [1, 2].

References

1. Wall JJ, Tay KY. Postoperative tonsillectomy hemorrhage. Emerg Med Clin North Am. 2018;36(2):415–26.
2. Windfuhr JP. Lethal post-tonsillectomy hemorrhage. Auris Nasus Larynx. 2003;30(4):391–6.
3. Gonçalves AI, Rato C, de Vilhena D, Duarte D, Lopes G, Trigueiros N. Evaluation of post-tonsillectomy hemorrhage and assessment of risk factors. Eur Arch Otorrinolaringol. 2020;277(11):3095–102.
4. Sarny S, Habermann W, Ossimitz G, Stammberger H. Significant post-tonsillectomy pain is associated with increased risk of hemorrhage. Ann Otol Rhinol Laryngol. 2012;121(12):776–81.
5. Akin RC, Holst R, Schousboe LP. Risk factors for post-tonsillectomy haemorrhage. Acta Otolaryngol. 2012;132(7):773–7.
6. Spektor Z, Saint-Victor S, Kay DJ, Mandell DL. Risk factors for pediatric post-tonsillectomy hemorrhage. Int J Pediatr Otorhinolaryngol. 2016;84:151–5.
7. Schrock A, Send T, Heukamp L, Gerstner AO, Bootz F, Jakob M. The role of histology and other risk factors for post-tonsillectomy haemorrhage. Eur Arch Otorrinolaringol. 2009;266(12):1983–7.
8. Patel PN, Arambula AM, Wheeler AP, Penn EB. Post-tonsillectomy hemorrhagic outcomes in children with bleeding disorders at a single institution. Int J Pediatr Otorhinolaryngol. 2017;100:216–22.
9. Witmer CM, Elden L, Butler RB, Manno CS, Raffini LJ. Incidence of bleeding complications in pediatric patients with type 1 von Willebrand disease undergoing adenotonsillar procedures. J Pediatr. 2009;155(1):68–72.
10. Baugh RF, Archer SM, Mitchell RB, Rosenfeld RM, Amin R, Burns JJ, Darrow DH, Giordano T, Litman RS, Li KK, Mannix ME, Schwartz RH, Setzen G, Wald ER, Wall E, Sandberg G, Patel MM, American Academy of Otolaryngology-Head and Neck Surgery Foundation. Clinical practice guideline: tonsillectomy in children. Otolaryngol Head Neck Surg. 2011;144(1 Suppl):S1–30.
11. Zuluaga Giraldo M. Management of perioperative bleeding in children. Step by step review. Colombian J Anesthesiol. 2013;41(1):50–6.
12. Thomson SJ, Cowan ML, Morgan R, Rahman TM. Gastrointestinal bleeding. Surg Intensive Care Med. 2010:455–69.
13. Bharadwaj A, Khandelwal M, Bhargava SK. Perioperative neonatal and paediatric blood transfusion. Indian J Anaesth. 2014;58(5):652–7.
14. Resuscitation Council (UK). European paediatric advanced life support. London: Resuscitation Council UK; 2016.
15. Murphy MF, Wallington TB, Kelsey P, Boulton F, Bruce M, Cohen H, Duguid J, Knowles SM, Poole G, Williamson LM, British Committee for Standards in Haematology, Blood Transfusion Task Force. Guidelines for the clinical use of red cell transfusions. Br J Haematol. 2001;113(1):24–31.
16. Abdelhamid AO, Sobhy TS, El-Mehairy HM, Hamid O. Role of antibiotics in post-tonsillectomy morbidities; a systematic review. Int J Pediatr Otorhinolaryngol. 2019;118:192–200.
17. Elinder K, Söderman AC, Stalfors J, Knutsson J. Factors influencing morbidity after paediatric tonsillectomy: a study of 18,712 patients in the National Tonsil Surgery Register in Sweden. Eur Arch Otorrinolaringol. 2016;273(8):2249–56.
18. Dhiwakar M, Clement WA, Supriya M, McKerrow W. Antibiotics to reduce post-tonsillectomy morbidity. Cochrane Database Syst Rev. 2012;12:CD005607.

Nasal Fracture

3

Paraskevi Karamitsou and Alexandros Poutoglidis

Abstract

Nasal bones are the most susceptible bones of the facial framework. Studies have shown a 2:1 ratio of male predominance. Children are also commonly affected. The primary symptoms include swelling, deformity, nasal obstruction, nosebleeds, bony crepitus, and bruising around the eyes. There are several types of nasal fractures, which can be classified as: (a) unilateral, (b) bilateral, (c) comminuted, (d) open-book (splayed), (e) impacted, and (g) greenstick. The presence of septal injury may also suggest a nasal fracture. If the fracture is nondisplaced and without defects, observation alone may be sufficient. Simple injuries may require closed nasal reduction, while more severe cases may necessitate an open approach for a satisfactory result. Ideally, intervention should be carried out within the first 10 days following the injury. However, it is also suggested that intervention could be performed up to 3 weeks after the injury. Furthermore, if an immediate reduction is not carried out, it is recommended to allow the swelling to decrease and reassess the integrity of the nasal bone and the need for intervention after the first 2 or 3 days. While a nasal injury typically does not require significant interventions, the undertreatment of a displaced fracture can lead to both cosmetic and functional issues, such as external nose deformity, nasal obstruction, septal perforation, and severe growth retardation in children.

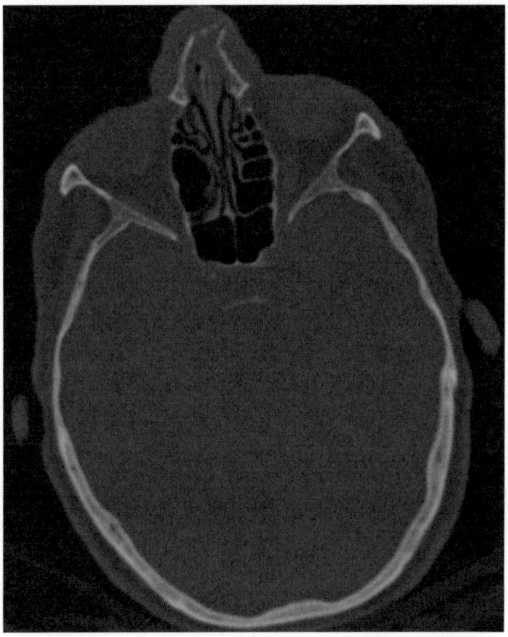

Fig. 3.1 Facial bone CT scan of the patient indicating nasal bone fractures

P. Karamitsou
ENT Head and Neck Surgery Department, "G. Papanikolaou" General Hospital of Thessaloniki, Thessaloniki, Greece

A. Poutoglidis (✉)
ENT Department, Lister Hospital, East and North Hertfordshire NHS Trust, Stevenage, UK

N. Tsetsos et al. (eds.), *Otolaryngology Study Guide*, https://doi.org/10.1007/978-3-031-77374-7_3

Case Presentation

A 40-year-old man presented to the Emergency ENT clinic, primarily complaining of left-sided epistaxis. He reported that he had sustained a head and nasal injury during a sports activity an hour earlier. Apart from this, his medical history was unremarkable. Upon his arrival, his vital signs were stable; however, he had two episodes of vomiting. A noticeable deviation of the nasal pyramid and significant asymmetry accompanied by substantial swelling were observed. The mobility of the nasal bones was evaluated by holding the dorsum between two fingers. Notable bony crepitus from the moving nasal bone fragments was detected. Clotted blood was cleared from the left nasal cavity and all mucosal surfaces were examined. A CT scan of the brain and the facial bones was requested that was clear for brain injury; however, indicated nasal bone fractures (Fig. 3.1). He was advised to apply cold packs around his nose to reduce the swelling and was given medication to manage the pain. He returned to the outpatient department 3 days later, where a closed nasal reduction was performed. No ongoing deformity was observed. The patient came back for a follow-up appointment 3 weeks later. The cosmetic and functional results were excellent, with no signs of nasal septal deviation or perforation.

Questions

1. Blood supply to the nose is provided by:
   A. Superficial temporal artery
   B. Anterior ethmoid artery
   C. Posterior ethmoid artery
   D. Sphenopalatine artery
   E. Greater palatine artery
2. Which of the following sentences is true for Stranc and Robertson's classification system?
   A. The categorization is based on the direction of the impact force.
   B. It is divided into three different planes.
   C. Each plane is associated with a lower likelihood of residual deformity after reduction.
   D. Plane 3 injury results in disruption of the naso-orbitoethmoidal complex.
   E. Surgery for plane 3 injury could completely restore the appearance and function of the nose.
3. The diagnosis of a nasal fracture should be based on:
   A. History
   B. Physical findings
   C. High-resolution ultrasound
   D. Computed tomography
   E. X-ray
4. Which is the most appropriate treatment for septal hematoma?
   A. Incision
   B. Incision and drainage
   C. Watchful waiting
   D. Use of antibiotics
   E. Incision, drainage, and use of antibiotics
5. Saddle nose deformity might be caused by:
   A. Nasal trauma
   B. Granulomatosis with polyangiitis
   C. Sarcoidosis
   D. Syphilis
   E. Lepromatous leprosy

Answers

1. **B, C, D, E**

   The nose receives a significant blood supply from both internal and external carotid arteries [1, 2]. The ophthalmic artery, a branch of the internal carotid artery, supplies both internal and external parts of the nose. The anterior and posterior ethmoid arteries supply the internal nasal cavity, while the dorsal and external nasal arteries supply the outer nose. The external carotid artery supplies the outer nose through the infraorbital (a branch of the maxillary artery), superior labial, and angular arteries (branches of the facial artery). The sphenopalatine artery, a branch of the external carotid artery, enters the nose through the sphenopalatine foramen and may provide up to ten branches. The greater palatine artery (a terminal branch of the maxillary artery) contributes to the lower part of the nasal septum through the incisive foramen.
2. **A, B, D**

   Stranc and Robertson's classification system [3] is a categorization based on the direction of the impact force. The classification consists of three different planes determined by the depth of injury from the nasal tip. Each plane is associated with a higher likelihood of residual deformity after reduction. Damages to the anterior nasal spine, the anterior septum, or the lower ends of the nasal bones are included in the plane 1 injury. Plane 2 injury includes more extensive damage to the nasal bones and ascending maxillary process but without the involvement of the orbital rims. Plane 3 injury results in disruption of the naso-orbitoethmoidal complex. Surgery for plane 3 injury is often unable to provide complete restoration of the appearance and function of the nose.

3. **A, B**

   The diagnosis of a nasal fracture is primarily based on history and physical findings. X-rays should not play a major role in the diagnosis or management of nasal fractures due to a 66% false–positive rate [4, 5]. Normal suture lines, developmental thinning of the nasal bones, and old fractures might mislead the clinician. Older patients tend to have osteopenic nasal bones prone to fractures, while pediatric patients tend to have more cartilaginous injuries. Cartilaginous fracture lines are not visible in X-rays. High-resolution ultrasound could potentially be used to diagnose bone and cartilage fractures that would not have been otherwise recognized due to soft tissue edema [5–8]. Compared to an X-ray, high-resolution ultrasound demonstrates better sensitivity and specificity [4, 5]. Computed tomography is recommended in more severe injuries, especially when other facial fractures are present [6–9].

4. **E**

   Septal hematoma is one of the most dangerous early complications of nasal trauma as it could lead to necrosis [10, 11]. Therefore, immediate treatment is necessary to prevent long-term complications. A wide incision to allow sufficient drainage is mandatory. Antibiotics are also required to prevent bacterial contamination. Additionally, splints or trans-septal sutures could be placed to obliterate the potential intermediate space and to prevent hematoma recurrence. If a septal infection is left untreated, it may lead to osteomyelitis, orbital or intracranial abscess, meningitis, and cavernous sinus thrombosis [11].

5. **A, B, C, D, E**

   Saddle nose deformity is a potential long-term complication of nasal trauma [12]. Granulomatosis with polyangiitis (formerly known as Wegener disease) is a systemic disease characterized by necrotizing granulomas and vasculitis of small and medium-sized vessels [13]. The nasal cavity and paranasal sinuses are the predominant sites of clinical manifestations. The anterior part of the nasal septum is one of the most frequently involved areas. The unregulated disease potentially causes deformities that range from loss of dorsal height to saddle nose deformity [13, 14]. Sarcoidosis is a systemic idiopathic granulomatous disease involving several organs in the body including the nose. Lesions in the nasal bones, cartilage, and subcutaneous tissues might lead to the widening of the nasal bridge and result in a saddle nose deformity [15]. Congenital syphilis is associated with many deformities, such as Hutchinson's teeth, saddle nose deformity, deafness, and interstitial keratitis [16]. In untreated lepromatous leprosy, the chronic ulceration of nasal mucosa makes the underlying components of nasal structures exposed to nonspecific infections, which leads to saddle nose deformity [17].

References

1. McKinney P, Johnson P, Walloch J. Anatomy of the nasal hump. Plast Reconstr Surg. 1986;77:404.
2. Oneal RM, Beil RJ, Schlesinger J. Surgical anatomy of the nose. Clin Plast Surg. 1996;23:195.
3. Stranc MF, Robertson GA. A classification of injuries of the nasal skeleton. Ann Plast Surg. 1979;2:468.
4. Chukwulebe S, Hogrefe C. The diagnosis and the management of facial bone structures. Emerg Med Clin North Am. 2019;37(1):137–51.
5. Gurkov R, Clevert D, Krause E. Sonography versus plain X-rays in diagnosis of nasal fractures. Am J Rhinol. 2008;22:613.

6. Javadrashid R, Khatoonabad M, Shams N. Comparison of ultrasonography with computed tomography in the diagnosis of nasal bone fractures. Dentomaxillofac Radiol. 2011;40:486.
7. Lee MH, Cha JG, Hong HS. Comparison of high-resolution ultrasonography and computed tomography in the diagnosis of nasal fractures. J Ultrasound Med. 2009;28:717.
8. Mohammadi A, Ghasemi-Rad M. Nasal bone fracture-ultrasonography or computed tomography. Med Ultrason. 2011;13:292.
9. Remmler D, Denny A, Gosain A, et al. Role of three-dimensional computed tomography in the assessment of naso-orbitoethmoidal fractures. Ann Plast Surg. 2000;44:553.
10. Lopez MA, Liu JH, Hartley BE, Myer CM. Septal hematoma and abscess after nasal trauma. Clin Pediatr. 2000;39(10):609–10.
11. Ali HM, Zavala H, Chinnadurai S, Roby B. Nasal septal hematoma in children: time to diagnosis and resulting complications. Int J Pediatr Otorhinolaryngol. 2021;145:110734.
12. Hwang K, Yeom SH, Hwang SH. Complications of nasal bone fractures. J Craniofac Surg. 2017;28:803.
13. Coordes A, Loose SM, Hofmann VM, Hamilton GS III, Riedel F, Menger DJ, Albers AE. Saddle nose deformity and septal perforation in granulomatosis with polyangiitis. Clin Otolaryngol. 2018;43(1):291–9.
14. Ezzat WH, Compton RA, Basa KC, Levi J. Reconstructive techniques for saddle nose deformity in granulomatosis with polyangiitis: a systematic review. JAMA Otolarygol Head Neck Surg. 2017;143:507–12.
15. Shimamura S, Yokogawa N, Murata K, Yamaguchi T, Uchida K, Eishi Y. Saddle nose with sarcoidosis: "a greater imitator" of relapsing polychondritis. Mod Rheumatol. 2018;28(6):1053–7.
16. Tsang SH, Sharma T. Syphilis. Adv Exp Med Biol. 2018;1085:219–21.
17. Ishida Y, Pecorini L, Guglielmelli E. A case of reconstruction of saddle nose deformity in leprosy. Nihon Hansenbyo Gakkai Zasshi. 1999;68(3):201–5.

4 Stridor

Konstantinos Garefis

Abstract

Stridor, a high-pitched, harsh respiratory noise, results from turbulent airflow through a restricted air passage, commonly observed during inhalation. It is more prevalent in pediatric cases than in adults. Notably, stridor is not a standalone diagnosis; rather, it serves as a key indicator of an underlying condition, which can vary from a chronic symptom present at birth or shortly after to an acute presentation at any age. Stridor can be attributed to both congenital malformations and acquired factors. Congenital stridor is commonly associated with conditions such as laryngomalacia, vocal cord paresis, subglottic stenosis, vascular ring, or glottic web. Conversely, acquired stridor may result from conditions like croup, epiglottitis, bacterial tracheitis, retropharyngeal abscess, or foreign body aspiration. The epidemiology of stridor relies on the specific underlying cause. The severity and origin of the stridor dictate the signs of respiratory distress, including dyspnea, nasal flaring, intercostal or subcostal retractions, grunting, cyanosis, somnolence, and periods of apnea. To establish a diagnosis, a comprehensive approach is necessary, involving a detailed history, thorough physical examination, and flexible fiber-optic endoscopy. In some cases, further evaluation with direct laryngoscopy and bronchoscopy under general anesthesia may be required. Management focuses on treating the underlying pathology responsible for the stridor.

Case Presentation

A 2-month-old male infant was brought to the Ear Nose Throat (ENT) Department with the chief complaint of stridor. The parents reported that the stridor had been present since birth and had gradually worsened over the past few weeks. The infant's medical history was unremarkable, with no significant respiratory illnesses or congenital anomalies reported. Symptoms noted by the parents included a high-pitched, inspiratory stridor that was more pronounced during periods of agitation or feeding (Fig. 4.1). Moreover, coughing, choking, and regurgitation are occasionally presented during feeding. Stridor subsides when the infant is in neck extension or when placed prone. Otherwise, his general health and weight gain were within normal limits. There were no signs of fever, cough, or hoarseness.

K. Garefis (✉)
2nd Academic ORL, Head and Neck Surgery Department, Aristotle University of Thessaloniki, Papageorgiou Hospital, Thessaloniki, Greece

N. Tsetsos et al. (eds.), *Otolaryngology Study Guide*, https://doi.org/10.1007/978-3-031-77374-7_4

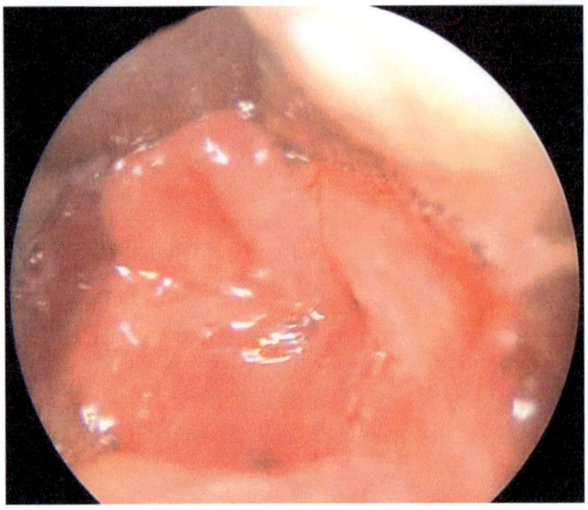

Fig. 4.1 Endoscopic image of the infant's larynx

Questions

1. Which of the following statements are true about stridor? (more than one correct answer possible)
   A. Retropharyngeal abscess can cause stridor
   B. It can be an expiratory sound
   C. It is associated with subglottic hemangioma
   D. Chronic stridor suggests a congenital cause
   E. All of the above
2. Which of the following is a probable diagnosis for the case described above and, at the same time, the most frequent cause of stridor?
   A. Croup
   B. Vocal cord palsy
   C. Subglottic stenosis
   D. Laryngomalacia
   E. Recurrent respiratory papillomatosis
3. Which is the most appropriate examination for the infant described above?
   A. Neck Magnetic resonance imaging (MRI)
   B. Airway fluoroscopy
   C. Flexible endoscopy
   D. Barium swallow
   E. Direct laryngoscopy with bronchoscopy
4. Stridor in children accompanied by a barking cough and low-grade fever is characteristic of which condition?
   A. Croup
   B. Laryngeal web
   C. Recurrent respiratory papillomatosis
   D. Retropharyngeal abscess
   E. Laryngeal tumor
5. The examination of the infant showed redundant supraarytenoid mucosa, arytenoid, postglottic edema, and erythema. Which is the appropriate treatment? (more than one correct answer possible)
   A. Epiglottopexy
   B. Proton pump inhibitor (PPI) therapy
   C. Supraglottoplasty
   D. Tracheostomy
   E. Ranitidine

Answers

1. **E**

   Stridor is typically heard during inspiration, but it can also occur during expiration and may even manifest as biphasic [1]. Inspiratory stridor results from turbulent airflow during inhalation, often due to a restricted larynx or upper trachea, resulting in a high-pitched respiratory noise. Conversely, expiratory stridor arises from turbulent airflow during exhalation, with obstruction typically located within the lower airway, such as the lower trachea or bronchi, leading to a harsh respiratory noise. Biphasic stridor, characterized by a harsh respiratory noise throughout the entire respiratory cycle, indicates a lesion in the mid-trachea, glottis, and subglottis [2]. Stridor can be either acute or chronic. Acute stridor is associated with various conditions, such as croup, epiglottitis, bacterial tracheitis, retropharyngeal abscess, foreign body aspiration, and acquired subglottic stenosis due to endotracheal intubation trauma. In contrast, chronic stridor often points to congenital causes, including laryngomalacia, vocal cord paresis, laryngeal webs or clefts, congenital subglottic stenosis, tracheomalacia, and subglottic hemangioma [2–4].
2. **D**

   Laryngomalacia stands as the predominant cause of stridor in neonates and infants (Table 4.1). Patients affected by laryngomalacia typically exhibit inspiratory stridor, which becomes more pronounced during feeding, agitation, and when placed in a supine posi-

Table 4.1 Common acquired and congenital causes of stridor

Acquired causes	Congenital causes
• Croup	• Laryngomalacia
• Epiglottitis	• Vocal cord paresis
• Bacterial tracheitis	• Laryngeal webs
• Retropharyngeal abscess	• Laryngeal cleft
• Foreign body aspiration	• Congenital subglottic stenosis
• Acquired subglottic stenosis due to endotracheal intubation trauma	• Tracheomalacia
• Reflux laryngitis	• Tracheal stenosis
• Recurrent respiratory papillomatosis	• Subglottic hemangioma
	• Congenital cysts

tion [2, 5]. Feeding difficulties are prevalent among these patients, with symptoms observed in approximately 50% of cases. They often experience issues such as delayed feeding, regurgitation, and coughing or choking during meals [5]. Symptoms typically emerge shortly after birth, with the average age of presentation being approximately 2 weeks; however, in some cases, symptoms may appear later during the neonatal period. Commonly associated conditions with laryngomalacia include obstructive sleep apnea and gastroesophageal reflux disorder. Stridor may diminish when the patient's neck is extended or when placed in a prone position [2, 5].

3. **C**

   The initial examination for these patients should involve flexible fiber-optic endoscopy while the child is awake and positioned upright to ensure a comprehensive view of the entire supraglottis and glottis [2, 6]. This safe procedure can be conducted in the office setting. The primary endoscopic findings of laryngomalacia include the following: Elongated epiglottis that prolapses posteriorly during inspiration, short aryepiglottic folds, and redundant supraarytenoid mucosa that prolapses anteriorly. The severity of the obstruction is determined by the visualization of the vocal cords [2, 7]. In cases where laryngomalacia is not detected or when mild disease observed during flexible endoscopy does not match clinical symptoms, the possibility of a synchronous lesion cannot be ruled out. In such instances, direct laryngoscopy with bronchoscopy becomes necessary [2]. The incidence of a synchronous lesion is approximately 15%, but only 5% exhibit a significant second lesion during bronchoscopy [5, 8, 9]. Radiologic studies like airway fluoroscopy and barium swallow have limited diagnostic utility due to their poor sensitivity [2, 10]. Although in children with stridor, dysphagia and aspiration may be observed, necessitating the use of airway fluoroscopy and barium swallow tests to evaluate swallowing function. Airway fluoroscopy offers a minimally invasive radiographic method to assess the upper airway, providing real-time dynamic images of airway patency and functionality [3].

4. **A**

   As one of the symptoms is fever, it is likely that infection is the etiology of this condition. Croup, also known as laryngotracheobronchitis, is the most common cause of acute airway obstruction in young children. It is defined as airway inflammation and edema that result in obstruction of the larynx, trachea, and bronchi, frequently as a result of viral infection. Low-grade fever, barky cough, stridor, hoarseness, and varying degrees of respiratory discomfort are its defining symptoms. Rhinorrhea and congestion of the nose usually occur 24–48 h before croup is experienced. The most frequent cause of viral or infectious croup is parainfluenza; however, croup can also be caused by infection with several different respiratory viruses. Viral croup usually manifests between the ages of 6 months and 3 years, peaking at 18 months. The symptoms of croup usually go away in 48 h, but they can linger for a week [11]. Although retropharyngeal abscesses can occur at any age, children under the age of 5 are most frequently affected. Children's retropharyngeal abscesses are mostly caused by infection and suppuration of the lymph nodes that make up the retropharyngeal chains. Fever, sore throat, dysphagia, odynophagia, neck pain, edema, restricted neck motion, and torticollis are common presenting symptoms. Most reports show a relatively small proportion of cases with airway obstruction symptoms like breathing difficulties and stridor. Airway obstruction primarily affects newborns and young children [12].

5. **B, E**

With conservative treatment, the majority of laryngomalacia patients usually experience symptom resolution by the time they become 1 year old. For the remaining children, resolution is often seen by the time they are 18–24 months old. Based on the medical history and examination, the patient has been diagnosed with moderate laryngomalacia. In such cases, the appropriate course of treatment is acid suppression medication, as acid reflux and laryngomalacia coexist. This may involve the use of a PPI, a histamine-2 blocker (H2RA), or a combination of both [5, 13]. The use of breast milk or formula that has been thickened, as well as slower feedings carried out while standing up, are examples of feeding interventions. However, in 10–15% of patients, severe laryngomalacia results in persistent stridor with failure-to-thrive symptoms [5]. Indications for surgery include stridor with respiratory distress, episodic cyanosis during feeding, dyspnea with retractions, recurrent aspiration pneumonia, pectus excavatum, failure to thrive, pulmonary hypertension, cor pulmonale, and severe obstructive sleep apnea. Currently, the preferred surgical technique is supraglottoplasty [5, 13]. In certain patients with blockage brought on by posterior epiglottis collapse, epiglottopexy may be required. Nowadays, tracheostomy is utilized in situations where supraglottoplasty proves ineffective or when patients exhibit other conditions necessitating a surgical airway [5].

References

1. Pfleger A, Eber E. Assessment and causes of stridor. Paediatr Respir Rev. 2016;18:64–72.
2. Zalzal HG, Zalzal GH. Stridor in the infant patient. Pediatr Clin N Am. 2022;69(2):301–17.
3. Clark CM, Kugler K, Carr MM. Common causes of congenital stridor in infants. JAAPA. 2018;31(11):36–40.
4. Garefis K, Garefi M, Tarazis K, Chatziavramidis A, Pervana S, Konstantinidis I. Postintubation hypopharyngeal granuloma causing stridor in an infant. Ear Nose Throat J. 2024;103(7):406–8.
5. Bedwell J, Zalzal G. Laryngomalacia. Semin Pediatr Surg. 2016;25(3):119–22.
6. Saravanam PK, Manimaran V. Flexible laryngoscopy in management of congenital stridor. Indian J Otolaryngol Head Neck Surg. 2017;69(4):509–13.
7. Zalzal GH, Anon JB, Cotton RT. Epiglottoplasty for the treatment of laryngomalacia. Ann Otol Rhinol Laryngol. 1987;96(1 Pt 1):72–6.
8. Dickson JM, Richter GT, Meinzen-Derr J, et al. Secondary airway lesions in infants with laryngomalacia. Ann Otol Rhinol Laryngol. 2009;118(1):37–43.
9. Schroeder JW Jr, Bhandarkar ND, Holinger LD. Synchronous airway lesions and outcomes in infants with severe laryngomalacia requiring supraglottoplasty. Arch Otolaryngol Head Neck Surg. 2009;135(7):647–51.
10. Berg E, Naseri I, Sobol SE. The role of airway fluoroscopy in the evaluation of children with stridor. Arch Otolaryngol Head Neck Surg. 2008;134(4):415–8.
11. Quraishi H, Lee DJ. Recurrent croup. Pediatr Clin N Am. 2022;69(2):319–28.
12. Tebruegge M, Curtis N. 28—Infections related to the upper and middle airways. In: Long SS, editor. Principles and practice of pediatric infectious diseases. 4th ed. Elsevier; 2012. p. 205–13.e6.
13. Carter J, Rahbar R, Brigger M, Chan K, Cheng A, Daniel SJ, De Alarcon A, Garabedian N, Hart C, Hartnick C, Jacobs I, Liming B, Nicollas R, Pransky S, Richter G, Russell J, Rutter MJ, Schilder A, Smith RJ, Strychowsky J, Ward R, Watters K, Wyatt M, Zalzal G, Zur K, Thompson D. International Pediatric ORL Group (IPOG) laryngomalacia consensus recommendations. Int J Pediatr Otorhinolaryngol. 2016;86:256–61.

Supraglottitis

5

Fotini Ieridou and Konstantinos Garefis

Abstract

Supraglottitis (SG) is a potentially life-threatening inflammatory condition of the supraglottic region, commonly caused by bacteria such as *Haemophilus influenzae* type b, *Streptococcus pneumoniae*, *Staphylococcus aureus*, etc. The incidence of SG has changed since the introduction of the *Haemophilus influenzae* vaccine. Symptoms and signs of this disease may be nonspecific. It commonly presents with symptoms such as sore throat, odynophagia, dysphagia, and drooling, while children more often present with stridor and fever. Diagnosis is usually made through clinical assessment, identifying signs of erythema and swelling in the supraglottic area, and/or may involve imaging studies. Treatment of SG depends on the severity of symptoms. For mild cases, it may include conservative therapy with intravenous antibiotics with possible additional steroids and closely monitoring the airway. In serious cases, interventions such as intubation, cricothyrotomy, or tracheostomy to secure the airway may be needed.

Case Presentation

A 45-year-old male presents to the emergency department with a severe sore throat, difficulty in swallowing his saliva, and a muffled voice persisting for approximately 2 days. The day before, he was examined by his GP and discharged home with a diagnosis of viral upper respiratory infection. He reports fever, chills, and a sensation of impending airway obstruction. He is currently breathing comfortably with no signs of respiratory distress. His neck is tender to palpation and refuses to lie flat. On endoscopy, there is a swollen, cherry-red epiglottis as well as mild arytenoid swelling (Fig. 5.1). The rest of the head and neck examination was normal.

Questions

1. Which of the following statements are true about supraglottitis (SG)? (more than one correct answer possible)
   A. It involves inflammation of arytenoids
   B. The peak incidence in adults occurs at 30 years of age
   C. The most commonly described pathogen in adults is *Haemophilus influenza* type b
   D. Currently, it is more frequent in children
   E. Treatment should be undertaken in a hospital
2. Which of the following are typical symptoms and signs of SG in adults? (more than one correct answer possible)

F. Ieridou
University Hospitals Plymouth NHS Trust, Plymouth, UK

K. Garefis (✉)
2nd Academic ORL, Head and Neck Surgery Department, Aristotle University of Thessaloniki, Papageorgiou Hospital, Thessaloniki, Greece

N. Tsetsos et al. (eds.), *Otolaryngology Study Guide*, https://doi.org/10.1007/978-3-031-77374-7_5

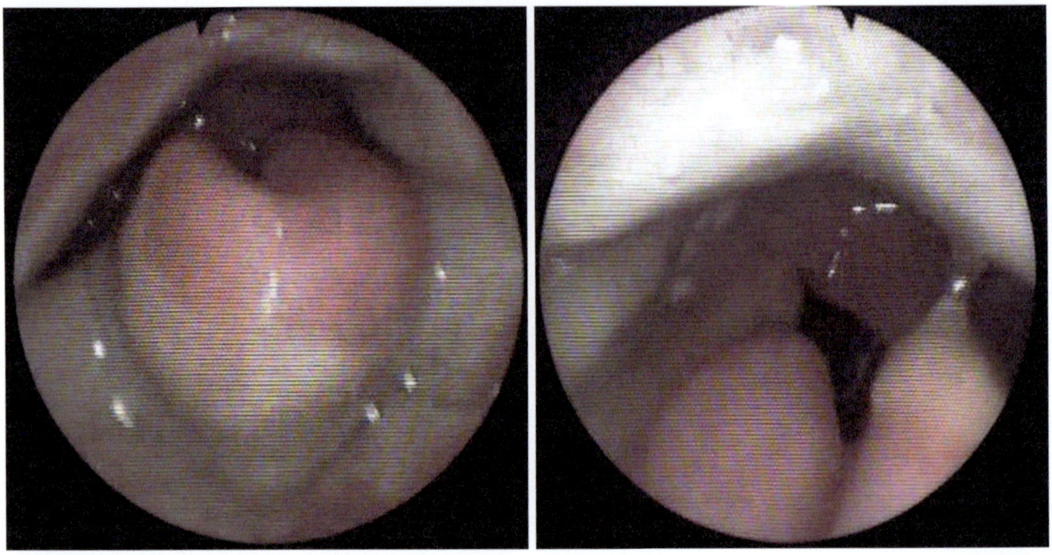

Fig. 5.1 Endoscopic images of the patient's larynx

A. Odynophagia
B. Cough
C. Sore throat with pain
D. Dysphagia
E. Tripod position

3. Which of the following examinations is most appropriate for establishing the diagnosis of SG?
   A. Lateral neck radiograph
   B. Oropharyngeal examination
   C. Neck ultrasonography
   D. Flexible laryngoscopy
   E. Computed tomography (CT)
4. Which of the following is NOT included in the differential diagnosis of SG? (more than one correct answer possible)
   A. Parapharyngeal abscess
   B. Ludwig angina
   C. Facial paralysis
   D. Angioedema
   E. Laryngeal papilloma
5. What treatment approach would you recommend as appropriate for the patient described above? (more than one correct answer possible)
   A. Tracheostomy
   B. Nebulized adrenaline
   C. Intravenous ceftriaxone
   D. Intravenous corticosteroids
   E. Intubation

Answers

1. **A, E**

   Supraglottitis (SG) involves inflammation of the supraglottic part of the larynx, including the arytenoids, false vocal cords, laryngeal ventricles, aryepiglottic folds, and epiglottis [1]. SG was historically viewed as primarily affecting children aged 2–6 years old [2]. However, following the introduction of the *Haemophilus influenzae* type b (HiB) vaccine, cases of SG are now more frequently diagnosed in adults [3]. The incidence rate in adults is approximately 1–2.9 cases per 100,000 per year, which is 2.5 times higher than that observed in children [4]. The typical age of onset falls between 42 and 48 years, with a male-to-female ratio of about 2.5–1 [3]. Although *Streptococcus pneumoniae* is commonly cited as the predominant pathogen in adults, other bacteria such as Hib, *Staphylococcus aureus*, and *Neisseria meningitidis* also play significant roles [1, 2].

2. **A, C, D**

   The presentation and clinical progression of SG in adults often differ from those observed in pediatric cases [4]. In adults, the onset of SG is typically slower compared to children, with fewer severe respiratory symptoms and a higher prevalence of pharyngeal symptoms [1]. Common initial symptoms include sore throat and pain while swallowing, seen in over 90% of cases, followed by muffled voice, drooling, dyspnea, stridor, and cough, which are reported in less than 50% of cases. Stridor and dyspnea are indicators of an increased likelihood of requiring airway intervention [5]. Although odynophagia and dysphagia are common symptoms, they may not always be present, particularly in the early stages [1]. Clinical signs include elevated temperature and respiratory rate, lymphadenopathy, and tenderness of the anterior neck, specifically over the hyoid bone [1, 4]. In contrast, children typically exhibit tripod positioning, fever, and stridor that worsen gradually over hours. However, less than half of adults with epiglottitis display tripod positioning and cough [6].

3. **D**

   Flexible laryngoscopy is the preferred diagnostic procedure, revealing an inflamed and swollen supraglottis, while a routine oropharyngeal examination may not reliably exclude epiglottitis [1, 4]. Abnormalities visible on lateral neck radiographs include thickening of the epiglottis (referred to as the "thumb sign"), arytenoid and aryepiglottic fold swelling, a pencil-thin airway, and swelling of the prevertebral soft tissues. In situations where flexible laryngoscopy is unavailable, a plain X-ray may offer diagnostic value. Neck ultrasonography as a diagnostic modality for SG lacks sufficient evaluation of its accuracy [7]. CT and magnetic resonance imaging (MRI) can aid in assessing complications such as the spread of infection and abscess formation. Radiological signs commonly seen in epiglottic abscess include thickening of the epiglottis, subcutaneous tissues, and muscles, as well as loss of preepiglottic fat [4]. Blood and throat cultures provide limited diagnostic utility. Laboratory tests typically lack specificity [6]. White blood cell counts are usually elevated in 65–90% of cases, with an average value of 15×10^9/L [4].

4. **C, E**

   Various infectious causes affecting the upper airways can present symptoms similar to SG. These include pharyngitis, infectious mononucleosis, lingual tonsillitis, peritonsillar abscess, Ludwig angina, and laryngitis. Additionally, non-infectious diseases such as angioedema, gastroesophageal reflux disease, laryngeal tumors or trauma, and injuries from chemical inhalation or ingestion can also mimic SG [4]. Approximately 90% of adult patients diagnosed with epiglottitis may exhibit a normal oropharyngeal examination. Therefore, clinicians should not disregard the possibility of epiglottitis or other potentially serious conditions solely based on a normal oropharyngeal assessment. These conditions may include a foreign body in the inferior oropharynx, Lemierre's syndrome, infection in the parapharyngeal space, retropharyngeal abscess, or tracheitis [6].

5. **B, C, D**

   The patient of case description has mild supraglottitis without respiratory distress. Therefore, it is crucial to promptly initiate intravenous antibiotic treatment using a broad-spectrum antibiotic effective against Gram-positive organisms Hib. Given the rising prevalence of beta-lactamase-resistant Hib, third-generation cephalosporins or amoxicillin/clavulanic acid are now preferred as first-line agents. Metronidazole may be considered as an addition if anaerobic bacteria are anticipated. The use of corticosteroids remains a topic of debate. Administering a short course of steroids, unless there are specific contraindications, might reduce airway inflammatory edema, potentially lowering the need for intubation and reducing hospital stay duration [4]. Moreover, the use of supplemental oxygen and nebulized adrenaline (1:1000 dilution) will aid the patient [1]. Typically, the disease resolves within 36–48 h [4]. Starting treatment promptly usually halts the disease's progression. However, if the patient's airway deteriorates, leading to acute airway obstruction (characterized by dyspnea, stridor, and cyanosis), immediate interventions such as intubation or emergency tracheostomy are necessary [1, 4]. In the postvaccine era, clinicians should anticipate the need to ensure airway stability in approximately 10.9% of instances [2].

References

1. Navaratnam AV, Smith ME, Majeed A, McFerran DJ. Adult supraglottitis: a potential airway emergency that can present in primary care. Br J Gen Pract. 2015;65(631):99–100.
2. Sideris A, Holmes TR, Cumming B, Havas T. A systematic review and meta-analysis of predictors of airway intervention in adult epiglottitis. Laryngoscope. 2020;130(2):465–73.
3. Sobol SE, Zapata S. Epiglottitis and croup. Otolaryngol Clin N Am. 2008;41(3):551–66, ix.
4. Al-Qudah M, Shetty S, Alomari M, Alqdah M. Acute adult supraglottitis: current management and treatment. South Med J. 2010;103(8):800–4.
5. Eskander A, de Almeida JR, Irish JC. Acute upper airway obstruction. N Engl J Med. 2019;381(20):1940–9.
6. Bridwell RE, Koyfman A, Long B. High risk and low prevalence diseases: adult epiglottitis. Am J Emerg Med. 2022;57:14–20.
7. Fujiwara T, Miyata T, Tokumasu H, Gemba H, Fukuoka T. Diagnostic accuracy of radiographs for detecting supraglottitis: a systematic review and meta-analysis. Acute Med Surg. 2016;4(2):190–7.

6 Complications of Rhinosinusitis

Yazan Kanaan

Abstract

Acute and chronic rhinosinusitis, if left untreated, can lead to complications that can be life-threatening on rare occasions. Due to the close anatomical relationship between the orbital cavity and the paranasal sinuses, orbital complications are the most common ones. The orbital complications of rhinosinusitis have been classified by Chandler et al. Pott's puffy tumour is not an actual tumour, but osteomyelitis of the frontal bone associated with subperiosteal abscess causing swelling and oedema over the forehead and scalp. Intracranial complications occur either due to direct extension or venous drainage. These complications include meningitis, epidural, subdural, brain abscess, and dural venous sinus thrombosis. Cavernous sinus thrombosis is a rare but life-threatening complication of sinusitis.

Case Presentation

A 15-year-old boy presented to the emergency department with a 2-day history of progressively worsening left periorbital swelling and pain; he has a recent history of nasal discharge that was being treated conservatively. On examination, there is left periorbital swelling, chemosis, painful eye movement, and purulent nasal discharge. The neurological exam was unremarkable. Swab cultures were taken and sent for analysis. CT scan with contrast was obtained (Fig. 6.1).

Questions

1. Which of the following is the most common complication of acute sinusitis?
   A. Orbital complication
   B. Meningitis
   C. Brain abscess
   D. Pott's puffy tumour
   E. Epidural abscess
2. Which of the following is not one of the orbital complications of sinusitis described in Chandler's classification?
   A. Pre-septal cellulitis
   B. Orbital cellulitis
   C. Orbital abscess
   D. Dacryocystitis
   E. Cavernous sinus thrombosis
3. Which of the following statements about Pott's puffy tumour are false (more than one answer can be chosen)?
   A. Mostly a complication of infection in the ethmoid sinuses.
   B. 15% are malignant.
   C. Can be associated with trauma.

Y. Kanaan (✉)
University Hospitals Plymouth NHS Trust,
Plymouth, UK

N. Tsetsos et al. (eds.), *Otolaryngology Study Guide*, https://doi.org/10.1007/978-3-031-77374-7_6

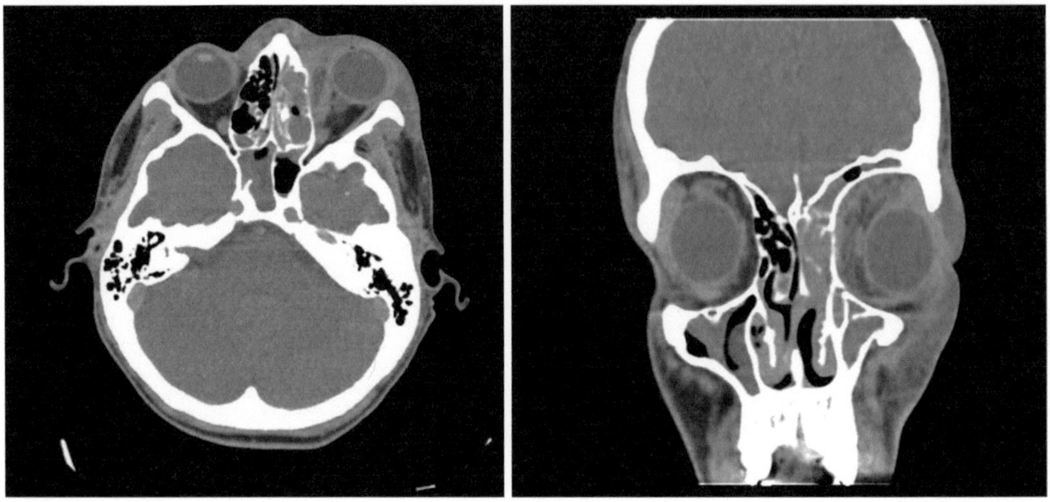

Fig. 6.1 CT scan

   D. Patients can present with forehead swelling, fever, headache, and periorbital swelling.
   E. Can be associated with intracranial complications including meningitis, brain abscess, and dural venous sinus thrombosis.
4. The most common microorganism associated with cavernous sinus thrombosis is:
   A. *Streptococcus pneumoniae*
   B. *Haemophilus influenzae*
   C. *Staphylococcus aureus*
   D. *Aspergillus*
   E. *Escherichia coli*
5. Which of the following statements is/are false regarding osteomyelitis as a complication of rhinosinusitis?
   A. The most common sinus involved is the sphenoid sinus.
   B. Usually occurs either due to direct extension or through thrombophlebitis of the diploic veins.
   C. Osteomyelitis of the frontal bone is more common in adults than in children and adolescents.
   D. Can lead to subperiosteal abscess or frontocutaneous fistula.
   E. Treatment required surgical drainage and antibiotics.

Answers

1. **A**

   Acute and chronic rhinosinusitis, if left untreated, can lead to complications that can be life-threatening on rare occasions. Due to the close anatomical relationship between the orbital cavity and the paranasal sinuses, orbital complications are the most common ones [1]. Intracranial complications are rare, and the incidence is about 4% in patients with acute or chronic sinusitis [1, 2]. The common presenting symptoms of intracranial involvement are altered mental state, headache, fever, seizure, vomiting, unilateral weakness, or cranial nerve involvement. Whenever intracranial complications are suspected, urgent magnetic resonance imaging (MRI) or computed tomography (CT) scans are needed to assess the extent of intracranial involvement and whether urgent neurosurgical interventions are needed [3].

2. **D**

   The orbital complications of rhinosinusitis have been classified by Chandler et al. into five categories: (1) Preseptal cellulitis, (2) orbital cellulitis, (3) subperiosteal abscess, (4) orbital abscess, and (5) cavernous sinus thrombosis [4, 5]. Chandler 1, 2, and some cases of 3 are primarily treated with intravenous antibiotics. However, additional surgical intervention is needed if the patient develops vision loss or does not show evidence of clinical improvement within 24–48 h. Chandler 4 and 5 are treated with intravenous antibiotics as well as surgical drainage by functional endoscopic sinus surgery and orbital drainage [4, 6].

3. **A, B**

Pott's puffy tumour is not an actual tumour; it is an osteomyelitis of the frontal bone associated with subperiosteal abscess causing swelling and oedema over the forehead and scalp. It is a complication of frontal sinusitis or trauma [7, 8]. Patients can present with headache, forehead and periorbital swelling, fever, and sometimes signs of intracranial involvement. Intracranial complications occur either due to direct extension or venous drainage. These complications include meningitis, epidural, subdural, brain abscess, and dural venous sinus thrombosis [7, 9].

4. **C**

Cavernous sinus thrombosis is a rare but life-threatening condition that can result from infections in the face, paranasal sinuses, orbits, or ears. It can also result from severe trauma or surgery. Fever, headache, periorbital oedema, and ophthalmoplegia are some of the most common symptoms [10]. Different infectious organisms can cause cavernous sinus thrombosis, but in most cases, they are bacterial. *Staphylococcus aureus* may be associated with two-thirds of cases, and methicillin resistance should always be considered [11, 12].

5. **A, C**

Osteomyelitis, as a complication of frontal sinusitis, usually occurs due to direct extension of the infection to the frontal bone or through thrombophlebitis of the diploic veins. It usually affects children and adolescents and is considered to be rare in adults. Osteomyelitis due to other paranasal sinusitis is rare. It can lead to the development of a subperiosteal abscess of the frontal bone (Pott's puffy tumour) or the formation of a frontocutaneous fistula [13]. A recent literature review has shown that performing intranasal sinus surgery along with simple percutaneous drainage is effective in treating this condition [14].

References

1. Pradhan P, Samal DK, Preetam C, Parida PK. Intraorbital and intracranial complications of acute rhinosinusitis: a rare case report. Iran J Otorhinolaryngol. 2018;30(100):301–4.
2. Clayman GL, Adams GL, Paugh DR, Koopmann CF Jr. Intracranial complications of paranasal sinusitis: a combined institutional review. Laryngoscope. 1991;101(3):234–9. https://doi.org/10.1288/00005537-199103000-00003.
3. Jones NS, Walker JL, Bassi S, Jones T, Punt J. The intracranial complications of rhinosinusitis: can they be prevented? Laryngoscope. 2002;112(1):59–63. https://doi.org/10.1097/00005537-200201000-00011.
4. Dankbaar JW, van Bemmel AJ, Pameijer FA. Imaging findings of the orbital and intracranial complications of acute bacterial rhinosinusitis. Insights Imaging. 2015;6(5):509–18. https://doi.org/10.1007/s13244-015-0424-y. Epub 2015 Aug 8.
5. Chandler JR, Langenbrunner DJ, Stevens ER. The pathogenesis of orbital complications in acute sinusitis. Laryngoscope. 1970;80(9):1414–28. https://doi.org/10.1288/00005537-197009000-00007.
6. Coenraad S, Buwalda J. Surgical or medical management of subperiosteal orbital abscess in children: a critical appraisal of the literature. Rhinology. 2009;47(1):18–23.
7. Sharma P, Sharma S, Gupta N, Kochar P, Kumar Y. Pott puffy tumor. Proc (Bayl Univ Med Cent). 2017;30(2):179–81. https://doi.org/10.1080/08998280.2017.11929575.
8. ur Rehman A, Muhammad MN, Moallam FA. Pott puffy tumor: a rare complication of sinusitis. Ann Saudi Med. 2013;33(1):79–80. https://doi.org/10.5144/0256-4947.2012.26.5.1116.
9. Ketenci I, Unlü Y, Tucer B, Vural A. The Pott's puffy tumor: a dangerous sign for intracranial complications. Eur Arch Otorrinolaringol. 2011;268(12):1755–63. https://doi.org/10.1007/s00405-011-1660-5.
10. Ali S. Cavernous sinus thrombosis: efficiently recognizing and treating a life-threatening condition. Cureus. 2021;13(8):e17339. https://doi.org/10.7759/cureus.17339.
11. Plewa MC, Tadi P, Gupta M. Cavernous sinus thrombosis. In: StatPearls. Treasure Island, FL: StatPearls Publishing; 2022.
12. Branson SV, McClintic E, Yeatts RP. Septic cavernous sinus thrombosis associated with orbital cellulitis: a report of 6 cases and review of literature. Ophthalmic Plast Reconstr Surg. 2019;35(3):272–80. https://doi.org/10.1097/IOP.0000000000001231.

13. Al Yaeesh I, AlOmairin A, Al Shakhs A, Almomen A, Almomen Z, AlBahr A, AlNaim A, Al Abdulgader A, Alawadh A. The serious complications of frontal sinusitis, a case series and literature review. J Surg Case Rep. 2020;2020(12):rjaa474. https://doi.org/10.1093/jscr/rjaa474.
14. Tatsumi S, Ri M, Higashi N, Wakayama N, Matsune S, Tosa M. Pott's puffy tumor in an adult: a case report and review of literature. J Nippon Med Sch. 2016;83(5):211–4. https://doi.org/10.1272/jnms.83.211.

7 Mastoiditis

Konstantinos Garefis

Abstract

Mastoiditis is an infection of the mastoid bone's cell system, caused by bacteria. It can present in various forms such as acute, coalescent, chronic, and masked mastoiditis. It is the most frequent complication of acute otitis media, affecting up to 0.4% of cases, predominantly in young children. The primary pathogen causing acute mastoiditis is *Streptococcus pneumoniae*, followed by *Streptococcus pyogenes*, *Staphylococcus aureus*, *Pseudomonas aeruginosa*, *Haemophilus influenzae*, *Escherichia coli*, and *Proteus mirabilis*. Typical symptoms include fever, ear pain, post-auricular erythema, tenderness, protrusion of the pinna, acute otitis media, and sagging of the posterior-superior external auditory canal (EAC) wall visible on otoscopy or a subperiosteal abscess. Patients may also exhibit leukocytosis, a low-grade or septic fever, and occasionally chills. Computed tomography (CT) scanning is the most commonly used imaging technique, which can show loss of mastoid air cell trabeculations, local bone destruction, and the presence of soft tissue within the mastoid cavity and middle ear cleft. Complications can be intratemporal (such as facial nerve palsy and labyrinthitis), extracranial (such as subperiosteal abscess and Bezold's abscess), or intracranial (such as meningitis and subdural/brain abscess). Treatment options for acute mastoiditis range from intravenous antibiotics alone or in combination with myringotomy or tympanostomy tube placement, to subperiosteal incision and drainage, or mastoidectomy.

Case Presentation

You are called to examine a 5-year-old boy. The information provided indicates that the boy experienced an acute otitis media in his left ear 12 days prior. A fever of 39 °C and ear pain on the same side began 2 days ago. At present, there is redness behind the ear, tenderness, and outward displacement of the ear. An otoscopic examination revealed a sagging of the posterior-superior ear canal and signs of acute otitis media.

Figure 7.1 shows intraoperative image of mastoidectomy showing pus into the left mastoid cavity.

Questions

1. Which of the following statements are true about acute mastoiditis? (more than one correct answer possible)
   A. It is a common complication of acute otitis media in pediatric population

K. Garefis (✉)
2nd Academic ORL, Head and Neck Surgery Department, Aristotle University of Thessaloniki, Papageorgiou Hospital, Thessaloniki, Greece

N. Tsetsos et al. (eds.), *Otolaryngology Study Guide*, https://doi.org/10.1007/978-3-031-77374-7_7

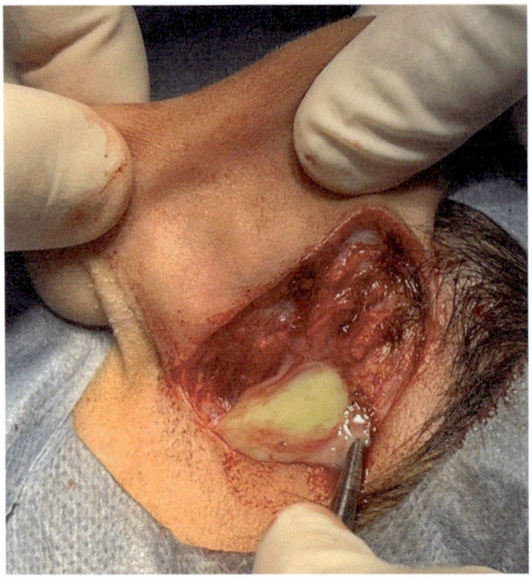

Fig. 7.1 Intraoperative image of mastoidectomy showing pus into the left mastoid cavity

B. *Streptococcus pneumoniae* is the most frequently isolated pathogen
C. *Pseudomonas aeruginosa* is the most frequently isolated pathogen
D. It is more common in neonates
E. As children grow up, it becomes more frequent

2. All of the following are clinical signs of mastoiditis except from?
   A. Sagging of posteroinferior deep part of EAC wall
   B. Reservoir sign
   C. Tenderness on mastoid tip
   D. Subperiosteal abscess
   E. Protrusion of the pinna
3. CT scanning is superior to magnetic resonance imaging (MRI) in establishing which one of the following diagnoses?
   A. Bezold's abscess
   B. Coalescent mastoiditis
   C. Epidural abscess
   D. Cerebellar abscess
   E. Subdural empyema
4. Which of the following statements about treatment of pediatric acute mastoiditis are true? (more than one correct answer possible)
   A. Intravenous antibiotics are always necessary
   B. Treatment with antibiotics alone can be effective in complicated cases
   C. Myringotomy is required in subperiosteal abscess
   D. Mastoidectomy is a first-line treatment in complicated cases
   E. All of the above
5. All of the following are complications of mastoiditis except from?
   A. Facial palsy
   B. Thrombosis of the cavernous sinus
   C. Labyrinthitis
   D. Bezold's abscess
   E. Petrous apicitis

Answers

1. **A, B**

Acute mastoiditis is the most frequent intratemporal complication of otitis media in children [1]. The bacteria causing acute mastoiditis are similar to those causing acute otitis media, including *Streptococcus pneumoniae* (10–43%), *Streptococcus pyogenes* (9–18%), *Staphylococcus aureus* (9–10%), *Pseudomonas aeruginosa* (8–11%), *Haemophilus influenzae* (3–4%), *Escherichia coli*, and *Proteus mirabilis* [2–4]. The highest incidence of acute mastoiditis is seen in the second to third year of life, with a twofold increase in children under 2 years old [1]. As children age, the incidence of acute mastoiditis decreases, with a rate of 13.5–16.8 per 100,000 in children under 2 years old and 4.3–7.1 per 100,000 in those aged 2–16 years [5].

2. **E**

The clinical manifestations of mastoiditis include a sagging of the posterosuperior deep part of the EAC wall, redness, sensitivity, outward displacement of the ear, fever, and ear pain [4, 6]. A quick recollection of pus in the EAC, known as the reservoir sign, is a potential clinical indicator of mastoiditis [7].

3. **B**

Coalescent mastoiditis is marked by the destruction of the bony septae within the mastoid air cells [8]. The most reliable imaging technique is contrast-enhanced high-resolution CT scanning of the temporal bone [8–10]. A CT scan can identify bone destruction caused by inflammation, as seen in coalescent mastoiditis. MRI has demonstrated greater sensitivity than CT in assessing vascular and intracranial complications (such as meningitis, subdural/epidural/brain abscess) of mastoiditis [9, 10].

4. **A, C, D**

While mastoidectomy may be the ultimate treatment, prior research indicates that using intravenous antibiotics alone, or in combination with myringotomy with or without tube placement (particularly in patients under 2 years old), is highly effective as initial therapy in uncomplicated cases of acute mastoiditis [1, 5, 11]. Indications for surgical intervention include the presence of complications, no improvement after 48 h, or disease progression. If a subperiosteal abscess is present, it should be managed either through incision and drainage or needle aspiration, along with concurrent myringotomy with or without tube placement [5, 11]. If less invasive methods are unsuccessful, a mastoidectomy may be necessary, which has a near 100% success rate [5]. Antibiotics are necessary in all cases of acute mastoiditis [11].

5. **B**

Potential complications of mastoiditis can be divided into extracranial and intracranial categories. Extracranial complications encompass subperiosteal abscess and Bezold's abscess, which is an abscess that spreads into the neck muscles due to mastoid bone destruction [12]. Intracranial complications include meningitis, brain abscess, and sigmoid sinus thrombosis. The latter can occur when infection from the middle ear and/or mastoid cavity spreads to the sigmoid sinus via small emissary veins or through a bone dehiscence of the mastoid process [12].

References

1. Loh R, Phua M, Shaw CL. Management of paediatric acute mastoiditis: systematic review. J Laryngol Otol. 2018;132(2):96–104.
2. Choi SS, Lander L. Pediatric acute mastoiditis in the post-pneumococcal conjugate vaccine era. Laryngoscope. 2011;121:1072–80.
3. Luntz M, Brodsky A, Nusem S, Kronenberg J, Keren G, Migirov L, et al. Acute mastoiditis—the antibiotic era: a multicenter study. Int J Pediatr Otorhinolaryngol. 2001;57:1–9.
4. Martin C, Sterkers O, Arnold W. Acute mastoiditis. In: Otorhinolaryngology, head and neck surgery. Berlin: Springer; 2010. p. 62–4.
5. Anne S, Schwartz S, Ishman SL, Cohen M, Hopkins B. Medical versus surgical treatment of pediatric acute mastoiditis: a systematic review. Laryngoscope. 2019;129(3):754–60.
6. van den Aardweg MT, Rovers MM, de Ru JA, Albers FW, Schilder AG. A systematic review of diagnostic criteria for acute mastoiditis in children. Otol Neurotol. 2008;29(6):751–7.
7. Asherson N. An early clinical sign of acute mastoiditis: the reservoir sign. Lancet. 1935;225(5812):150–1.
8. Fullmer T, Sweeney AD. Coalescent mastoiditis. Oper Tech Otolaryngol Head Neck Surg. 2017;28(4):270–6.
9. Antonelli PJ, Garside JA, Mancuso AA, Strickler ST, Kubilis PS. Computed tomography and the diagnosis of coalescent mastoiditis. Otolaryngol Head Neck Surg. 1999;120:350–4.
10. Saat R, Kurdo G, Laulajainen-Hongisto A, Markkola A, Jero J. Detection of coalescent acute mastoiditis on MRI in comparison with CT. Clin Neuroradiol. 2021;31(3):589–97.
11. Chesney J, Black A, Choo D. What is the best practice for acute mastoiditis in children? Laryngoscope. 2014;124(5):1057–8.
12. Ulanovski D, Yacobovich J, Kornreich L, Shkalim V, Raveh E. Pediatric otogenic sigmoid sinus thrombosis: 12-year experience. Int J Pediatr Otorhinolaryngol. 2014;78(6):930–3.

8 Sudden Sensorineural Hearing Loss

Konstantinos Garefis and Vasilios Nikolaidis

Abstract

Sudden sensorineural hearing loss (SSNHL), also known as sudden deafness, is an audiological emergency characterized by a swift decrease of over 30 dB in sensorineural hearing loss across at least three consecutive frequencies in less than 3 days. SSNHL can be idiopathic in cases with an unknown cause or non-idiopathic. The reported occurrence of SSNHL varies widely, with rates of 27 and 60 per 100,000 people per year in the United States and the European Union, respectively. The incidence of SSNHL does not differ between sexes. Clinical presentation typically includes unilateral sensorineural hearing loss, often accompanied by tinnitus and, in some cases, vertigo. Diagnosis is established through a comprehensive evaluation, including history taking, physical examination, and audiometric assessment. Corticosteroids alone or in combination with hyperbaric oxygen may be offered as treatment options. Corticosteroids can be given either systemically or locally via the middle ear. However, a significant percentage of patients' hearing will spontaneously recover. SSNHL patients with residual hearing loss and/or tinnitus should be counseled about the possible benefits of audiologic rehabilitation and other supportive interventions.

K. Garefis (✉) · V. Nikolaidis
2nd Academic ORL, Head and Neck Surgery Department, Aristotle University of Thessaloniki, Papageorgiou Hospital, Thessaloniki, Greece

Case Presentation

A 52-year-old male presents to the otolaryngology clinic with sudden onset hearing loss in his right ear over the past 48 h. He describes waking up with a sensation of muffled hearing and ringing in the affected ear. There is no history of preceding upper respiratory tract infection, trauma, or exposure to loud noise. The patient denies any history of vertigo or imbalance. Otoscopic examination reveals a normal tympanic membrane with no signs of infection or obstruction. His tympanogram was type A. Pure-tone audiometry shows sensorineural hearing loss in the affected ear, with an average threshold of 65 decibels (Fig. 8.1). There are no significant findings on neurological examination. The patient is otherwise healthy, with no known medical conditions or medication use, and he reports prior equally hearing from both ears.

Questions

1. Most cases of SSNHL are caused by:
   A. Temporal bone trauma

N. Tsetsos et al. (eds.), *Otolaryngology Study Guide*, https://doi.org/10.1007/978-3-031-77374-7_8

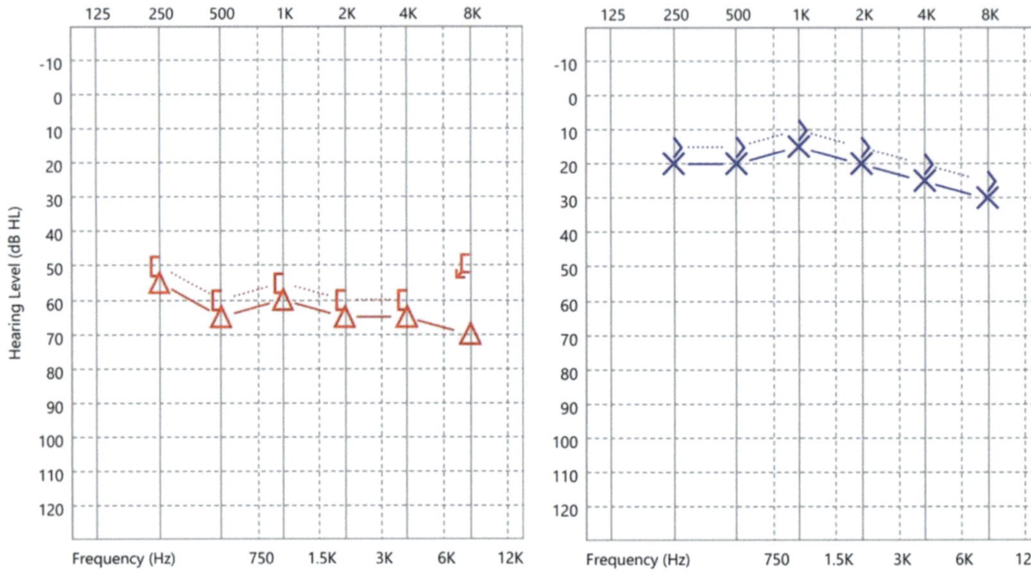

Fig. 8.1 Audiogram of the patient

B. Genetic predisposition
C. Vestibular schwannoma
D. No identifiable source\Idiopathic
E. Vascular insufficiency

2. Which of the following are probable symptoms of SSNHL? (more than one correct answer possible)
   A. Tinnitus
   B. Vertigo
   C. Ear pain
   D. Fullness in the ear
   E. All of the above
3. Which of the following statements are true about SSNHL? (more than one correct answer possible)
   A. It can affect both ears
   B. The peak age of occurrence is 30–40
   C. Routine laboratory tests are needed
   D. Computed tomography of the head should not be performed in the initial evaluation
   E. Pure-tone audiometry is essential as soon as possible to confirm the diagnosis
4. Treatment of SSNHL includes (more than one correct answer possible):
   A. Vitamin E
   B. Famvir
   C. Hyperbaric oxygen
   D. Intratympanic methylprednisolone
   E. Prednisone orally
5. Spontaneous hearing recovery after SSNHL, if it is to occur, usually occurs within what time frame?
   A. 5 days
   B. 2 weeks
   C. 2 months
   D. 6 months
   E. None of the above

Answers

1. **D**

   SSNHL can result from various factors such as viral infections, vascular insufficiency, autoimmune disorders, neoplasms (like vestibular schwannoma), stroke, radiation, head trauma, and ototoxicity. However, approximately 90% of SSNHL cases are idiopathic, as no specific cause can be identified despite thorough investigation [1–4].
2. **A**, **B**, **D**

   The primary symptom of SSNHL is sudden hearing loss. The degree of severity can vary from mild hearing loss to total deafness.

SSHNL is often, but not always, accompanied by additional symptoms such as ringing in the ears (tinnitus), dizziness (vertigo), a sensation of spinning, balance issues, and/or a feeling of fullness, pressure, or blockage in the ear. Patients experience dizziness in a range of 30–60% of cases. In more severe cases of SSNHL, dizziness or vertigo at the time of onset is usually observed, and it is generally linked to a worse prognosis for hearing recovery [3]. Tinnitus occurs in about 80% of patients and might persist, causing significant economic and psychological disturbance to the patient [1, 3]. If hearing is recovered, tinnitus often improves as well. Sudden SSNHL, especially when combined with tinnitus and dizziness, can lead to further declines in the quality of life [3].

3. **A, D, E**

Bilateral SSNHL is a rare condition. It can be caused by various systemic diseases, including neoplasms (such as neurofibromatosis type 2 with bilateral vestibular schwannomas), stroke, infections (viral infections such as herpes simplex virus, varicella-zoster virus, HIV; bacterial infections; syphilis; mycoplasma; tuberculosis; fungal infections; Lyme disease), and autoimmune disorders such as sarcoidosis or Cogan's syndrome [3]. Bilateral SSNHL occurring simultaneously is uncommon, representing only 0.4–3.4% of all cases. Despite prompt treatment, the prognosis for hearing recovery is typically poor [2]. SSNHL exhibits a broad age range, with an average occurrence observed between the ages of 50 and 60, while there is no predilection for gender [1]. Routine laboratory tests should not be ordered in patients with SSNHL due to the associated costs and potential harms related to false-positive and/or false-negative results. Furthermore, evidence indicates that these tests will not lead to changes in the diagnosis, treatment, or prognosis. Nonetheless, specific serologic testing should be conducted based on clinical assessment, such as when Lyme disease is suspected. CT of the head should not be routinely ordered during initial evaluation due to its low diagnostic yield, significant cost, and radiation exposure. However, it can be beneficial for patients with specific findings on history or physical examination, such as focal neurologic deficits, a history of trauma, or chronic ear disease. MRI is a valuable tool for assessing SSNHL patients for retrocochlear pathologies such as vestibular schwannoma. Auditory brainstem response (ABR) is also helpful in diagnosing such pathologies. MRI has largely replaced CT as the preferred imaging modality for detecting cerebellopontine angle tumors. Additionally, because CT lacks the resolution to detect brainstem infarcts in their early stages, emergent MRI is preferred when immediate imaging is necessary based on clinical presentation. Audiometry should be conducted promptly (within 14 days of symptom onset) to confirm the diagnosis. It is essential for definitive diagnosis and determines frequency-specific hearing thresholds and word recognition ability. SSNHL is defined as a hearing loss of 30 dB at three consecutive frequencies within a 72-h period. This assumes either normal hearing in each ear just before the SSNHL episode or symmetrical hearing loss in each ear prior to the SSNHL [3].

4. **C, D, E**

According to recent Clinical Practice Guideline, clinicians may prescribe corticosteroids (oral, intravenous, intramuscular, and/or intratympanic) as the initial treatment within 2 weeks of SSNHL onset. While oral administration is common, intratympanic injections may be used, especially for patients who cannot take oral steroids [1, 5]. The recommended corticosteroids for systemic administration include prednisone (max dose of 60 mg/day), methylprednisolone (48 mg/day), or dexamethasone (10 mg/day), taken at full dose for 7–14 days with no divided doses, followed by a taper over a similar period.

Moreover, intratympanic steroid therapy (injecting 0.4–0.8 mL into the middle ear space, up to four injections over a 2-week period) is recommended for salvage within 2–6 weeks after symptom onset. Hyperbaric oxygen therapy is considered a treatment option, but it should only be used in conjunction with steroid therapy, whether for initial treatment or salvage therapy. Initial treatment should begin within 2 weeks of onset, while salvage therapy should be initiated within 1 month. Antivirals, thrombolytics, vasodilators, or vasoactive substances should not be routinely recommended. Multiple trials have failed to show any benefit from adding antiviral drugs. Additionally, antioxidants have been removed from the list of interventions for SSNHL. However, patients with residual hearing loss and/or tinnitus should be counseled about the potential benefits of audiological rehabilitation and further supportive measures such as hearing aids, cochlear implants, and osseointegrated implants if appropriate [3].

5. **B**

Approximately half of patients experience full spontaneous recovery, typically occurring within 2 weeks [1, 6]. Partial recovery may occur in approximately one-third to two-thirds of patients within the same timeframe. Although the most significant improvement usually happens during this initial period, late recovery has been documented but is rare. Those who regain at least half of their hearing within the first 2 weeks generally have a more favorable prognosis, contrasting with patients who exhibit minimal change during this period, who are less likely to undergo significant improvement [3].

References

1. Schreiber BE, Agrup C, Haskard DO, Luxon LM. Sudden sensorineural hearing loss. Lancet. 2010;375(9721):1203–11.
2. Young YH. Contemporary review of the causes and differential diagnosis of sudden sensorineural hearing loss. Int J Audiol. 2020;59(4):243–53.
3. Chandrasekhar SS, Tsai Do BS, Schwartz SR, Bontempo LJ, Faucett EA, Finestone SA, Hollingsworth DB, Kelley DM, Kmucha ST, Moonis G, Poling GL, Roberts JK, Stachler RJ, Zeitler DM, Corrigan MD, Nnacheta LC, Satterfield L. Clinical practice guideline: sudden hearing loss (update). Otolaryngol Head Neck Surg. 2019;161(1_Suppl):S1–S45.
4. Chau JK, Lin JR, Atashband S, Irvine RA, Westerberg BD. Systematic review of the evidence for the etiology of adult sudden sensorineural hearing loss. Laryngoscope. 2010;120(5):1011–21.
5. Mirsalehi M, Ghajarzadeh M, Farhadi M, Akbarnejad Z, Ahmadi S, Salem MM. Intratympanic corticosteroid injection as a first-line treatment of the patients with idiopathic sudden sensorineural hearing loss compared to systemic steroid: a systematic review and meta-analysis. Am J Otolaryngol. 2022;43(5):103505.
6. Chaushu H, Ungar OJ, Abu Eta R, Handzel O, Muhanna N, Oron Y. Spontaneous recovery rate of idiopathic sudden sensorineural hearing loss: a systematic review and meta-analysis. Clin Otolaryngol. 2023;48(3):395–402.

9 Neck Wounds

Konstantinos Geronatsios

Abstract

Neck wounds are quite common ENT emergencies. Proper clinical evaluation and management is vital, as they can be life-threatening. The reason for this is that the neck is a region of the body which contains many vital structures, such as major blood vessels, nerves, muscles, the larynx, the trachea, and the esophagus. Neck traumas can be blunt including strangulation, penetrating, or both blunt and penetrating. The neck is divided into three anatomical zones, and this division has anatomic, diagnostic, and management purposes. Zone I is the area between the clavicles and cricoid cartilage, Zone II between the cricoid cartilage and the angle of the mandible, and Zone III between the angle of the mandible and the skull base. Vascular injuries are the most common in cases of penetrating neck wounds. In cases of carotid artery and internal jugular vein rupture, or airway injury, time is critical, and we should act immediately. In cases of non-life-threatening injuries, we should perform a detailed clinical and neurological examination, combined with a detailed history of the trauma, and imaging studies (neck CT scan, CT angiography, conventional angiography, ultrasound, and esophagography), before any surgical intervention.

K. Geronatsios (✉)
ENT Head and Neck Surgery Department,
424 General Military Hospital, Thessaloniki, Greece

Case Presentation

You are called from A&E at 01:30 am for two cases of neck wounds, which were transferred 5 min apart by ambulances. Case A involves a stab wound to the neck that occurred 20 min ago, and case B involves a blunt neck wound as a result of a horse bite 3 h ago. Both patients are stable and oriented. Patient A's neck (Fig. 9.1) was packed with gauze by paramedics due to active bleeding before the emergency ambulance transport to A&E. After carefully removing the packs, you notice that there is no active bleeding. Patient B (Fig. 9.2) complains of worsening swelling, a hematoma, but there are no signs of airway compromise or subcutaneous emphysema.

Questions

1. Which structures could be damaged in Case A? (more than one correct answer possible)
   A. External jugular vein
   B. Brachiocephalic artery
   C. Main trunk of the facial nerve
   D. Larynx
   E. Common carotid artery
2. Which scans would you request urgently for both cases? (more than one correct answer possible)
   A. MRI neck scan with contrast
   B. CT neck scan with contrast

N. Tsetsos et al. (eds.), *Otolaryngology Study Guide*, https://doi.org/10.1007/978-3-031-77374-7_9

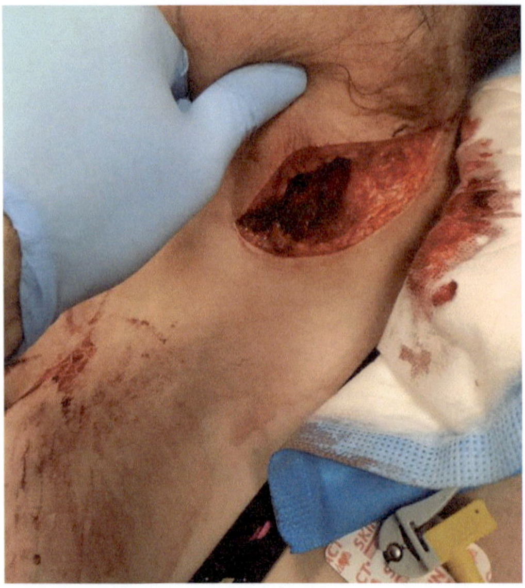

Fig. 9.1 Case A: Stab neck wound on the left side of the neck

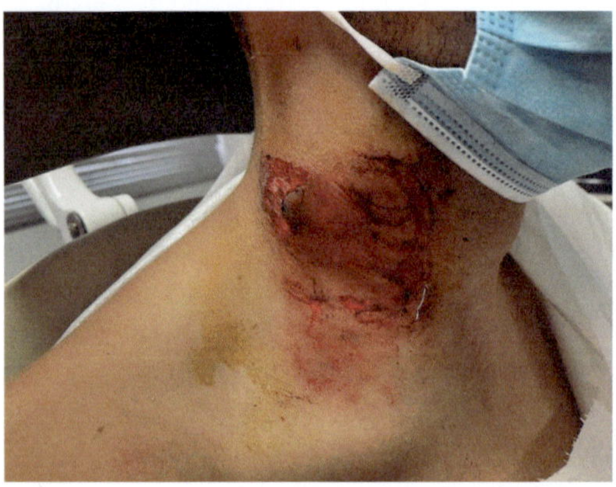

Fig. 9.2 Case B: Horse bite—blunt neck wound on the right side of the neck. Platysma is intact. Please notice the haematoma and the mild edema

C. Neck spine X-ray
D. CT neck angiography
E. CT head with contrast

3. There is a slot available for an urgent CT scan now. You have to prioritize your patients and choose one for a scan immediately. Which of the following you would choose first?
   A. A 3-year-old with otorrhea and possible mastoiditis, admitted a few hours ago and started on IV antibiotics. The cranial nerve examination is unremarkable
   B. Case A
   C. A 40-year-old with mild trismus and possible parapharyngeal abscess, no airway compromise, no signs of sepsis
   D. Case B
   E. A 72-year-old patient with hoarseness of voice and mild stridor with possible laryngeal malignancy on endoscopy, improved with steroids and adrenaline nebulizers
4. Which of the following would you do in A&E for both patients? Patients are both fully orientated with GCS = 15, stable and can communicate properly (more than one correct answer possible)
   A. Cranial nerve examination
   B. Cervical spine immobilization
   C. Flexible nasolaryngoscopy
   D. Exploration of the trauma in A&E
   E. Assessment of swallowing for solids and fluids in A&E
5. How would you treat both cases of neck wound? (more than one correct answer possible)
   A. Both cases should be treated surgically under anesthesia in theater for wound exploration and closure
   B. Case A should be treated surgically under anesthesia for wound exploration and closure
   C. Case B should be treated conservatively only
   D. Case A should be treated surgically under local anesthesia in A&E for wound closure
   E. Case B should be treated surgically or conservatively, depending on the clinical and radiological findings

Answers

1. **A, D, E**

   In case A, Zone II of the left side of the neck is involved. The neck is divided into three anatomical zones for anatomic, diagnostic, and management purposes. Zone I is the area between the clavicles and cricoid cartilage, Zone II is between the cricoid cartilage and the angle of the mandible, and Zone III is between the angle of the mandible and the skull base

[1]. The left external jugular vein, left common carotid artery, and larynx could be damaged in this case [1, 2]. The cervical branch of the facial nerve can also be damaged in this case, but the marginal mandibular branch is also in Zone II, but it is impossible to be traumatized in this case (the wound is more than 1.5 cm below the lower margin of the mandible). The brachiocephalic artery is on the right side of the neck. Even though part of the trachea is in Zone II, it is impossible for it to be ruptured in this case, because the level of the wound is above the cricoid cartilage [1–4].

2. **B, D**

In an emergency setting, a CT neck scan with contrast and CT angiography (the gold standard) are the indicated imaging studies for neck wounds. An MRI scan is not indicated and usually it is not available in A&E. An ultrasound and triplex of the neck may also be helpful, if available and if the patient is stable. A CT head scan and other investigations should be requested in cases of multi-trauma patients [5].

3. **D**

The correct answer is that we should perform a neck CT scan with contrast and CT angiography as soon as possible for case B. The reason for this is the presence of an expanding hematoma following a blunt neck injury (with an intact platysma) [1, 5]. We should immediately rule out any vessel rupture, pseudoaneurysm, dissection, or thrombosis. An expanding hematoma can cause airway compromise, requiring immediate action. Blunt traumas can also cause laryngeal fractures and esophageal rupture, so we should examine the patient for signs of subcutaneous emphysema, inquire about possible hemoptysis, and carefully evaluate any retrosternal pain or pain on swallowing [3, 5, 6].

4. **A, C**

We should thoroughly examine both patients, including a cranial nerve examination, and document our findings [3, 5]. This is very important in awake patients, especially pre-operatively. Flexible fiberoptic nasolaryngoscopy should be performed to evaluate any possible submucosal swelling—hematomas, vocal cord mobility, airway patency, and signs of hemorrhage. Trauma exploration in A&E is not indicated, as proper equipment is usually not available. It should be done in the theater for safety reasons and to avoid any hemorrhage and patient discomfort. Assessment of swallowing in A&E should not be done, especially if the patient is planned to have general anesthesia for surgical exploration of the wound. Cervical spine immobilization should be avoided, except in cases where cervical spine injury is potential [2, 6, 7].

5. **B, E**

Case A should be treated under general anesthesia for wound exploration and closure. We don't recommend closure under local anesthesia in A&E, because it is not well tolerated, there is no proper equipment available, and major bleeding may occur during the exploration [1, 4, 8]. The only case in which a penetrating wound could be treated in A&E under local anesthesia and the patient could be discharged after wound closure is when the platysma is intact [2, 7]. We should also mention that stab wounds, compared to gunshot wounds, usually cause less extensive damage, because damage is only found in the injury trajectory. Case B can be treated conservatively, if the hematoma is not worsening, and there are no signs of vessel injury, airway or esophageal trauma, or nerve damage [1–3].

References

1. Paul W, Flint MD. Penetrating and blunt trauma to the neck. In: Cummings otolaryngology: head and neck surgery. Elsevier; 2021.
2. Ernest E, Burnett A, Frascone RJ. High index of suspicion. Recognizing & managing traumatic neck injuries. JEMS. 2014;39(4):50–4.
3. Verdonck P, de Schoutheete J-C, Monsieurs KG, Van Laer C, Vander Poorten V, Vanderveken O. Penetrating and blunt trauma to the neck: clinical presentation, assessment and emergency management. B-ENT. 2016;12(Suppl 26/2):69–85.
4. Nowicki JL, Stew B, Ooi E. Penetrating neck injuries: a guide to evaluation and management. Ann R Coll

Surg Engl. 2018;100(1):6–11. https://doi.org/10.1308/rcsann.2017.0191. Epub 2017 Oct 19.
5. Offiah C, Hall E. Imaging assessment of penetrating injury of the neck and face. Insights Imaging. 2012;3(5):419–31. https://doi.org/10.1007/s13244-012-0191-y. Epub 2012 Sep 4.
6. Alao T, Waseem M. Neck trauma. In: StatPearls. Treasure Island, FL: StatPearls Publishing; 2022.
7. Sperry JL, Moore EE, Coimbra R, Croce M, Davis JW, Karmy-Jones R, McIntyre RC Jr, Moore FA, Malhotra A, Shatz DV, Biffl WL. Western Trauma Association critical decisions in trauma: penetrating neck trauma. J Trauma Acute Care Surg. 2013;75(6):936–40. https://doi.org/10.1097/TA.0b013e31829e20e3.
8. Tisherman SA, Bokhari F, Collier B, Cumming J, Ebert J, Holevar M, Kurek S, Leon S, Rhee P. Clinical practice guideline: penetrating zone II neck trauma. J Trauma. 2008;64(5):1392–405. https://doi.org/10.1097/TA.0b013e3181692116.

10 Tracheostomy Complications

Vaios Kaminiotis and Marios Stavrakas

Abstract

Tracheostomy is considered one of the oldest surgical procedures, as archaeological data dates back to ancient Egypt (3600 BC). The indications for tracheostomy are for emergency and elective reasons. The most common indication is airway management in critically ill patients, especially in ICU (70%), while the indication of emergency airway obstruction falls within a small percentage. Deficits in quality of care of a tracheostomy have led to adverse events in 20–30% of all in-patients in UK hospitals. It's been reported that around 50% of all airway-related deaths and hypoxic brain damage were caused by tracheostomy incidents. The safety of care delivery in tracheostomies depends on education, training, staffing, equipment provision, and infrastructure. Adverse events in adult patients with a new tracheostomy include accidental decannulation, tracheostomy-related haemorrhage, tube obstruction, skin breakdown, failed decannulation, cuff-related airway injury/hypoxaemia, and infection.

V. Kaminiotis
Harefield Hospital, Guy's and St Thomas' NHS Foundation Trust, London, UK

M. Stavrakas (✉)
ENT Head and Neck Surgery Department, University Hospitals Plymouth NHS Trust, Plymouth, UK

Case Presentation

You are called in the ICU because an intubated, obese patient with a recent tracheostomy is desaturating fast. The nurse in charge noticed that the tracheostomy tube is pulled approximately 1–2 cm away from the stoma and can't be pushed again as she meets resistance. Eventually, she manages to put it back in place, but the patient still desaturates, and there is significant resistance against manual ventilation (Fig. 10.1).

Questions

1. Which is the most possible cause of the first desaturation in the case presented?
   A. Tube obstruction
   B. Cuff-related hypoxaemia
   C. Skin breakdown
   D. Tracheoesophageal fistula
   E. Accidental decannulation/dislodgement
2. Which is the most possible cause for the patient to keep desaturating, even if the tracheostomy tube is placed back?
   A. Wrong pulse oximeter readings
   B. False passage anterior to the trachea
   C. Pneumonia
   D. Stroke
   E. Myocardial infarction
3. Which of the following represent late tracheostomy complications?
   A. Tracheo-innominate artery blowout
   B. Tracheal stenosis

N. Tsetsos et al. (eds.), *Otolaryngology Study Guide*, https://doi.org/10.1007/978-3-031-77374-7_10

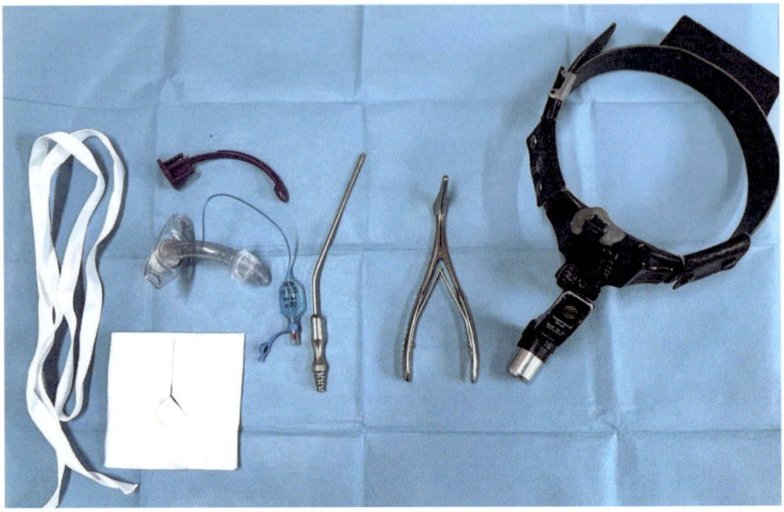

Fig. 10.1 Equipment for routine tracheostomy assessment and tracheostomy tube change

C. Tracheocutaneous fistula
D. Tracheoesophageal fistula
E. All the above

4. Which of the following statements are true?
   A. Tracheostomy is a clean-contaminated procedure
   B. Routine antibiotics are required
   C. Pneumonia and lung abscess are immediate complications
   D. Transient tracheitis and stomal cellulitis may occur
   E. A and D
5. What are the key differences in emergency oxygenation between the paediatric and adult populations?
   A. Bespoke paediatric bedhead signs reflecting paediatric tracheostomy indications and pathologies
   B. Recognition of (almost) exclusively surgical tracheostomies with stay sutures and maturation sutures available to aid emergency management
   C. Initial management includes up to three attempts at emergency tracheostomy tube changes
   D. Use of suction catheters to guide re-insertion
   E. All the above

Answers

1. **E**

   Global Tracheostomy Collaborative found that among 3443 adults, there were 167 cases where accidental decannulation occurred (4.85%), making it the most common adverse event. The second most common was tracheostomy-related bleeding (3.69%), and the third most common was tracheostomy tube obstruction (2.09%) [1].
2. **B**

   For the tracheostomy tube to be inserted directly into the trachea, the cutaneous and tracheal stoma should be aligned. Other signs of malposition in an intubated patient are high airway pressure ventilator alarms, the suction catheter not passing beyond the tracheostomy tube, and subcutaneous emphysema due to positive pressure ventilation [2].
3. **E**

   Massive bleeding is usually due to erosion of the innominate artery and formation of a tracheoinnominate artery fistula in 0.4% of tracheotomies and carries a mortality rate of 80–90%. Predisposing factors are long-term tracheal intubation and ventilation with a cuffed tracheotomy tube, which may result in cartilage necrosis. A "sentinel" bleed can occur 3 days to 3 weeks and precede the massive bleeding. Subglottic stenosis is predisposed by previous endotracheal tube intubation, high tracheostomy or cricothyroidotomy, and trauma to the airway. Children and patients tracheotomized for closed head trauma are at increased risk for tracheal stenosis. Tracheoesophageal fistula is rare, with a reported incidence of 0.01–1% but high mortality (70–80%). It is thought to result from damage to the posterior tracheal wall at the time of surgery or a combination of two factors: an overinflated and improperly fitted cuffed tube that puts pressure on the posterior tracheal wall together with a nasogastric tube in the oesophagus. Tracheocutaneous fistula is a late complication, which is more common because the stomal tract is epithelialized with long-term cannulation [3].

4. **E**

Tracheostomy is a clean-contaminated procedure, and routine administration of antibiotics is not indicated. Transient tracheitis and stomal cellulitis may occur. These infections are associated with mucosal injury, and aggressive local wound care is mandatory, even in seemingly mild local infections. Pulmonary complications, such as pneumonia or lung abscess, represent intermediate complications (hours—days in the post-operative period) and may arise due to aspiration of infected secretions. The causative organisms in most infections related to tracheostomy are *Staphylococcus aureus*, *Pseudomonas*, and other mixed flora. In more severe infections, such as necrotizing fasciitis, the organisms involved in 90% of cases are β-haemolytic streptococci or coagulase-positive staphylococci [3].

5. **E**

According to the National Tracheostomy Safety Project (Paediatric Working Party), all the statements represent differences in oxygenation and airway management attempts. It is essential to mention the stay sutures and stoma maturation sutures that aid re-insertion by widening the stoma and bringing the trachea closer to the skin. We should remember the different pathologies and tracheostomy indications in children and the differences in anatomy between children and adults [4].

References

1. Brenner MJ, Pandian V, Milliren CE, Graham DA, Zaga C, Morris LL, Bedwell JR, et al. Global Tracheostomy Collaborative: data-driven improvements in patient safety through multidisciplinary teamwork, standardisation, education, and patient partnership. Br J Anaesth. 2020;125(1):e104–18.
2. Morris LL, Afifi MS. The dreaded false passage: management of tracheostomy tube dislodgement. Emerg Med News. 2011;33(8):1. https://doi.org/10.1097/01.EEM.0000399883.10405.3d.
3. Goldenberg D, Ari EG, Golz A, Danino J, Netzer A, Joachims HZ. Tracheotomy complications: a retrospective study of 1130 cases. Otolaryngol Head Neck Surg. 2000;123(4):495–500.
4. Doherty C, Neal R, English C, Cooke J, Atkinson D, Bates L, Moore J, Monks S, Bowler M, Bruce IA, Bateman N. Multidisciplinary guidelines for the management of paediatric tracheostomy emergencies. Anaesthesia. 2018;73(11):1400–17.

Deep Neck Space Infections

11

Alexandros Poutoglidis and Paraskevi Karamitsou

Abstract

Deep neck infections are urgent and common conditions that can be life-threatening for people of all ages. To prevent serious complications, it is important to follow a thorough and quick algorithm in every case. The neck fasciae divide the head and neck into compartments, which determine the risk of inflammation spreading to nearby or distant areas.

The deep neck spaces are complex and have a predictable pattern of communication. The infected compartment provides information about the possible site of the original infection and guides the management of the condition. In children, acute Waldeyer's ring inflammations and dental infections (biofilms) are the main causes, and in adults, dental infections are more common. It is worth noting that methicillin-resistant *Staphylococcus aureus* (MRSA) is the most common pathogen in children under 24 months of age.

Although surgical management with drainage is usually the preferred treatment, the first priority should secure a threatened or potentially threatened airway through formal intubation or an emergent tracheostomy. Therefore, a computed tomography (CT) scan and its valuable information may not always be feasible. Conservative management with antibiotics and without drainage should only be considered in cases where there is involvement of a single neck space and an abscess cavity measuring less than 2.5 in. in its highest dimension. The presence of acute or progressive neurological symptoms is a worrisome sign and indicates the spread of infection throughout the body.

A. Poutoglidis (✉)
ENT Department, Lister Hospital, East and North Hertfordshire NHS Trust, Stevenage, UK

P. Karamitsou
ENT Head and Neck Surgery Department, "G. Papanikolaou" General Hospital of Thessaloniki, Thessaloniki, Greece

Case Presentation

A 69-year-old man visited the emergency otolaryngology department with a main complaint of a gradually increasing swelling in the left submandibular region. He had a small movable lump in that area for several years, but it had never caused any complications. However, he noticed that it had been getting larger over the past 5 days. He also experienced pain and difficulty swallowing, but had no trouble breathing or any abnormal breathing sounds.

During a physical examination using a flexible endoscope, it was observed that the airway was not blocked, but it was slightly shifted toward the unaffected side. An urgent CT scan revealed a large cyst in the left submandibular region (see Fig. 11.1). The patient was intubated and under-

N. Tsetsos et al. (eds.), *Otolaryngology Study Guide*, https://doi.org/10.1007/978-3-031-77374-7_11

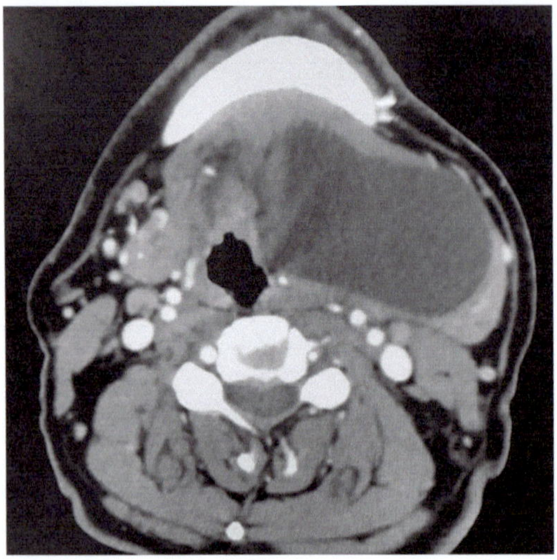

Fig. 11.1 A computed tomography demonstrates the presence of a huge cyst in the left submandibular area

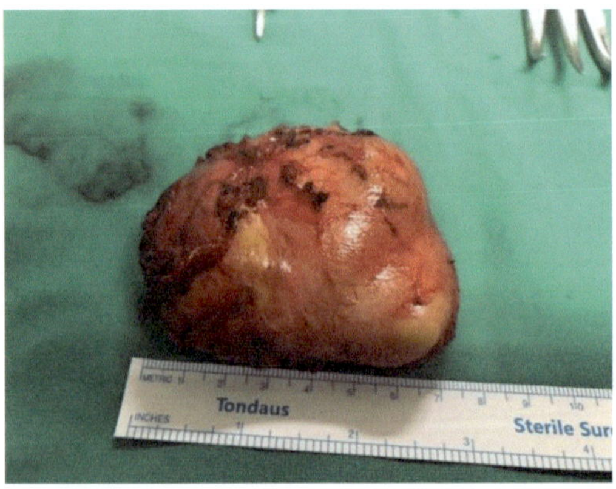

Fig. 11.2 Surgical specimen after excision of the inflamed cyst. Its highest dimension is 7.5 cm

went a surgical removal of the cyst. The cyst was successfully extracted without damaging its infected walls (see Fig. 11.2). To prevent the formation of pus again, three penrose drains were inserted. The histopathology results indicated that it was a dermoid cyst with inflamed walls and pus inside. After 6 days, the patient was discharged without any complications and was prescribed oral antibiotics.

Questions

1. The first step in a patient with Ludwig angina is:
   A. Secure the airway with intubation or tracheostomy
   B. Surgical drainage
   C. Antibiotic coverage for the most suspected bacteria
   D. Computed tomography
   E. Watchful waiting
2. Deep neck infections etiology includes:
   A. Dental infections
   B. Sialadenitis
   C. Infected congenital or acquired cysts
   D. Trauma
   E. Iatrogenic penetrations of upper aerodigestive tract
3. Thoracic involvement of deep neck infections may happen primarily through spreading from:
   A. Parapharyngeal space
   B. Retropharyngeal space
   C. Danger space
   D. Carotid sheath
   E. Masseter space
4. An intubated patient with deep neck infection will undergo imaging. Which modality is the most useful for his further investigation and management?
   A. Magnetic resonance imaging (MRI)
   B. Computed tomography (CT)
   C. Ultrasound (US)
   D. Plain radiograph
   E. Positron emission tomography (PET)
5. Lethal complications of deep neck infections include:
   A. Lemierre's syndrome
   B. Mediastinitis
   C. Carotid rupture
   D. Cavernous sinus thrombosis
   E. Malignant degeneration

Answers

1. **A**

Ludwig angina is a life-threatening condition characterized by the simultaneous involvement of both the submandibular and submental spaces. Infection can spread to secondary spaces and is primarily caused by dental infections, followed by inflammations of the submandibular gland [1]. The most common pathophysiologic sequelae include tenderness in the suprahyoid neck and elevation of the tongue. CT scan imaging is not recommended due to the patient's inability to tolerate the supine position, which can also delay treatment. Untreated patients may experience trismus, difficulty managing oral secretions, and eventually dyspnea. Emergent intubation is crucial, and if not possible, a tracheostomy or cricothyrotomy should be performed to secure the airway. Additionally, wide surgical drainage should be conducted to open all suprahyoid spaces and drain any collections. Infected teeth cannot be saved with endodontic treatment, and extraction is strongly recommended [2].

2. **A, B, C, D, E**

   The etiology of deep neck infections is closely related to the age of the patient. Dental infections are the most common cause in adults, particularly when combined with periodontitis and comorbidities such as diabetes mellitus [2]. Tooth decay and plaque serve as breeding grounds for bacteria, which can potentially disseminate and form abscesses in deep neck spaces. In contrast, children are susceptible to deep neck infections following acute tonsillitis, rhinosinusitis, or other viral or bacterial inflammations in the head and neck region [3]. Understanding the lymphatic drainage pattern is crucial for determining the origin of the inflammation and providing valuable information for patient management. It is important for clinicians to consider that even cysts, whether congenital or acquired, can become inflamed and result in deep neck infections. Additionally, both iatrogenic and non-iatrogenic trauma in the upper aerodigestive tract can serve as potential entry points for microorganisms that may be established and spread through the ruptured mucous barrier. Finally, immunosuppression favors the development of deep neck infections and so immunocompromised patients should be treated aggressively to avoid lethal complications [4].

3. **B, C, D**

   Dissemination of the inflammation to the thoracic cavity consists of a major complication with very high mortality [5]. However not so often in the antibiotic era, upper mediastinum is sometimes infected secondary to a deep head and neck infection. Parapharyngeal space is an inverted pyramid space extending from the skull base to the lesser horn of the hyoid bone. It does not communicate straightforward to thorax, but parapharyngeal space infections can easily spread to retropharyngeal space. Retropharyngeal space extends from skull base superiorly to the second vertebra inferiorly, between the buccal fascia of pharynx anteriorly and the alar fascia posteriorly. Alar fascia is the barrier to the danger space. Danger space is extended from the skull base to the diaphragm, and any involvement may lead to mediastinitis. Finally, the carotid sheath shapes a space which communicates straightforward with the great vessels of thorax and heart. Transmission of the infection from carotid sheath to thorax is well known as the "Lincoln highway" [6].

4. **B**

   Deep neck infections are treated more effectively after imaging. When possible (intubated patients or stable with no obstruction), a computed tomography is of great value. However, even patients with no stridor or dyspnea and normal oxygen saturation are not always eligible for imaging. Oxygen saturation is not a reliable index of obstruction. Decrease of oxygen saturation happens in a very late stage and so a normal value should not be considered a mark of safety [7].

   Computed tomography with contrast enhancement remains the gold standard for diagnosis and surgical plan in patients with deep neck infections. Hypodense collections with peripheral enhancement are the most common presentation. However, in a 25% of cases surgical drainage will not confirm the presence of pus due to the inability of CT to distinguish inflammatory collections and pure abscess [8].

   Plain film radiography is a rapid examination which provides information about a retropharyngeal abscess or epiglottis involvement (but results are not always reliable). MRI is a time-consuming test and may be used complementary to CT scan when great vessels involvement is suspected. US is of great value to perform an imaging-guided drainage of a superficial abscess, but it has limitations in deeper spaces and does not provide detailed images.

5. **A, B, C, D**

Untreated deep neck infections can lead to serious conditions with high mortality rates. Lemierre syndrome, associated with the gram-negative bacterium *Fusobacterium necrophorum*, causes thrombophlebitis of the internal jugular vein. A contrast-enhanced CT scan can confirm a deficit in the vein [9]. Carotid sheath involvement can result in local complications such as pseudoaneurysm formation, rupture, and Horner syndrome, as well as distant complications like mediastinitis. Additionally, the cavernous sinus may be affected through retrograde venous dissemination.

References

1. Pak S, Cha D, Meyer C, Dee C, Fershko A. Ludwig's angina. Cureus. 2017;21(9):1588.
2. Cousin GC, Yousaf I. Ludwig's angina: infected teeth must be extracted. BMJ. 2020;8(371):4466.
3. Huang CM, Huang FL, Chien YL, Chen PY. Deep neck infections in children. J Microbiol Immunol Infect. 2017;50:627–33.
4. Chang GH, Ding MC, Chen YC, et al. Real-world evidence for increased deep neck infection risk in patients with rheumatoid arthritis. Laryngoscope. 2020;130:1402–7.
5. Hsu RF, Wu PY, Ho CK. Transcervical drainage for descending necrotizing mediastinitis may be sufficient. Otolaryngol Head Neck Surg. 2011;145:742–7.
6. Gavid M, Dumollard JM, Habougit C, et al. Anatomical and histological study of the deep neck fasciae: does the alar fascia exist? Surg Radiol Anat. 2018;40:917–22.
7. Chen SL, Young CK, Tsai TY, et al. Factors affecting the necessity of tracheostomy in patients with deep neck infection. Diagnostics (Basel). 2021;25:1536.
8. Smith JL II, Hsu JM, Chang J. Predicting deep neck space abscess using computed tomography. Am J Otolaryngol. 2006;27:244–7.
9. Lee WS, Jean SS, Chen FL, Hsieh SM, Hsueh PR. Lemierre's syndrome: a forgotten and re-emerging infection. J Microbiol Immunol Infect. 2020;53:513–7.

Laryngeal Fracture 12

Vaios Kaminiotis and Marios Stavrakas

Abstract

Laryngeal trauma is a rare injury that accounts for <1% of all traumas but remaining undiagnosed can be a life-threatening situation. Blunt injury is more frequent than penetrating trauma and can be caused mainly by motor vehicle accidents. Other causes are sports, firearm, falls, assaults, and strangulation (Sethi et al. Laryngoscope. 129(10):2341–6, 2019). Due to the mechanism of injury, the patient commonly presents with accompanying injuries, which leave laryngeal fracture undiagnosed. The most common symptoms include hoarseness, stridor, neck pain, dysphagia, dysphonia, and hemoptysis. On examination, flattening of thyroid cartilage protuberance, neck crepitus, and reduction in breathing sounds may be present. Some patients may remain asymptomatic though (Bourdillon et al. J Voice, 2022). Laryngeal injuries are most commonly classified according to Schaefer Fuhrman's classification from Group I to Group V. Other existing classifications are Legacy Emanuel Hospital and Health Center (LEHHC) by Verscheuren et al. and anatomical location of injury (supraglottic, glottic, and subglottic injury) (Moroco et al. Craniomaxillofac Trauma Reconstruct. 16(1):62–69, 2023).

V. Kaminiotis
Harefield Hospital, Guy's and St Thomas' NHS Foundation Trust, London, UK

M. Stavrakas (✉)
ENT Head and Neck Surgery Department, University Hospitals Plymouth NHS Trust, Plymouth, UK

Case Presentation

A 42-year-old male patient presented to the emergency department following a blunt trauma to the neck while he was surfing. He reported mild pain, hoarse voice, and some difficulty in swallowing. On inspection, there is mild ecchymosis on the anterior neck and tenderness on palpation. Flexible nasendoscopy demonstrated mild edema and bruising but mobile vocal cords. The patient underwent CT neck (Fig. 12.1) and received conservative treatment, with uneventful recovery.

Questions

1. According to Schaefer Fuhrman's classification what does injury group IV include?
   A. Complete laryngotracheal separation
   B. Minor endolaryngeal hematoma
   C. Minor mucosal disruption without exposed cartilage
   D. Exposed cartilage and vocal fold immobility
   E. Two or more fracture lines or massive trauma to laryngeal mucosa

N. Tsetsos et al. (eds.), *Otolaryngology Study Guide*, https://doi.org/10.1007/978-3-031-77374-7_12

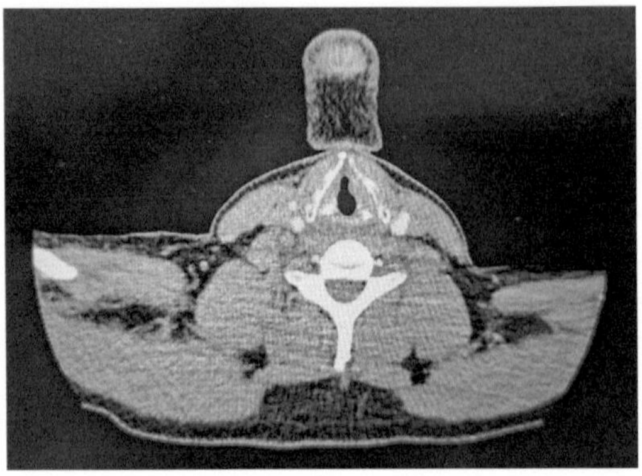

Fig. 12.1 Undisplaced left laryngeal fracture, with associated posterior hematoma (contrecoup mechanism)

2. Which group of injury according to Schaefer Fuhrman's classification should be treated conservatively?
   A. Group I
   B. Group III
   C. Group I and II
   D. Group III and IV
   E. Group IV
3. Which is the most common cause of laryngeal fracture?
   A. Intubation
   B. Assaults
   C. Motor vehicle accidents
   D. Falls
   E. Hanging
4. The first step in treating laryngeal fractures is to secure patient's airway. What is/are the next step(s) for the assessment of laryngeal trauma?
   A. CT scan
   B. Flexible laryngoscopy
   C. Esophagoscopy
   D. Chest X-ray
   E. All of the above
5. What is the most appropriate treatment in the case presented above?
   A. Monitoring and conservative treatment
   B. Endotracheal stent
   C. Esophagoscopy
   D. Direct laryngoscopy
   E. None of the above

Answers

1. **E**

   Group IV includes disruption of anterior larynx, unstable fractures, two or more fracture lines, or massive trauma to laryngeal mucosa. More specifically, Table 12.1 describes the laryngeal fracture classification in association with the severity and the structures involved. Consequently, it dictates the appropriate management for each group. [4]
2. **C**

   Group I and II of laryngeal injury are recommended to be treated conservatively. Effectiveness is around 100% to this population, whereas surgical intervention is advised for Groups III and IV [5]. Conservative treatment varies depending on local protocols and includes observation, head of the bed elevation, steam inhalation, voice rest, IV corticosteroid, adrenaline nebulizers, and anti-reflux treatment. Surgical treatment depends on the injury and can involve direct laryngoscopy or open exploration with manipulation of fractures, plating, stents, and tracheostomy.
3. **C**

   One study found that almost 45% of the mechanisms of injury are owed to motor vehicle trauma, 14% due to firearm, and 12% to falls.

   Blunt trauma is responsible for around 80% of the injuries while penetrating trauma for about 20%; 67% of the patients who pres-

Table 12.1 Laryngeal fracture classification

Group I	Minor endolaryngeal hematoma with undetectable fracture
Group II	Extreme edema, hematoma, minor mucosal disruption without exposed cartilage, and undisplaced fractures
Group III	Massive edema, mucosal disruption, exposed cartilage, vocal cord immobility, and displaced fracture
Group IV	Disruption of anterior larynx, unstable fractures, two or more fracture lines, or massive trauma to laryngeal mucosa
Group V	Complete laryngotracheal separation

ent with laryngeal fractures suffer from other injuries as well [1].

4. **E**

Flexible laryngoscopy can be used to assess the interior mucosal tissues of the larynx, detect any exposed vocalis muscles and range of motion of vocal cords. CT scan will benefit the patients with stable airway but with a strong suspicion of laryngeal injury that remains undetected. About 4–6% of laryngeal injuries are accompanied by esophageal injury, and esophagoscopy should be performed after stabilizing the patient under general anesthesia. In a polytrauma patient with a neck trauma, a portable chest X-ray may be used to clarify the existence of a laryngeal fracture [3].

5. **A**

In case of impending airway compromise, the clinician must ensure patent airway creating a cricothyrotomy, tracheostomy or intubating the patient. After that laryngoscopy and esophagoscopy should be performed [6]. According to the results:

Injury	Management
Normal endolarynx or fracture with minor trauma of mucosa	Monitoring
Fracture of thyroid or cricoid with uninjured endolarynx	Throat examination, ORIF of skeletal fractures of the larynx with plating without thyrotomy
Unsteady fractures/ anterior commissure interruption/major mucosal lacerations	ORIF of fractures, correction of laceration of mucosa, and stent of endolarynx
Steady fractures of the larynx, uninterrupted anterior commissure, change of mucosa which is less severe	Throat examination, ORIF of skeletal fractures of the larynx with plating thyrotomy, primary closure of lacerations

ORIF Open reduction and internal fixation

In case of stable airway, the clinician should perform flexible laryngoscopy and neck CT scan. If there are available, laryngeal electromyography and videostroboscopy should also be considered [7]. According to the results:

	Management
Normal endolarynx ± reversible mucosal trauma without fracture	Monitoring
Cartilage or endolarynx interruption	Tracheostomy/ intubation, direct laryngoscopy and esophagoscopy, throat examination, and treatment as in impending airway compromise

Generally, the best results are noted when airway injuries are treated within the first 24 h.

References

1. Sethi RK, Khatib D, Kligerman M, Kozin ED, Gray ST, Naunheim MR. Laryngeal fracture presentation and management in United States emergency rooms. Laryngoscope. 2019;129(10):2341–6.
2. Bourdillon AT, Kafle S, Salehi PP, Steren B, Pei KY, Azizzadeh B, Lee YH. Characterization of laryngotracheal fractures and repairs: a TQIP study. J Voice; 2022.
3. Moroco AE, Patel VA, Saadi RA, Gniady JP, Lighthall JG. Systematic review of laryngeal fractures and trends in operative management. Craniomaxillofac Trauma Reconstruct. 2023;16(1):62–9.
4. Moonsamy P, Sachdeva UM, Morse CR. Management of laryngotracheal trauma. Ann Cardiothorac Surg. 2018;7(2):210.
5. Bent JP III, Porubsky ES. The management of blunt fractures of the thyroid cartilage. Otolaryngol Head Neck Surg. 1994;110(2):195–202.
6. Abhinav M, Shraddha J. Laryngeal trauma, its types, and management. Cureus. 2022;14(10)
7. Schaefer SD. Management of acute blunt and penetrating external laryngeal trauma. Laryngoscope. 2014;124(1):233–44.

Part II

Otology/Audiology

13 Acute Otitis Media

Konstantinos Garefis

Abstract

Acute otitis media (AOM) is an inflammation of the middle ear, most commonly seen between the ages of 6 months and 2 years, and its incidence decreases after the age of 5. This condition is typically caused by bacterial or viral infections. Depending on the age-group, symptoms can include ear discomfort (manifested as tugging, rubbing, or holding of the ear), fever, hearing loss, excessive crying, and changes in sleep or behavior patterns, as observed by parents. These symptoms can often be non-specific. Factors that increase the risk of AOM include upper respiratory infections, exposure to second-hand smoke, attending day-care, and allergies. Diagnosis is made based on the presence of acute symptoms and findings from a physical examination, which may show redness, reduced mobility, bulging of the tympanic membrane (TM), and fluid in the middle ear. Pneumatic otoscopy and tympanometry are useful tests to confirm the diagnosis. Potential complications of AOM include TM perforation, mastoiditis, labyrinthitis, facial nerve paralysis, meningitis, among others. The treatment approach for AOM includes managing pain and administering antibiotics, and in some cases, a watchful waiting strategy may be adopted depending on the severity of the infection. Amoxicillin is the first-choice antibiotic for uncomplicated AOM, with alternative antibiotics being considered in cases of treatment failure or allergies.

Case Presentation

A 2-year-old boy is brought to the emergency ENT clinic, exhibiting symptoms of right ear pain and fever for the past 2 days. The parents report that the child has been pulling at his ear and crying. Both the child and his older sister have recently been dealing with runny noses. During the examination, the child has a fever of 39 °C, and the right tympanic membrane (TM) shows moderate bulging, erythema, and reduced mobility. The left ear appears normal. Based on the symptoms and clinical findings (Fig. 13.1), a diagnosis of acute otitis media (AOM) is made. The child is prescribed amoxicillin, and the parents are instructed to administer acetaminophen or ibuprofen to alleviate the pain. A follow-up appointment is scheduled in the coming days to monitor the response to treatment.

K. Garefis (✉)
2nd Academic ORL, Head and Neck Surgery Department, Aristotle University of Thessaloniki, Papageorgiou Hospital, Thessaloniki, Greece

N. Tsetsos et al. (eds.), *Otolaryngology Study Guide*, https://doi.org/10.1007/978-3-031-77374-7_13

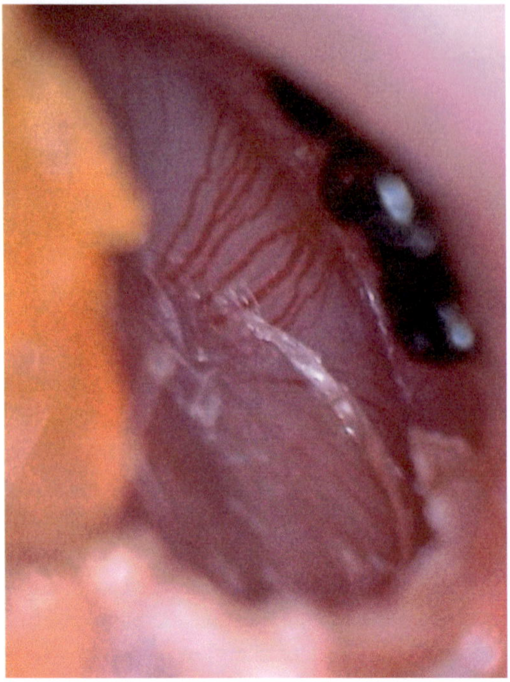

Fig. 13.1 Bulging and erythema of the right tympanic membrane

Questions

1. Which of these are the most common pathogens causing acute otitis media?
   A. *Streptococcus pyogenes*, *Moraxella catarrhalis*, nontypeable *Haemophilus influenzae*
   B. *Staphylococcus aureus*, nontypeable *Haemophilus influenzae*, *Pseudomonas aeruginosa*
   C. *Streptococcus pneumoniae*, nontypeable *Haemophilus influenzae*, *Moraxella catarrhalis*
   D. *Streptococcus pneumoniae*, *Staphylococcus aureus*, *Pseudomonas aeruginosa*
   E. *Staphylococcus aureus*, *Moraxella catarrhalis*, nontypeable *Haemophilus influenzae*
2. Which of the following is a risk factor for acute otitis media in infants and children? (more than one correct answer possible)
   A. Bottle feeding
   B. Second-hand smoke exposure
   C. Day-care attendance
   D. Early introduction of solid foods
   E. All of the above
3. Which of the following scenario is not a criterion to diagnose AOM? (more than one correct answer possible)
   A. Moderate to severe bulging of the TM alone
   B. Middle ear effusion or new onset of otorrhea due to acute otitis externa
   C. Mild bulging of the TM and recent onset of holding, tugging, rubbing of the ear in a nonverbal child
   D. Severe bulging of the TM and intense erythema of it
   E. Children who do not have middle ear effusion, based on pneumatic otoscopy and/or tympanometry
4. Which of the following statements about treatment of AOM are true? (more than one correct answer possible)
   A. If the pain persists for a minimum of 48 h, then the clinician should recommend pain-relieving treatment
   B. Children aged between 6 and 23 months with bilateral AOM without severe signs or symptoms should be treated with antibiotics
   C. Children 24 months or older with unilateral AOM without severe signs and symptoms must not be treated with antibiotics immediately
   D. Amoxicillin is the first-line antibiotic for AOM and simultaneous concurrent purulent conjunctivitis
   E. Reevaluation of patient if caregiver reports worsening symptoms or no response to initial antibiotics in 48–72 h.
5. During the follow-up appointment 48 h later, the child's fever persists, and there is minimal improvement in his pain. A repeat examination reveals that the erythema and bulging of the tympanic membrane remain largely unchanged. In light of these findings, what would be your next course of action?
   A. Placement of a tympanostomy tube in the right TM
   B. Continue amoxicillin for 2 days more and reexamine

C. Change the antibiotic to amoxicillin-clavulanate and reexamine after 48 h
D. Change the antibiotic to trimethoprim-sulfamethoxazole and reexamine after 48 h
E. Perform tympanocentesis/drainage

Answers

1. **C**

The presence of bacteria and respiratory viruses has been detected in the middle ear during AOM [1–3]. AOM is primarily caused by a viral upper respiratory tract infection, which leads to inflammation and dysfunction of the Eustachian tube, resulting in negative pressure in the middle ear cavity [4, 5]. As a result, secretions containing the virus and bacteria from the nasopharynx are forced into the middle ear, causing infection. The most commonly identified bacterial pathogens in AOM include *Streptococcus pneumoniae*, nontypeable *Haemophilus influenzae*, and *Moraxella catarrhalis*. *Streptococcus pyogenes* (group A *β-Hemolytic streptococci*) is responsible for less than 5% of AOM cases and is more prevalent in older children, causing more pronounced inflammation in the middle ear [3, 4, 6]. Additionally, nontypeable Haemophilus influenzae is more likely to cause AOM associated with conjunctivitis (otitis-conjunctivitis syndrome) than other bacteria. This bacterium has been linked to bilateral AOM and more severe inflammation of the tympanic membrane [6].

2. **A, B, C**

Multiple risk factors contribute to the development of AOM in infants and children. The use of pacifiers and bottle feeding has been associated with an increased risk of AOM, and it is recommended to limit or avoid their use after the first 6 months of life to reduce this risk [7, 8]. Studies have shown that breastfeeding for a minimum of 4–6 months can also lower the incidence of AOM [6, 9, 10]. Exposure to second-hand smoke has been linked to an increased likelihood of AOM [6, 11]. Similarly, children who attend day-care centers, especially during their first year, are at an elevated risk of developing AOM [6, 12]. Modifying the attendance patterns of children at day-care centers during infancy and early childhood can significantly decrease the recurrence of AOM by reducing the incidence of upper respiratory tract infections [6].

3. **B, E**

When diagnosing AOM in children, clinicians should consider specific criteria. A diagnosis of AOM should be made if children exhibit moderate to severe bulging of the TM or new onset of otorrhea that is not caused by acute otitis externa. AOM can also be diagnosed in children with mild bulging of the TM and recent onset of ear pain (such as holding, tugging, or rubbing of the ear in a nonverbal child) or intense erythema of the TM within the past 48 h. However, it is important not to diagnose AOM in children who do not have middle ear effusion, which can be determined through pneumatic otoscopy and/or tympanometry [6].

4. **B, E**

The American Academy of Pediatrics has set forth particular guidelines for handling and treating AOM. Evaluating pain and administering treatment to alleviate it when present are crucial part of managing AOM. For children aged 6 months and older who exhibit severe signs or symptoms of AOM, such as moderate to severe otalgia or otalgia persisting for at least 48 h, or a temperature of 39 °C or higher, antibiotics should be administered. For younger children between 6 and 23 months with non-severe bilateral AOM, antibiotics should be given for mild otalgia that lasts less than 48 h and a temperature below 39 °C. For non-severe unilateral AOM in this age group, either antibiotics or observation with close monitoring can be considered, based on a joint decision with the parent(s)/caregiver. For older children aged 24 months or older with non-severe AOM, either antibiotics or observation with close monitoring can also be considered. If observation is chosen, it's essential to have a system in place that allows for tracking and prompt initiation of antibiotic treatment if the child's condition worsens or does not improve within 48–72 h from the onset of symptoms [6]. Amoxicillin is the preferred antibiotic for treating AOM unless the child is allergic to it, has taken it in the past 30 days, or has concurrent purulent conjunctivitis [6, 13]. In the latter two scenarios, therapy should be started with amoxicillin-clavulanate [6, 14].

5. **C**

In the event that a caregiver observes a lack of improvement or worsening of the child's symptoms within 48–72 h of initial antibiotic treatment, it is crucial for healthcare professionals to reassess the patient and determine if a modification in treatment is required [6]. If the child's condition did not improve with initial amoxicillin treatment, amoxicillin-clavulanate should be considered. For those who were initially treated with amoxicillin-clavulanate or oral third-generation cephalosporins, intramuscular ceftriaxone may be administered [6, 15]. Previously, trimethoprim-sulfamethoxazole and erythromycin-sulfisoxazole were used for AOM treatment, but due to significant resistance found in pneumococcal surveillance studies, they are no longer recommended. If a series of antibiotics fail to improve the condition, tympanocentesis and culture of the middle ear fluid should be conducted. If tympanocentesis is not feasible, clindamycin, possibly combined with an antibiotic effective against nontypeable *Haemophilus influenzae, Moraxella catarrhalis*, such as cefdinir, cefixime, or cefuroxime, may be utilized. Tympanostomy tubes may be suggested for recurrent AOM. Specifically, a child should have experienced either three AOM episodes within 6 months or four episodes within a year, with at least one episode in the six months preceding the diagnosis [6].

References

1. Pitkäranta A, Virolainen A, Jero J, Arruda E, Hayden FG. Detection of rhinovirus, respiratory syncytial virus, ând coronavirus infections in acute otitis media by reverse transcriptase polymerase chain reaction. Pediatrics. 1998;102(2 pt 1):291–5.
2. Heikkinen T, Thint M, Chonmaitree T. Prevalence of various respiratory viruses in the middle ear during acute otitis media. N Engl J Med. 1999;340(4):260–4.
3. Chonmaitree T. Acute otitis media is not a pure bacterial disease. Clin Infect Dis. 2006;43(11):1423–5.
4. Chonmaitree T, Heikkinen T. Role of viruses in middle-ear disease. Ann N Y Acad Sci. 1997;830:143–57.
5. Chonmaitree T, Revai K, Grady JJ, et al. Viral upper respiratory tract infection and otitis media complication in young children. Clin Infect Dis. 2008;46(6):815–23.
6. Lieberthal AS, Carroll AE, Chonmaitree T, Ganiats TG, Hoberman A, Jackson MA, Joffe MD, Miller DT, Rosenfeld RM, Sevilla XD, Schwartz RH, Thomas PA, Tunkel DE. The diagnosis and management of acute otitis media. Pediatrics. 2013;131(3):e964–99. https://doi.org/10.1542/peds.2012-3488. Epub 2013 Feb 25. Erratum in: Pediatrics. 2014 Feb;133(2):346
7. Brown CE, Magnuson B. On the physics of the infant feeding bottle and middle ear sequela: ear disease in infants can be associated with bottle feeding. Int J Pediatr Otorhinolaryngol. 2000;54(1):13–20.
8. Niemelä M, Pihakari O, Pokka T, Uhari M. Pacifier as a risk factor for acute otitis media: a randomized, controlled trial of parental counseling. Pediatrics. 2000;106(3):483–48.
9. Duncan B, Ey J, Holberg CJ, Wright AL, Martinez FD, Taussig LM. Exclusive breast feeding for at least 4 months protects against otitis media. Pediatrics. 1993;91(5):867–72.
10. Duffy LC, Faden H, Wasielewski R, Wolf J, Krystofik D. Exclusive breastfeeding protects against bacterial colonization and day care exposure to otitis media. Pediatrics. 1997;100(4)
11. Ilicali OC, Keles N, Deger K, Savas I. Relationship of passive cigarette smoking to otitis media. Arch Otolaryngol Head Neck Surg. 1999;125(7):758–62.
12. Prins-van Ginkel AC, Bruijning-Verhagen PC, Uiterwaal CS, van der Ent CK, Smit HA, de Hoog ML. Acute otitis media during infancy: parent-reported incidence and modifiable risk factors. Pediatr Infect Dis J. 2017 Mar;36(3):245–9.
13. Piglansky L, Leibovitz E, Raiz S, et al. Bacteriologic and clinical efficacy of high dose amoxicillin for therapy of acute otitis media in children. Pediatr Infect Dis J. 2003;22(5):405–13.
14. Hoberman A, Paradise JL, Burch DJ, et al. Equivalent efficacy and reduced occurrence of diarrhea from a new formulation of amoxicillin/clavulanate potassium (Augmentin) for treatment of acute otitis media in children. Pediatr Infect Dis J. 1997;16(5):463–70.
15. Leibovitz E, Piglansky L, Raiz S, Press J, Leiberman A, Dagan R. Bacteriologic and clinical efficacy of one day vs. three day intramuscular ceftriaxone for treatment of nonresponsive acute otitis media in children. Pediatr Infect Dis J. 2000;19(11):1040–5.

14 Malignant Otitis Externa

Konstantinos Garefis

Abstract

Malignant otitis externa (MOE) also known as necrotizing otitis externa, is a rare but potentially fatal infection that impacts the external auditory canal and nearby structures, associated with skull base soft tissue infection and osteomyelitis. This condition is most commonly seen in diabetic or immunocompromised individuals, especially those aged 65 and above. *Pseudomonas aeruginosa* is the most frequently identified pathogen, although other bacteria and fungi have been found as well. Symptoms of NOE include persistent ear pain, chronic ear discharge, sensation of fullness in the ear, hearing loss, headaches, and involvement of the cranial nerves. The diagnosis is usually made through a combination of patient history, physical examination, lab tests, and imaging studies. An otoscopic examination may show inflammation in the external auditory canal, along with polyps or granulation tissue. Inflammatory markers such as white blood cell count, C-reactive protein (CRP), or erythrocyte sedimentation rate (ESR) may be elevated. Imaging studies like Computed tomography (CT) and Magnetic resonance imaging (MRI) scans can help identify involvement of bone and soft tissue, respectively. A positive result on a methylene diphosphonate (MDP)-technetium-99 m (Tc99m) bone scan and Gallium-67 (Ga67) scan can further support the diagnosis of NOE. Complications can include osteomyelitis, meningitis, brain abscess, and cranial nerve palsy. The primary treatment is long-term systemic antibiotics targeting Pseudomonas, but in aggressive or advanced cases, or those not responding to antibiotics, surgical debridement may be necessary.

K. Garefis (✉)
2nd Academic ORL, Head and Neck Surgery Department, Aristotle University of Thessaloniki, Papageorgiou Hospital, Thessaloniki, Greece

Case Presentation

An 85-year-old man with diabetes presented to the emergency Ear, Nose, and Throat (ENT) clinic, reporting a three-week duration of intense pain in his left ear that worsened at night, accompanied by a foul-smelling discharge, hearing loss, and severe headaches. Despite several rounds of antibiotics prescribed by his primary care doctor, the patient stated that his symptoms had not improved. Upon physical examination, redness and swelling were observed in the left external auditory canal, along with a polyp on the canal floor. There was no evidence of facial nerve paralysis. A CT scan (Fig. 14.1) was conducted, which identified osteomyelitis at the base of the skull.

N. Tsetsos et al. (eds.), *Otolaryngology Study Guide*, https://doi.org/10.1007/978-3-031-77374-7_14

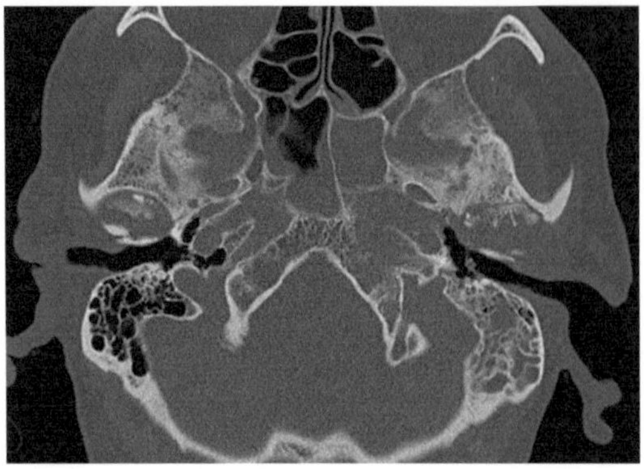

Fig. 14.1 CT scan showing skull base osteomyelitis on the left side

Questions

1. Which of the following statements are true about MOE? (more than one correct answer possible)
   A. The most frequent risk factor is diabetes mellitus
   B. Typically starts in the stylomastoid foramen
   C. The most commonly nerve involved is the trigeminal nerve
   D. It can cause skull base osteomyelitis
   E. Otitis media is a risk factor
2. What is the most common causative pathogen of MOE?
   A. *Hemophilus influenza*
   B. *Pseudomonas aeruginosa*
   C. *Methicillin-resistant Staphylococcus aureus (MRSA)*
   D. *Aspergillus fumigatus*
   E. *Streptococcus pneumoniae*
3. Which of the following symptoms and findings are not typically associated with MOE? (more than one correct answer possible)
   A. Otorrhea
   B. Facial palsy
   C. Elevated CRP
   D. Tinnitus
   E. Hypokalemia
4. Which of the following is not a component of MOE management? (more than one correct answer possible)
   A. Antibiotic therapy with clarithromycin
   B. Mastoidectomy
   C. Hyperbaric oxygen therapy
   D. Glycemic control in patients with diabetes
   E. Corticosteroid therapy
5. After 6 weeks of antibiotic therapy for the patient described above, which examination can determine whether to continue or stop the therapy?
   A. Serum glucose level
   B. Tc99 scan
   C. Ga67 scan
   D. MRI
   E. Relief of symptoms

Answers

1. **A, D**

   Literature suggests that between 90 and 100% of patients with MOE also have diabetes mellitus. This correlation is due to the fact that diabetes can lead to microangiopathy, hinder the healing of wounds, and compromise the immune system, thereby increasing the susceptibility to MOE. Another major risk factor for MOE is immunosuppression [1]. Conditions such as HIV infection, AIDS, neoplasia, leukemia, lymphoma, splenectomy, and immunosuppression post-transplantation can heighten the risk of MOE, regardless of whether the patient has diabetes or not [2, 3]. The typical progression of MOE starts in the external auditory canal and then spreads to the stylomastoid foramen, mastoid tip, and jugular foramen. Eventually, the infection progresses to affect the petrous apex and the middle cranial fossa [4]. The facial nerve is often involved due to its close proximity to the external auditory canal and the stylomastoid foramen. Subsequently, the glossopharyngeal, vagal, and spinal accessory nerves at the jugular foramen are the next most frequently affected nerves. If the disease progresses further medially, the petrous apex involvement can affect the abducens and trigeminal nerves, as well as the optic nerve [3, 4].
2. **D**

   The most common pathogen causing MOE is *Pseudomonas aeruginosa*, a gram-negative, obligate aerobe that is typically absent from the external auditory canal [1–5]. Pseudomonas accounts for a significant percentage of MOE cases, with an incidence ranging from 50% to 90% [5]. Other bacteria, such as *MRSA, Proteus mirabilis, Klebsiella oxytoca*, and *Staphylococci*, have also been identified [1–5]. Clinicians should be alert to the presence of unusual organisms like *MRSA* or fungal infections when diagnosing MOE in patients without diabetes [5]. *Aspergillus fumigatus* is the most frequently reported causative organism of fungal MOE, often found in HIV patients, particularly those with advanced AIDS [3, 4].

3. **D, E**

   MOE typically causes severe, persistent ear pain and can lead to cranial nerve involvement, particularly affecting the facial nerve (25% of patients) [1, 3]. The common symptoms of MOE include nighttime pain, chronic ear discharge, headache, conductive hearing loss, and temporomandibular joint pain. Fever is usually absent. Some patients may recall minor trauma to the ear canal in the past [1, 3]. During examination, a tender and swollen external auditory canal with purulent discharge is commonly observed. Granulation tissue or exposed bone is often seen in the floor of the canal at the bony-cartilaginous junction, but the middle ear and tympanic membrane typically appear healthy [1, 3–5]. If MOE is not diagnosed or inadequately treated, it can spread to the base of the skull and lead to serious complications such as meningitis, thrombosis of the lateral sinus or internal jugular vein, and Bezold's abscess [5]. Inflammatory markers such as ESR, CRP, or white blood cell count may be elevated in patients with MOE [1, 5].

4. **A, E**

   Effective management of MOE requires several key strategies such as rigorous control of diabetes, enhancement of immunocompetency, and reversal of acidosis when feasible [3]. The cornerstone of treatment is prolonged antibiotic therapy, which should be directed by culture-specific therapy [3, 5, 6]. Fluoroquinolones, especially oral ciprofloxacin, are the first-line therapy of choice due to their superior bone penetration and coverage against *Pseudomonas aeruginosa* [1–3]. In instances of ciprofloxacin resistance, third-generation cephalosporins can serve as an alternative [5]. Although surgery is no longer the standard treatment, it may be required in advanced cases, facial nerve paralysis, deep tissue sterile culture, or refractory MOE [3, 5]. Surgical interventions like mastoidectomy can decrease the local infection load, remove necrotic tissue, and stimulate new tissue growth, thereby increasing local blood flow and aiding systemic antibiotics to reach the affected area [5]. Hyperbaric oxygen therapy could be a potential treatment for refractory or advanced MOE; however, its effectiveness lacks robust scientific evidence. This therapy enhances the partial pressure of oxygen, aiding in the improvement of hypoxia and oxidative bacterial destruction [1, 3, 7].

5. **C**

   A Ga67 scan can help determine the duration of antimicrobial treatment for malignant external otitis (Fig. 14.2). This scan, or 111In-labeled leukocyte scintigraphy with SPECT/CT, can distinguish between healing bone and active infection in the hard-to-reach skull base area. If the scans indicate active infection, antimicrobial treatment should persist, and the scans should be repeated every 2–4 weeks until they normalize. A minimum of 6 months follow-up for MOE is recommended, with a low threshold for additional imaging, given that recurrence rates are reported to be around 15–20% [8]. While MRI and CT provide excellent anatomical resolution, their sensitivity, along with that of the Tc99 scan, for detecting treatment-related changes in MOE is limited [6, 8]. The combined imaging technique of 18F-FDG-PET/CT shows promise for both diagnosing and monitoring treatment response in MOE [6]. ESR has been suggested as a potentially good marker of treatment response [5]. As per recommendations for treating osteomyelitis, bac-

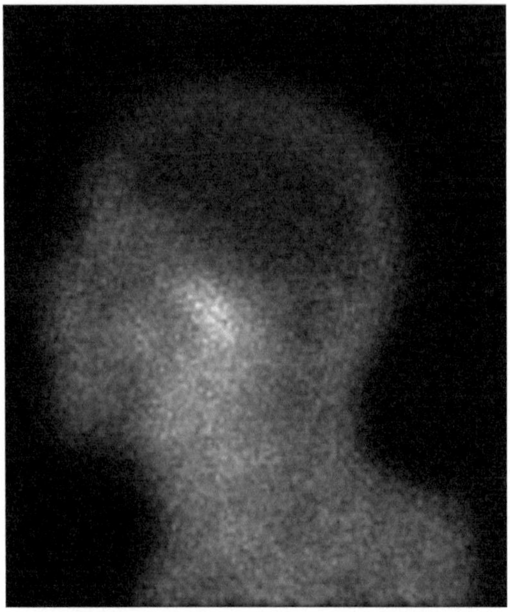

Fig. 14.2 Ga67 scan indicating the presence of osteomyelitis

terial MOE should be treated with a minimum of 6 weeks of antibiotics, even if clinical resolution is achieved [8].

References

1. Long DA, Koyfman A, Long B. An emergency medicine-focused review of malignant otitis externa. Am J Emerg Med. 2020;38(8):1671–8.
2. Hollis S, Evans K. Management of malignant (necrotising) otitis externa. J Laryngol Otol. 2011;125(12):1212–7.
3. Carfrae MJ, Kesser BW. Malignant otitis externa. Otolaryngol Clin North Am. 2008;41(3):537–49. viii–ix
4. Rubin Grandis J, Branstetter BF 4th, Yu VL. The changing face of malignant (necrotising) external otitis: clinical, radiological, and anatomic correlations. Lancet Infect Dis. 2004;4(1):34–9.
5. Treviño González JL, Reyes Suárez LL, Hernández de León JE. Malignant otitis externa: an updated review. Am J Otolaryngol. 2021;42(2):102894.
6. Sturm JJ, Stern Shavit S, Lalwani AK. What is the best test for diagnosis and monitoring treatment response in malignant otitis externa? Laryngoscope. 2020;130(11):2516–7.
7. Byun YJ, Patel J, Nguyen SA, Lambert PR. Hyperbaric oxygen therapy in malignant otitis externa: a systematic review of the literature. World J Otorhinolaryngol Head Neck Surg. 2020;7(4):296–302.
8. Courson AM, Vikram HR, Barrs DM. What are the criteria for terminating treatment for necrotizing (malignant) otitis externa? Laryngoscope. 2014;124(2):361–2.

Cholesteatoma

15

Adamantios Kilmpasanis and Nikolaos Tsetsos

Abstract

Cholesteatoma refers to a buildup of squamous epithelium in the middle ear. Although it's not a tumor, it can erode bones as it grows, making early treatment crucial. There are two primary types of cholesteatoma: congenital and acquired. Congenital cholesteatoma occurs due to epithelial growth in the middle ear during embryological development, while acquired cholesteatoma is further divided into primary and secondary types. The disease typically presents with symptoms such as otorrhea and hearing loss. If not treated promptly, cholesteatoma can lead to serious complications, categorized as either intracranial (like meningitis, abscesses, and sigmoid sinus thrombosis) or extracranial (like facial nerve palsy or labyrinthitis). These complications require immediate and aggressive treatment. High-resolution computed tomography (HRCT) of the temporal bone is the preferred imaging method for cholesteatoma, as it accurately depicts bone erosions. In cases where differential diagnosis is challenging or intracranial complications are present, an MRI can provide useful additional information. The standard treatment for cholesteatoma is a surgical procedure known as a mastoidectomy. Depending on the extent of the lesion, either an open or closed technique may be used. The primary objective is to fully eliminate the inflammation, achieve a dry ear, and, if feasible, restore the patient's hearing.

Case Presentation

A 40-year-old patient has been experiencing recurring foul-smelling discharge from his right ear for the past nine months. He was previously diagnosed with chronic otitis media due to a perforation in his right tympanic membrane, which occurred 6 years ago during a sea diving incident. He has tried various antibiotic ear drops, which have only provided temporary relief, and he was advised to keep his ear dry and avoid water. Currently, he is experiencing a sensation of fullness in his ear, foul-smelling ear discharge, and dizziness. An otomicroscopy examination revealed significant central retraction of the tympanic membrane, inflammation, and a white, pearly mass in the epitympanic area. The stapes bone was visible, but the incus bone was missing. A CT scan of the temporal bone showed a large lesion in the middle ear that extended into the mastoid cavity and confirmed the absence of the incus (Fig. 15.1).

A. Kilmpasanis
Private Practice, Thessaloniki, Greece

N. Tsetsos (✉)
ENT Head and Neck Surgery Department,
424 General Military Hospital, Thessaloniki, Greece

N. Tsetsos et al. (eds.), *Otolaryngology Study Guide*, https://doi.org/10.1007/978-3-031-77374-7_15

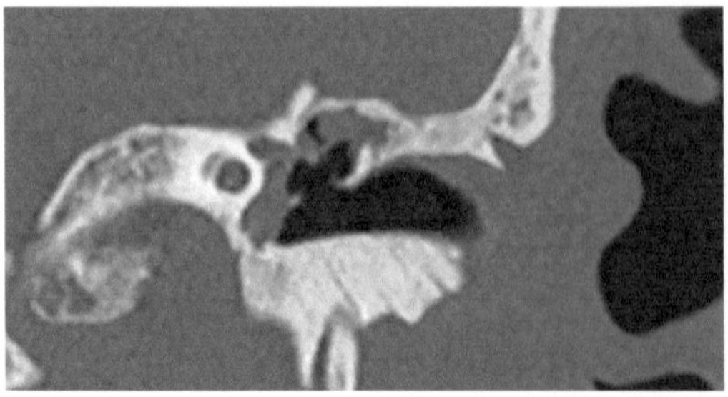

Fig. 15.1 A CT scan of the temporal bone showed a large lesion in the middle ear that extended into the mastoid cavity and confirmed the absence of the incus

Questions

1. Which of the following are true about congenital cholesteatoma? (more than one correct answer possible).
   A. It appears as a "whitish mass" behind an intact tympanic membrane
   B. Congenital cholesteatoma is the result of a middle ear inflammation due to a tympanic membrane perforation
   C. It appears after middle ear surgery
   D. Otorrhea is usually the first symptom
   E. Many cases of congenital cholesteatoma may be asymptomatic
2. Which of the following are considered symptoms or signs of cholesteatoma? (more than one correct answer possible).
   A. Smelly discharge from the affected ear
   B. Hearing loss
   C. Sensation of ear fullness
   D. Recurrent ear infections
   E. All the above
3. Which of the following are possible complications of cholesteatoma? (more than one correct answer possible).
   A. Meningitis and brain abscess
   B. Labyrinthitis
   C. Facial nerve paralysis
   D. Sigmoid sinus thrombosis
   E. All the above
4. Which of the following are true about the imaging of cholesteatoma? (more than one correct answer possible)
   A. High-resolution computed tomography (HRCT) of temporal bone has high sensitivity as far as the imaging of middle ear lesions is concerned
   B. HRCT can differentiate a cholesteatoma from granulation tissue
   C. Contrast-enhanced T1-weighted imaging can differentiate a cholesteatoma from granulation tissue
   D. MRI and HRCT of temporal bone are complementary examinations for diagnosis of cholesteatoma
   E. HRCT has high negative prognostic value when the middle ear and mastoid are free of lesions.
5. Which of the following are true about the treatment of cholesteatoma? (more than one correct answer possible)
   A. Conservative treatment with antibiotic ear drops is usually sufficient
   B. The type of surgery depends on the location and the extension of the cholesteatoma
   C. After a canal wall down technique, the patient should avoid water exposure
   D. Canal wall up mastoidectomy has higher recurrence rates than canal wall down mastoidectomy
   E. Canal wall down technique is preferred in revision surgery

Answers

1. **A, E**

   Cholesteatomas can be categorized into two groups: congenital and acquired. Congenital cholesteatomas in the middle ear typically manifest as a white, pearly lesion behind an intact tympanic membrane, without any symptoms of otorrhea, pain, or a history of previous ear surgery [1, 2]. In some cases, the only indication of a congenital cholesteatoma is conductive hearing loss, resulting from damage to the ossicular chain [3]. These cholesteatomas are often incidentally discovered during an MRI or CT scan. Acquired cholesteatomas are further divided into primary and secondary. The origin of primary acquired cholesteatoma has multiple theories, but the most widely accepted one suggests that it originates from a retracted tympanic membrane into the middle ear cavity [2, 4]. On the other hand, secondary acquired cholesteatoma occurs when a perforated tympanic membrane is caused by trauma, infection, or previous otologic surgery, leading to the entrapment of epithelium in the middle ear [4].

2. **E**

The primary symptoms associated with cholesteatoma include otorrhea (ear discharge) and hearing loss [2]. Otorrhea occurs as a result of chronic inflammation in the ear and a perforated eardrum [4]. Patients typically experience recurrent smelly drainage from the ear and a sensation of fullness in the affected ear. Pain may or may not be present [2, 4]. In the early stages of cholesteatoma, hearing loss is primarily conductive, but as the condition progresses and the labyrinth is affected, the hearing loss becomes mixed [5]. Tinnitus may also be present in these cases [6]. Congenital cholesteatomas can remain asymptomatic for many years, as they are estimated to grow at a rate of approximately 1mm per year [6]. They are usually discovered incidentally during routine ENT examinations [6].

3. **E**

Cholesteatoma has the potential to aggressively expand and erode bones, leading to serious complications. The destruction of bone is caused by the activation of osteoclasts, and when inflammation is present, the erosion occurs at an even faster rate [2, 4]. Complications of cholesteatoma can be divided into two categories: intracranial and extracranial [7–9]. The most common intracranial complications include meningitis, brain abscess, and sigmoid sinus thrombosis [7–9]. Clinical doctors should be vigilant if they observe symptoms such as otorrhea, headache, and fever [7]. These conditions have a high mortality rate and require prompt treatment, often involving neurosurgeons [7, 8]. Less common intracranial lesions include perisinus and epidural abscesses, as well as hydrocephalus [7]. In terms of extracranial (temporal bone) complications, labyrinthitis, labyrinthine fistula, mastoid abscess, and facial nerve paralysis are the most frequently encountered [7, 9]. Aggressive treatment is necessary for all of these conditions. Fortunately, the incidence of these potentially fatal complications is decreasing due to the widespread use of antibiotics [7, 8].

4. **A, C, D, E**

High-resolution computed tomography (HRCT) is the preferred imaging method for a suspected cholesteatoma [2, 10]. It effectively illustrates the middle ear bones and the damage caused by the cholesteatoma [11]. However, HRCT is unable to distinguish between a cholesteatoma and granulation tissue [10]. Typical signs of cholesteatoma, such as scutum erosion (the top wall of the external auditory canal), tegmen or ossicle destruction, are visible through HRCT [10, 11]. Furthermore, HRCT has a high negative predicted value (NPV) when imaging a clear middle ear and mastoid cavity [10]. MRI offers more information about the soft tissues [10, 12]. For instance, it can differentiate between granuloma tissue and a cholesteatoma, as the former shows contrast enhancement in contrast-enhanced T1-weighted imaging, while the latter does not [10, 12]. This is due to the fact that a cholesteatoma is a collection of keratinized squamous epithelium and lacks vascularization [10, 12]. Recent research using diffusion-weighted MR imaging indicates its sensitivity to cholesteatoma tissue. When combined with conventional MR imaging, diffusion-weighted MR imaging can verify the presence of remaining or recurring cholesteatoma in patients who have had middle ear surgery by revealing a lesion with high signal intensity [13]. In summary, HRCT of the temporal bone and MRI are the primary imaging techniques for cholesteatoma, as they complement each other [14].

5. **B, C, D, E**

The only method to completely eliminate cholesteatoma is through surgical management [6, 12]. Antibiotic ear drops are typically used to dry the ear as much as possible prior to surgery [15]. Mastoidectomy is the most commonly used type of ear surgery [15, 16]. There are two primary types of mastoidectomy: canal wall up (CWU) and canal wall down (CWD), each with its own advantages and disadvantages, and the choice of approach depends on the surgeon's preference [15]. The choice of approach is also influenced by the location and extent of the cholesteatoma [4]. The primary objective is to achieve a dry ear, with secondary aim being the restoration of the patient's hearing [15, 16]. Many surgeons prefer the CWU technique, where the posterior canal wall is preserved, when disease control is possible, as it offers certain benefits [15]. With this method, patients are not required to avoid water exposure and the healing process is quicker [14]. However, the recurrence rates are higher than with the CWD technique [4, 16, 17]. The CWD mastoidectomy offers a higher likelihood of cholesteatoma eradication, but it has the downside of an open cavity and typically results in poorer hearing [18]. In revision surgeries, the CWD approach is usually preferred.

References

1. Gilberto N, Custódio S, Colaço T, Santos R, Sousa P, Escada P. Middle ear congenital cholesteatoma: systematic review, meta-analysis and insights on its pathogenesis. Eur Arch Otorhinolaryngol. 2020;277:987–98.
2. Gulati M, Gupta S, Prakash A, et al. HRCT imaging of acquired cholesteatoma: a pictorial review. Insights Imaging. 2019;10:92.
3. Giannuzzi AL, Merkus P, Taibah A, Falcioni M. Congenital mastoid cholesteatoma: case series, definition, surgical key points, and literature review. Ann Otol Rhinol Laryngol. 2011;120(11):700–6.
4. Kennedy KL, Singh AK. Middle ear cholesteatoma. [Updated 2022 Jul 4]. In: StatPearls. Treasure Island (FL): StatPearls Publishing; 2022.
5. Khdim M, Douimi L, Choukry K, Oukessou Y, Rouadi S, Abada R, et al. Hearing loss in cholesteatoma. Am J Otolaryngol Head Neck Surg. 2020;3(8):1115.
6. Castle JT. Cholesteatoma pearls: practical points and update. Head Neck Pathol. 2018;12(3):419–29.
7. Wu J-F, Jin Z, Yang J-M, Liu Y-H, Duan M-L. Extracranial and intracranial complications of otitis media: 22-year clinical experience and analysis. Acta Otolaryngol. 2012;132(3):261–5.
8. Sun J, Sun J. Intracranial complications of chronic otitis media. Eur Arch Otorhinolaryngol. 2013;271(11):2923–6.
9. Martins GSQ, Hausen-pinna M, Tsuji RK, Brito Neto RV, Bento RF. Description of 34 patients with complicated cholesteatomatous chronic otitis media. Int Arch Otorhinolaryngol. 2008;12(3):370–6.
10. Baráth K, Huber AM, Stämpfli P, Varga Z, Kollias S. Am J Neuroradiol. 2011;32(2):221–9.
11. Ayache D, Darrouzet V, Dubrulle F, Vincent C, Bobin S, Williams M, Martin C. Imaging of non-operated cholesteatoma: clinical practice guidelines. Eur Ann Otorhinolaryngol Head Neck Dis. 2012;129(3):148–52.
12. Cimsit NC, Cimsit C, Baysal B, Ruhi IC, Ozbilgen S, Aksoy EA. Diffusion-weighted MR imaging in post-operative follow-up: reliability for detection of recurrent cholesteatoma. Eur J Radiol. 2010;74(1):121–3.
13. Aikele P, Kittner T, Offergeld C, Kaftan H, Hüttenbrink KB, Laniado M. Diffusion-weighted MR imaging of cholesteatoma in pediatric and adult patients who have undergone middle ear surgery. AJR Am J Roentgenol. 2003;181(1):261–5.
14. Corrales CE, Blevins NH. Imaging for evaluation of cholesteatoma: current concepts and future directions. Curr Opin Otolaryngol Head Neck Surg. 2013;21(5):461–7.
15. Nikolopoulos TP, Gerbesiotis P. Surgical management of cholesteatoma: the two main options and the third way—atticotomy/limited mastoidectomy. Int J Pediatr Otorhinolaryngol. 2009;73(9):1222–7.
16. Blanco P, González F, Holguín J, Guerra C. Surgical management of middle ear cholesteatoma and reconstruction at the same time. Colombia Méd. 2014;45(3):127–31.
17. Nadol JB. Revision mastoidectomy. Otolaryngol Clin North Am. 2006;39(4):723–40.
18. Karamert R, Eravci FC, Cebeci S, Düzlü M, Zorlu ME, Gülhan N, et al. Canal wall down versus canal wall up surgeries in the treatment of middle ear cholesteatoma. Turkish J Med Sci. 2019;49(5):1426–32.

16 Tympanoplasty

Adamantios Kilmpasanis and Nikolaos Tsetsos

Abstract

Tympanoplasty is a surgical procedure designed to repair a ruptured eardrum, potentially including the reconstruction of the ossicular chain. The dual objectives of tympanoplasty are to ensure the ear remains dry and to enhance the patient's hearing. The overlay and underlay techniques are the most frequently employed methods for repairing a ruptured tympanic membrane. The choice of technique and graft for the perforation repair is influenced by the size of the perforation and the surgeon's expertise. Various grafts, such as temporalis fascia, perichondrium/cartilage island, veins, and canal skin, are utilized in tympanoplasty. Conducting ossiculoplasty to enhance hearing presents a challenge for the surgeon. In recent times, endoscopic ear surgery has increasingly been preferred over the traditional microscope method due to its minimally invasive nature and lower complication rate. However, like all surgeries, tympanoplasty carries some risks. Patients considering tympanoplasty should be informed of potential complications, including residual perforation, taste disturbances, facial nerve damage, and auditory chain damage.

Case Presentation

A patient aged 25 reports frequent bouts of otorrhea and diminished hearing in his left ear. He recalls an incident involving a cotton swab a decade ago that resulted in a perforated tympanic membrane. Upon clinical examination, a large near-total perforation was observed, accompanied by a foul-smelling ear discharge. The patient was prescribed antibiotic ear drops for a 10-day period. Post-treatment, the patient returned for a follow-up, at which point no active otorrhea was detected (Fig. 16.1). An audiological examination was conducted, revealing a conductive hearing loss of 35–40 db. Consequently, a tympanoplasty was arranged. The procedure was carried out using a surgical microscope, with the underlay technique selected. A posterior incision was made, and the tympanomeatal flap was elevated. The middle ear condition was found to be poor, with granulation tissue present. Given the size of the perforation and the state of the middle ear, a conchal cartilage harvest was deemed the best option. The graft was applied and fully covered the perforation. The patient's recovery post-surgery was smooth. A follow-up conducted a month after the surgery showed an

A. Kilmpasanis
Private Practice, Thessaloniki, Greece

N. Tsetsos (✉)
ENT Head and Neck Surgery Department, 424 General Military Hospital, Thessaloniki, Greece

N. Tsetsos et al. (eds.), *Otolaryngology Study Guide*, https://doi.org/10.1007/978-3-031-77374-7_16

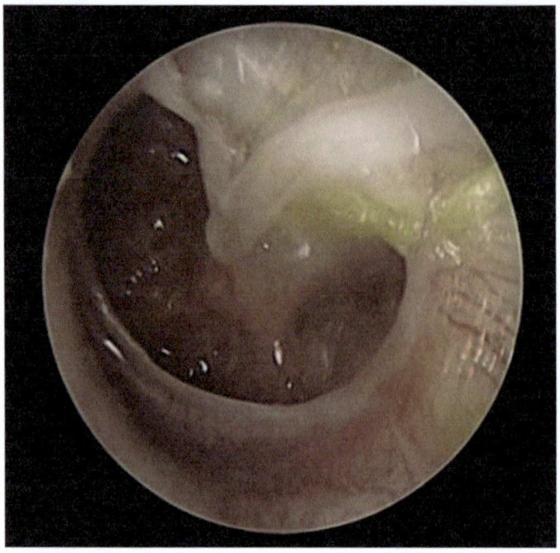

Fig. 16.1 Otoscopic view of the perforated left tympanic membrane.

intact tympanic membrane and improved audiogram, with conductive hearing measured at 25 db.

Questions

1. Which of the following are true about tympanoplasty (more than one correct answer possible)
   A. Repair of the tympanic membrane perforation is the major goal
   B. Hearing improvement is one of the goals of tympanoplasty
   C. The overlay technique has the risk of potential iatrogenic cholesteatoma
   D. An uncontrolled cholesteatoma is not a contraindication for tympanoplasty
   E. All the above
2. Which of the following are considered complications of tympanoplasty?
   A. Failure of the graft
   B. Abnormal taste in mouth
   C. Damage of the facial nerve
   D. Ossicular chain damage
   E. All the above
3. What types of graft are used in tympanoplasty?
   A. Temporalis fascia
   B. Perichondrium/cartilage island
   C. Veins
   D. Canal skin
   E. All the above
4. Which of the following are true about ossicular reconstruction in tympanoplasty?
   A. The skills of the surgeon and the right technique chosen are essential.
   B. Titanium and hydroxyapatite implants are widely used and are shown to have stability and better hearing results
   C. The post-operative ABG in a successful surgery is equal or lower than 30db
   D. A common cause of surgical failure is the remaining middle ear disease
   E. All the above
5. Which of the following are true about endoscopic tympanoplasty?
   A. Endoscopic approach offers a wider and angled view of the middle ear
   B. Bleeding is a major problem as the surgeon cannot use both hands
   C. The heat of the endoscope's light cannot harm the middle ear structures
   D. It is a minimal invasive technique with less postoperative pain
   E. All the above

Answers

1. **A, B, C**

   Tympanoplasty is a surgical intervention designed to address a perforated eardrum, potentially including the rebuilding of the ossicular chain [1]. The surgery aims to maintain a dry, safe ear and enhance the patient's auditory capacity by minimizing the air-bone gap [2]. Certain conditions, such as malignant tumors, unmanaged cholesteatomas, and complications from chronic otitis media like meningitis and intracranial abscesses, are specific contraindications to tympanoplasty [1]. The "underlay" and "overlay" methods are the most commonly employed surgical techniques [3, 4]. While the underlay technique is often favored by surgeons, it's generally agreed that the choice is dependent on the size and nature of the perforation [4, 5]. The underlay technique is straightforward, with the graft positioned medial to the remaining tympanic membrane [4]. In contrast, the overlay tympanoplasty requires careful removal of the squamous layer, with the graft placed lateral to the tympanic annulus. The overlay technique carries a higher risk of iatrogenic cholesteatoma and graft lateralization [3, 6].

2. **E**

Tympanoplasty, an ear surgery, boasts high success rates [7]. Nevertheless, all surgical procedures carry inherent risks. It's crucial for surgeons to be cognizant of the potential complications associated with tympanoplasty and to communicate these to their patients prior to surgery. Graft failure can occur due to incorrect surgical technique or limited surgeon experience [1, 7, 8]. However, even highly experienced surgeons can encounter graft lateralization or failure due to an active or postoperative ear infection [7]. During ear surgery, ossicles may be damaged, necessitating careful handling by the surgeon and readiness to reconstruct the chain if required [7]. Additionally, instrument manipulation should be gentle to avoid the rare but possible iatrogenic direct facial nerve injury reported in tympanoplasty [9]. During post-tympanoplasty, some patients may experience taste disturbances due to chorda tympani nerve (CTN) injury. The nerve's location in the middle ear and its proximity to the ossicular chain render the CTN susceptible to injuries [10, 11].

3. **E**

Various graft types are utilized in tympanoplasty. Autologous grafts, including temporalis fascia, perichondrium/cartilage island, palisade cartilage, fat, and skin, are frequently cited in literature [12, 13]. Additionally, numerous allografts such as veins, peritoneum, and dura mater are also used [13]. In recent times, the use of synthetic grafts has been on the rise, aligning with the trend toward minimally invasive procedures and reduced postoperative hospital stays [14]. The criteria for graft selection are diverse, with the choice largely dependent on the surgeon's experience, the size of the perforation, and the existence of hearing loss. Temporalis fascia is the most commonly selected graft by ear surgeons [12, 15], given its similarity to the tunica propria of the absent eardrum [15]. However, for large perforations or revision surgeries, cartilage/perichondrium is typically preferred due to its superior resistance [12]. Conversely, chondroperichondrium grafts may result in suboptimal hearing improvement, depending on the thickness of the cartilage [16].

4. **A, B, D**

Ossiculoplasty, which can be incorporated into tympanoplasty, is a surgical intervention aimed at restoring the ossicular chain and enhancing air-conduction (AC) thresholds [17, 18]. The operation's success hinges not only on the surgeon's expertise but also on the middle ear's condition, the Eustachian tube's functionality, and the chosen prosthesis [17–19]. The primary cause of osteoplasty failure is the presence of active disease in the middle ear [17, 19]. However, the selection of the right prosthesis and technique is also vital [17]. Prostheses made of hydroxyapatite and titanium are known for their rigidity, stability, and excellent results in hearing improvement [19, 20]. Yet, many surgeons favor autologous materials, citing concerns over high long-term extrusion rates associated with synthetic implants [21]. Research has demonstrated that interposing cartilage between the graft and the tympanic membrane makes the graft more stable and less prone to dislocation, particularly in plastipore and titanium implants [19]. Most experts deem an osteoplasty successful when the postoperative ABG is 20 db or less [17, 18].

5. **A, B, D**

Technological advancements have significantly transformed (the medical field) of middle ear surgery. Endoscopic surgery, long utilized in various surgical specialties including otorhinolaryngology, primarily for nasal and sinus surgery, has recently begun to gain traction in middle ear surgery [22, 23]. While endoscopic surgery offers several benefits over traditional microscope use, it also presents certain challenges that necessitate experience and familiarity with endoscopes [23, 24].

Endoscopic ear surgery is a minimally invasive procedure, leading to shorter patient recovery time [23]. It also results in less postoperative discomfort and superior cosmetic outcomes [23, 25]. The use of endoscopes allows surgeons to more effectively visualize the middle ear's anatomy, even at an angle, while also recording surgical maneuvers and techniques [24, 25]. However, operating with one hand without ear suction can be challenging, especially if bleeding obscures the surgical field and impairs the surgeon's vision [23, 25]. Additionally, there have been rare reports of thermal damage to middle ear structures due to the endoscope's light [26, 27].

References

1. Brar S, Watters C, Winters R. Tympanoplasty. [Updated 2022 Jul 1]. In: StatPearls. Treasure Island (FL): StatPearls Publishing; 2022.
2. Tshifularo M. Tympanoplasty success based on surgeon and patient-reported outcomes perspectives: a 10-year review in a tertiary center. Egypt J Otolaryngol. 2022;38:15.
3. Sergi B, Galli J, De Corso E, Parrilla C, Paludetti G. Overlay versus underlay myringoplasty: report of outcomes considering closure of perforation and hearing function. Acta Otorhinolaryngol Ital. 2011;31(6):366–71.
4. Kalsotra P, Gupta R, Gupta N, Kotwal S, Suri A, Kanotra S. Overlay versus underlay myringoplasty: a comparative study. Indian J Otolaryngol. 2014;20(4):183.
5. Ricciardiello F, Pisani D, Petruzzi G, Viola P, Palladino R, Sequino G, Raucci AF, Motta G, Coppola C, Cavaliere M, Astorina A, Di Nola C, Oliva F, Scarpa A, Chiarella G. Comparison between overlay and underlay primary myringoplasty: retrospective analysis on anatomical and functional results in 497 adult patients. Acta Biomed. 2022;93(4):e2022072.
6. Glasscock ME. Tympanic membrane grafting with fascia: overlay vs. undersurface technique. Laryngoscope. 1973;83(5):754–70.
7. Grosso JJ, Pensak ML. Complications in tympanoplasty. Oper Tech Otolaryngol Head Neck Surg. 1992;3(4):279–84.
8. Dispenza F, Battaglia AM, Salvago P, Martines F. Determinants of failure in the reconstruction of the tympanic membrane: a case-control study. Iran J Otorhinolaryngol. 2018;30(101):341–6.
9. Green JD Jr, Shelton C, Brackmann DE. Iatrogenic facial nerve injury during otologic surgery. Laryngoscope. 1994;104(8 Pt 1):922–6.
10. Michael P, Raut V. Chorda tympani injury: operative findings and postoperative symptoms. Otolaryngol Head Neck Surg. 2007;136(6):978–81.
11. Iynen I, Dundar R. Chorda Tympani nerve injury during tympanoplasty. Comparison of endoscopic and microscopic methods. Ann Ital Chir. 2021;10:S0003469X2102813X.
12. Bayram A, Bayar Muluk N, Cingi C, Bafaqeeh SA. Success rates for various graft materials in tympanoplasty: a review. J Otolaryngol. 2020;15(3):107–11.
13. De Freitas MR, de Oliveira TC. The role of different types of grafts in tympanoplasty. Braz J Otorhinolaryngol. 2014;80(4):275–6.
14. Ghanad I, Polanik MD, Trakimas DR, Knoll RM, Castillo-Bustamante M, Black NL, et al. A systematic review of nonautologous graft materials used in human tympanoplasty. Laryngoscope. 2020;131(2):392–400.
15. Singh BJ, Sengupta A, Das SK, Ghosh D, Basak B. A comparative study of different graft materials used in myringoplasty. Indian J Otolaryngol Head Neck Surg. 2009;61(2):131–4.
16. Shechy JL, Anderson RG. Myringoplasty. A review of 472 cases. Ann Otol Rhinol Laryngol. 1980;89:331–4.
17. Yung M. Long-term results of ossiculoplasty: reasons for surgical failure. Otol Neurotol. 2006;27(1):20–6.
18. Castro Sousa A, Henriques V, Rodrigues J, Fonseca R. Ossiculoplasty in chronic otitis media: Surgical results and prognostic factors of surgical success. Acta Otorrinolaringol Esp. 2017;68(3):131–7.
19. Javia LR, Ruckenstein MJ. Ossiculoplasty. Otolaryngol Clin N Am. 2006;39(6):1177–89.
20. Lahlou G, Sonji G, De Seta D, Mosnier I, Russo FY, Sterkers O, Bernardeschi D. Anatomical and functional results of ossiculoplasty using titanium prosthesis. Acta Otorhinolaryngol Ital. 2018;38(4):377–83.
21. Nagenahlli Siddappa P, Poojar Jayakumar P, Jonnalagadda DK. A study of use of autologous cartilage in ossicular reconstruction. Indian J Otolaryngol Head Neck Surg. 2019;71(Suppl. 2):1431–5.
22. Moneir W, Elkahwagi M. Endoscopic ear surgery: then and now, review article. Egypt J Otolaryngol. 2022;38:115.
23. Akyigit A, Sakallıoglu O, Karlidag T. Endoscopic tympanoplasty. J Otolaryngol. 2017;12(2):62–7.
24. Ridge SE, Shetty KR, Lee DJ. Current trends and applications in endoscopy for otology and neurotology. World J Otorhinolaryngol Head Neck Surg. 2021;7(2):101–8.
25. Emre IE, Cingi C, Bayar Muluk N, Nogueira JF. Endoscopic ear surgery. J Otolaryngol. 2020;15(1):27–32. https://doi.org/10.1016/j.joto.2019.11.004.
26. Badr-El-Dine M, James AL, Panetti G, Marchioni D, Presutti L, Nogueira JF. Instrumentation and technologies in endoscopic ear surgery. Otolaryngol Clin North Am. 2013;46(2):211–25.
27. Tu LJ, Fina M, Golub JS, Kazahaya K, Quesnel AM, Tawfik KO, Cohen MS. Current trends in endoscopic ear surgery. Otol Neurotol Open. 2022;2(4):e023.

17 Otosclerosis

Nikolaos Tsetsos

Abstract

Otosclerosis is a prevalent cause of adult-onset progressive hearing loss, typically beginning around the age of 30. This disease is marked by abnormal bone remodeling in the otic capsule, primarily affecting the stapes region, which results in conductive hearing loss. Approximately 10% of patients exhibit sensorineural hearing loss. In 70–80% of cases, it affects both ears, and half of the patients experience tinnitus, while vertigo is reported in 10% of cases. The medical approach to otosclerosis aims to prevent or at least decelerate the progression of the disease. Sodium fluoride and bisphosphonates are the preferred treatments for active lesions to curb the progressively degenerative activity of otospongiosis. Both stapedectomy and stapedotomy are highly successful surgical procedures for addressing the conductive hearing loss caused by otosclerosis. However, stapedotomy has become more popular in recent years due to its superior hearing outcomes at high frequencies and lower complication rates. Stapes surgery can be performed either microscopically or endoscopically. Potential complications of stapes surgery include sensorineural hearing loss, an increase in tinnitus, dizziness, taste disturbance, and in rare cases, facial nerve palsy and deafness.

Case Presentation

A 39-year-old female presented to the otology clinic with bilateral hearing loss that had been gradually worsening over the last few years. She reported that the hearing loss started in her right ear and progressively involved the left ear as well. She also mentioned mild tinnitus but had not experienced any episodes of dizziness. Interestingly, she pointed out improved speech understanding in noisy environments. Her past medical history was otherwise normal. On examination, both tympanic membranes were normal. The tuning fork test showed a negative Rinne test, while the Weber test lateralized to the right ear. The pure tone audiogram is shown below (Fig. 17.1). The tympanogram was depressed (type As), while the stapedial reflex could not be elicited. High-resolution computed tomography (CT) did not reveal any abnormal findings.

Questions

1. Which of the following are true for otosclerosis? (more than one correct answer possible)
   A. The average age of onset in the 40s
   B. The female: male prevalence is 2:1

N. Tsetsos (✉)
ENT Head and Neck Surgery Department,
424 General Military Hospital, Thessaloniki, Greece

N. Tsetsos et al. (eds.), *Otolaryngology Study Guide*, https://doi.org/10.1007/978-3-031-77374-7_17

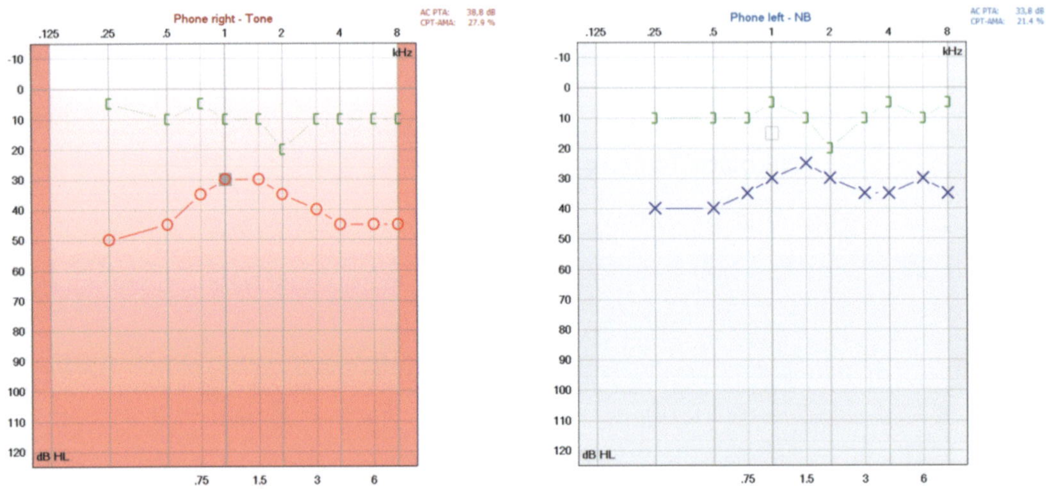

Fig. 17.1 A bilateral conductive hearing loss consistent with bilateral otosclerosis. Notice the Carhart notch in the bone conduction scores in both ears (2000 Hz)

   C. Otosclerosis occurs most commonly among Asians
   D. It occurs bilaterally in 30–40% of the cases
   E. The late phase of otosclerosis is called the otospongiotic phase
2. Which of the following are true for otosclerosis? (more than one correct answer possible)
   A. Tinnitus occurs in 20–30% of patients with otosclerosis
   B. Tinnitus is usually reduced following a successful surgery
   C. True vertigo is a common symptom
   D. Deterioration in hearing ability in noisy environments is a phenomenon known as Willis paracusis
   E. Schwartze sign is associated with the active phase of the disease
3. Which of the following are true for the diagnostic tests of otosclerosis? (more than one correct answer possible)
   A. The tuning fork test shows a positive Rinne test
   B. Weber's test is lateralized to the ear with severe conductive loss
   C. A bone conduction dip more pronounced at 3000 Hz is called Carhart notch
   D. Carhart notch remains after stapedotomy
   E. Magnetic resonance imaging is the imaging tool of choice
4. Which of the following statements are true regarding the management of otosclerosis? (More than one correct answer possible)
   A. Sodium fluoride and bisphosphonates have been used as a conservative treatment of otosclerosis
   B. The minimum air-bone gap in performing stapes surgery is 15 dB
   C. A stapedotomy is considered successful if an air-bone gap of 20 dB is achieved
   D. Either stapedotomy or stapedectomy may be used to address successfully the conductive hearing loss
   E. Excellent vision is the main advantage of endoscopic stapes surgery
5. Which of the following are true about post stapes surgery complications? (more than one correct answer possible)
   A. The incidence of dead ear following stapes surgery is 10%
   B. Reparative granuloma is one of the most common causes of dead ear
   C. Cerebrospinal fluid gusher is a common complication of stapes surgery
   D. Taste disturbance only rarely persists at 1 year after stapes surgery

E. Incus necrosis is among the most common causes of stapedectomy failure

Answers

1. **B**

   Otosclerosis is a prevalent cause of progressive hearing loss that begins in adulthood, typically around the age of 30 [1]. The condition is twice as common in women as in men [2]. It is most frequently found in Caucasians, with a clinical incidence of 0.3–0.4%, and is less common in Africans and Asians (0.03–0.1%) [3]. In the Caucasian population, histological otosclerosis is about ten times more prevalent than clinical otosclerosis [4]. The condition affects both ears in 70–80% of cases [5]. Otosclerosis progresses in two stages, starting with the otospongiotic phase and followed by the formation of dense sclerotic bone in areas where resorption previously occurred, marking the late phase of otosclerosis [5, 6]. Otosclerosis is typically viewed as an autosomal dominant condition with decreased penetrance [7].
2. **B, E**

   According to research, between 65% and 90% of otosclerosis patients also report experiencing tinnitus. This symptom often significantly decreases following successful stapes surgery [8, 9]. Vestibular symptoms are reported by 25–45% of otosclerosis patients, although true vertigo is uncommon. Vertigo is linked with cochlear otosclerosis and may therefore go undiagnosed. Vestibular symptoms are typically associated with the active stages of the disease [10, 11]. Many otosclerosis patients report improved hearing in noisy environments, a phenomenon known as Willis paracusis [12]. The Schwartze sign, also known as Flemingo's flush sign or Rising sun sign, is a reddish discoloration over the promontory visible during an otoscopic examination through the intact tympanic membrane. This sign is believed to be associated with otospongiosis, the active phase of the disease [13].
3. **B**

   Tuning fork tests can identify conductive hearing loss resulting from footplate fixation. The Rinne test, which should show bone conduction as superior to air conduction (a negative Rinne), is a valuable tool in determining if a patient could benefit from stapes surgery. The Weber test is expected to lateralize to the ear experiencing a higher degree of conductive hearing loss [14, 15]. The "Carhart notch," an increase in bone conduction thresholds (20–30 db) in patients with clinical otosclerosis, peaking at 2 kHz, disappears following successful stapes surgery [16, 17]. High-resolution computed tomography (CT) is the preferred imaging method for otosclerosis. CT scans may reveal a lucent or hypodense focus within the otic capsule, typically anterior to the oval window. Other CT findings may include a thickened footplate, a narrowed oval or round window niche, and a distinctive pericochlear hypodense double ring [18].
4. **A, D, E**

   The primary goal of otosclerosis medical treatment is to halt or at least decelerate the progression of the disease. Sodium fluoride and bisphosphonates are typically employed to curb the progressively degenerative activity of otospongiosis in instances of active lesions [19]. Stapes surgery is recommended when the air-bone gap reaches at least 25 dB for speech frequencies, and a Rinne test for the 512 tuning forks yields a negative result [20]. A stapedotomy is deemed successful if it results in an air-bone closure to 10 dB. Primary stapedotomy is generally a highly effective procedure, with success rates reported between 72% and 94%. However, the success rates for revision stapes surgery are more variable, ranging from 24% to 80% according to various studies [21]. Both stapedectomy and stapedotomy have proven their effectiveness and long-term stability. Yet, in recent years, stapedotomy has gained popularity due to its superior hearing outcomes at high frequencies and lower complication rates [22]. Endoscopic stapes surgery offers several advantages, including a magnified, wide-field view and enhanced illumination compared to the microscopic technique. However, the endoscopic approach has its drawbacks, such as the need for single-handed instrumentation and prosthesis placement, the absence of stereoscopic vision, and a learning curve [23, 24]. Throughout the years, stapedotomy fenestration techniques have progressed from utilizing microinstruments to microdrills, and most recently, laser technology. The primary benefits of using laser technology include its high precision during application and the reduced risk of footplate mobilization due to the no-touch principle employed in this technique. Reports suggest that patients undergoing conventional stapedotomy are more prone to experiencing footplate fractures or sensorineural hearing loss compared to those undergoing laser stapedotomy [25].

5. **B, D, E**

Dead ear is a severe adverse outcome of stapes surgery, with occurrence rates reported between 0.6% and 3% in large series [26]. The development of reactive granulation tissue around the prosthesis and the oval window is a well-documented phenomenon. The cause of reparative granuloma is still unclear, but one theory suggests it may be a foreign body reaction to fat or gelfoam when these materials were used to seal the oval window [27]. A cerebrospinal fluid (CSF) gusher, characterized by a sudden outflow of perilymph fluid upon entering the vestibule, is a rare event. It is thought that the underlying reason for gusher is the abnormal connection between perilymphatic and subarachnoid spaces [28]. Taste disturbances immediately after surgery are reported by nearly 60% of patients undergoing a stapedotomy, as the chorda tympani nerve is often damaged by traction, stretching, and cutting during the procedure. However, only 5% of these patients continue to experience taste disturbances after 1 year [29]. Incus necrosis is one of the most common reasons of stapedectomy failure, necessitating revision stapedectomy which is considered a challenging procedure. The incidence of incus necrosis in revision stapedectomy varies from 5% to 49%. The most plausible explanations for this include strong crimping, loss of blood supply, or a poorly fitting prosthesis that causes inflammation and bone erosion over time [30].

References

1. Ealy M, Smith RJH. Otosclerosis. Adv Otorhinolaryngol. 2011;70:122–9.
2. Fabbris C, Molteni G, Tommasi N, Marchioni D. Does pregnancy have an influence on otosclerosis? J Laryngol Otol. 2022;136(3):191–6.
3. Karosi T, Szekanecz Z, Sziklai I. Otosclerosis: an autoimmune disease? Autoimmun Rev. 2009;9(2):95–101.
4. Arnold W. Some remarks on the histopathology of otosclerosis. Adv Otorhinolaryngol. 2007;65:25–30.
5. Menger DJ, Tange RA. The aetiology of otosclerosis: a review of the literature. Clin Otolaryngol Allied Sci. 2003;28(2):112–20.
6. Rudic M, Keogh I, Wagner R, et al. The pathophysiology of otosclerosis: review of current research. Hear Res. 2015;330(Pt A):51–6.
7. Ealy M, Smith RJ. The genetics of otosclerosis. Hear Res. 2010;266(1–2):70–4.
8. Skarżyński H, Gos E, Dziendziel B, Raj-Koziak D, Włodarczyk EA, Skarżyński PH. Clinically important change in tinnitus sensation after stapedotomy. Health Qual Life Outcomes. 2018;16(1):208. Published 2018 Nov 6
9. Sobrinho PG, Oliveira CA, Venosa AR. Long-term follow-up of tinnitus in patients with otosclerosis after stapes surgery. Int Tinnitus J. 2004;10(2):197–201.
10. Yetişer S. Bilateral vestibulopathy due to severe cochlear otosclerosis: a well-known condition without any favorable solution. Turkish Arch Otorhinolaryngol. 2018;56(3):174–6.
11. de Vilhena D, Gambôa I, Duarte D, Lopes G. Vestibular disorders after stapedial surgery in patients with otosclerosis. Int J Otolaryngol. 2016;2016:6830648.
12. Dudok de Wit CA, van Dishoeck HA. Paracusis willisii. Int Audiol. 1964;3:43–53.
13. Isaacson B, Kutz JW Jr, Roland PS. Otosclerosis. In: Johnson JT, Rosen CA, editors. Bailey's head and neck surgery: otolaryngology. 5th ed. Philadelphia: Lippincott Williams & Wilkins; 2014. p. 2487–502.
14. Danesh AA, Shahnaz N, Hall JW 3rd. The audiology of otosclerosis. Otolaryngol Clin North Am. 2018;51(2):327–42.

15. Kelly EA, Li B, Adams ME. Diagnostic accuracy of tuning fork tests for hearing loss: a systematic review. Otolaryngol Head Neck Surg. 2018;159(2):220–30.
16. Wiatr A, Składzień J, Strek P, Wiatr M. Carhart Notch—a prognostic factor in surgery for otosclerosis. Ear Nose Throat J. 2021;100(4):NP193–7.
17. Carhart R. Clinical application of bone conduction audiometry. Arch Otolaryngol (1925). 1950;51(6):798–808.
18. Quesnel AM, Moonis G, Appel J, O'Malley JT, McKenna MJ, Curtin HD, Merchant SN. Correlation of computed tomography with histopathology in otosclerosis. Otol Neurotol. 2013;34(1):22–8.
19. de Oliveira PN, de Oliveira VA. Medical management of otosclerosis. Otolaryngol Clin North Am. 2018;51(2):441–52.
20. Velusamy A, Kavithadevi A, Hameed N, Anand A. Comparison of short-term hearing outcome in stapedotomy using either vein or fat (adipose tissue) as sealing material. Int Arch Otorhinolaryngol. 2023;27(2):e226–33. Published 2023 Mar 29
21. Blijleven EE, Wegner I, Tange RA, Thomeer HGXM. Revision stapes surgery in a tertiary referral center: surgical and audiometric outcomes. Ann Otol Rhinol Laryngol. 2019;128(11):997–1005.
22. Cheng HCS, Agrawal SK, Parnes LS. Stapedectomy versus stapedotomy. Otolaryngol Clin North Am. 2018;51(2):375–92.
23. Isaacson B, Hunter JB, Rivas A. Endoscopic stapes surgery. Otolaryngol Clin North Am. 2018;51(2):415–28.
24. Moneir W, Abd El-Fattah AM, Mahmoud E, Elshaer M. Endoscopic stapedotomy: merits and demerits. J Otolaryngol. 2018;13(3):97–100.
25. Wegner I, Kamalski DM, Tange RA, et al. Laser versus conventional fenestration in stapedotomy for otosclerosis: a systematic review. Laryngoscope. 2014;124(7):1687–93.
26. Vital V, Konstantinidis I, Vital I, Triaridis S. Minimizing the dead ear in otosclerosis surgery. Auris Nasus Larynx. 2008;35(4):475–9.
27. Tange RA, Schimanski G, van Lange JW, Grolman W, Zuur LC. Reparative granuloma seen in cases of gold piston implantation after stapes surgery for otosclerosis. Auris Nasus Larynx. 2002;29(1):7–10.
28. Satar B, Genc H, Meral SC. Why did we encounter gusher in a stapes surgery case? Was it enlarged medial aperture of the cochlear aqueduct? Surg Radiol Anat. 2021;43(2):225–9.
29. Berling Holm K, Knutsson J, Strömbäck K, et al. Taste disturbance after stapes surgery: an evaluation of frequency, severity, duration, and quality-of-life. Acta Otolaryngol. 2017;137(1):39–43.
30. Massimilla EA, Testa D, Nunziata M, Donadio A, Romano ML, Motta G. Long process incus necrosis in revision stapedotomy: retrospective clinical study. Ear Nose Throat J. 2023;102(1):58–63.

Temporal Bone Fracture

18

Dimitrios Daskalakis, Ram Vaidhyanath, and Peter Rea

Abstract

Temporal bone fractures are most commonly seen in patients involved in road traffic accidents and are commonest between the second and the fourth decade of life. There is a 3:1 male to female prevalence ratio in sustaining temporal bone fractures. Temporal bone fractures are traditionally classified as longitudinal, transverse, and mixed. Often these fractures are associated with other craniofacial fractures as well as brain injuries, and the management of the temporal bone fractures may vary depending on the coexisting injuries and the general condition of the patient. A hearing test is ultimately required to investigate for sensorineural and conductive hearing loss, although bedside tuning fork exam might be the only way to initially assess the patient's hearing depending on consciousness and comorbidities. The hearing test should be repeated 6–8 weeks later to allow for resolution of middle ear effusion if present.

D. Daskalakis (✉)
ENT Head and Neck Surgery Department, 424 General Military Hospital, Thessaloniki, Greece

R. Vaidhyanath · P. Rea
University Hospitals of Leicester NHS Trust, Leicester, UK

Case Presentation

You are going to see, a 15-year old boy who fell from an electric skateboard without a helmet and hit his head 3 months ago. His CT head scan organized by the emergency department showed an undisplaced right-sided longitudinal temporal bone fracture with partial opacification of the mastoid air cells along the fracture line due to bleeding. There was no evidence of intracranial bleeding. On otoscopy, bleeding into the ear canal was reported and fluid samples from the ear canal were sent for CSF leak analysis (beta 2 transferrin) which came back negative. The General Practitioner (GP) reports on their referral letter that following the injury the patient developed a new onset of right-sided conductive hearing loss. The audiogram undertaken in the audiology department on the day of your assessment revealed normal hearing on the left, but a conductive hearing loss on the right-hand side ranging from 25 dB in the low frequencies to 65 dB at 4 kHz. Tympanometry was type A bilaterally. Figure 18.1 is from the CT head which was performed after the initial trauma, whereas Figs. 18.2 and 18.3 are from the cone beam CT of the right temporal bone that followed the initial scan.

N. Tsetsos et al. (eds.), *Otolaryngology Study Guide*, https://doi.org/10.1007/978-3-031-77374-7_18

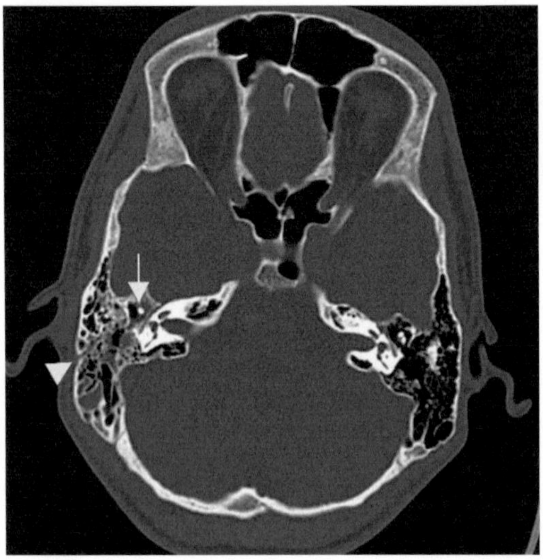

Fig. 18.1 CT Head performed after initial trauma. There is longitudinal fracture through the right petrous bone (arrow head). Head of the right malleus (small arrow). Body of the right incus is "missing"

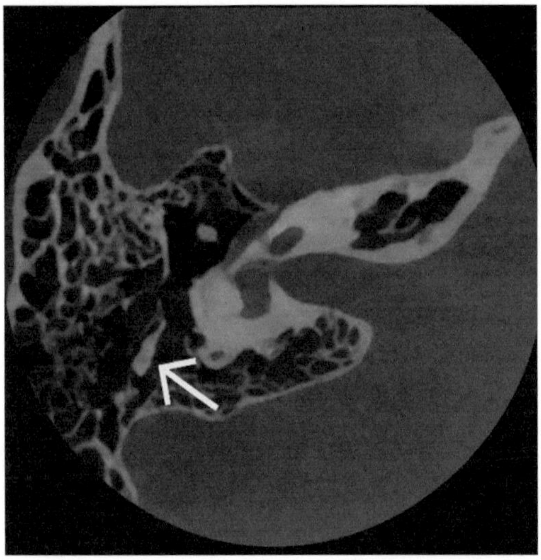

Fig. 18.2 Cone beam CT of the right temporal bone showing the displaced incus in the right mastoid (long arrow)

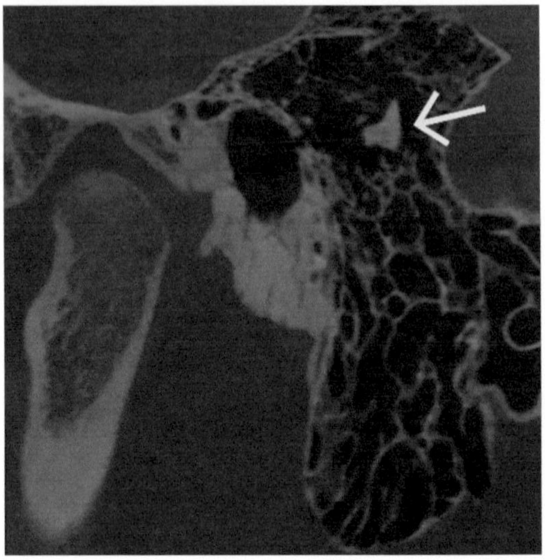

Fig. 18.3 Cone beam CT of the right temporal bone showing the displaced incus in the right mastoid (long arrow)

Questions

1. Temporal bone fractures (Multiple correct answers possible):
   A. Are more frequently transverse
   B. Rarely require CSF leak repair when CSF leak occurs
   C. Are also classified as "otic capsule violating" and "otic capsule sparing"
   D. Can lead to VII cranial nerve palsy in 50% of cases
   E. Can rarely be associated with VI cranial nerve palsy
2. CT head and cone beam CT of the right temporal bone showed ossicular chain injury in the middle ear. Please select which of the following types of ossicular dislocation in the middle ear is the most commonly encountered in temporal bone fracture cases?
   A. Dislocation of the malleoincudal complex
   B. Dislocation of the incus
   C. Dislocation of the malleus
   D. Dislocation of the incudostapedial complex
   E. Stapediovestibular dislocation
3. Profound hearing loss suggests:
   A. Hemotympanum
   B. Traumatic perforation of tympanic membrane
   C. Disruption of the ear ossicles
   D. Violation of otic capsule which is more frequent in longitudinal temporal bone fractures

   E. Violation of otic capsule which is more frequent in transverse temporal bone fractures
4. Emergency exploration of the middle ear may be considered following a temporal bone fracture when (Multiple correct answers possible):
   A. Acute onset of vertigo and high frequency sensorineural hearing loss occurs
   B. Acute onset of conductive hearing loss occurs
   C. CSF leak persists
   D. Uncomplicated tympanic membrane perforation has occurred
   E. Immediate and complete post-traumatic facial palsy occurs without other coexisting neurological trauma or brain injury.
5. Complete or incomplete peripheral facial nerve paralysis following a temporal bone fracture occurs in:
   A. Less than 1% of cases
   B. 5–10% of cases
   C. 30–50% of cases
   D. 50–70% of cases
   E. 70–90% of cases

Answers

1. **B, C, E**

   Transverse temporal bone fractures are rare [1–3]. The otic capsule is violated in only 5.8% of the temporal bone fractures [4]. Otic capsule violating versus otic capsule sparing temporal bone fractures is an alternative classification system introduced by Dahiya et al. [5]. Facial palsy may occur. This may be immediate or may develop after 2–12 days. It may be complete or incomplete and is reported to occur in 5–10% of cases. CSF fistulas are reported in 15–35% of cases but surgical management is infrequently required as these tend to resolve with conservative management including CSF diversion in almost 90% of cases [6]. Abducens nerve palsy is rare but may occur in 1% of cases [1]. Vascular injuries are also reported after temporal bone fracture (e.g., carotid-cavernous fistula, sigmoid sinus thrombosis, and internal carotid artery rupture).
2. **B**

   Middle ear ossicular injury following head injury, with temporal bone fracture, usually occurs as a bone dislocation or a joint separation. The most common type of dislocation encountered is the dislocation of the incus bone (62%) [7, 8].
3. **E**

   Violation of the otic capsule is more frequent in transverse temporal bone fractures and may manifest itself with severe sensorineural hearing loss, however, it has been suggested that otic capsule sparing temporal bone fractures may also cause sensorineural hearing loss due to intralabyrinthine hemorrhage and injury of the membranous labyrinth [4]. The otic capsule heals by fibrous union and therefore this puts the patient at lifelong risk for developing meningitis [2, 9].
4. **A, C, E**

   Emergency exploratory tympanotomy is advisable when perilymphatic fistula is suspected (vertigo, dizziness, sloping hearing levels) [1]. Surgical treatment of CSF fistulas is uncommon as they resolve with conservative management including CSF diversion within a week in more than 90% of cases [6]. Closure of a tympanic membrane perforation is not suggested as an urgent surgery, as most heal spontaneously [1]. All patients with post-traumatic facial nerve palsy should undergo a CT scan and should be evaluated with transcutaneous nerve excitability tests and electroneurography. Immediate and complete post-traumatic facial palsy with more than 90% denervation documented by electroneurography requires urgent surgical management, taking into account the general clinical condition of the patient and other coexisting neurological trauma [2].
5. **B**

   A peripheral facial nerve paralysis complete or incomplete occurs in 5–10% of cases of temporal bone fractures and can be immediate due to the injury or occur within 2–12 days as a consequence of neural edema or herpes virus being reactivated in the geniculate ganglion [10, 11].

References

1. Darrouzet V. Traumatisms of the temporal bone. In: Otorhinolaryngology, head and neck surgery; 2010. p. 85–91.
2. Katzen JT, Jarrahy R, Eby JB, Mathiasen RA, Margulies DR, Shahinian HK. Craniofacial and skull base trauma. J Trauma. 2003;54(5):1026–34.
3. Basavaraju U, Jayaramaiah SK, Turamari RU, Prakash V, Mankani S. Temporal bone fractures and its classification: retrospective study of incidence, causes, clinical features, complications and outcome. Int J Anat Radiol Surg. 2017;6(4):RO57–61. Available from: https://doaj.org/article/96f80c7479a340d790ba401a1e612cbd
4. Goddard J, McRackan T. Noninfectious disorders of the ear. In: KJLEE's essential otolaryngology, head and neck surgery. 11th ed; 2016. p. 424–35.
5. Dahiya R, Keller JD, Litofsky NS, Bankey PE, Bonassar LJ, Megerian CA. Temporal bone fractures: otic capsule sparing versus otic capsule violating clinical and radiographic considerations. J Trauma. 1999;47(6):1079–83.
6. Prosser JD, Vender JR, Solares CA. Traumatic cerebrospinal fluid leaks. Otolaryngol Clin North Am. 2011;44(4):857–73. https://doi.org/10.1016/j.otc.2011.06.007.
7. Meriot P, Veillon F, Garcia JF, Nonent M, Jezequel J, Bourjat P, et al. CT appearances of ossicular injuries. Radiographics. 1997;17(6):1445–54.
8. Oozeer N, Crowther J. Otological trauma. In: Logan Turner's diseases of the nose, throat and ear, head and neck surgery; 2015. Chapter 51 (14 pages).
9. Fisch U, Mattox D. Microsurgery of the skull base. New York: Thieme; 1988. p. 4–53.
10. Gordin E, Lee TS, Ducic Y, Arnaoutakis D. Facial nerve trauma: evaluation and considerations in management. Craniomaxillofac Trauma Reconstr. 2015;8(1):1–13.
11. Vajpayee D, Mallick A, Mishra AK. Post temporal bone fracture facial paralysis: strategies in decision making and analysis of efficacy of surgical treatment. Indian J Otolaryngol Head Neck Surg. 2018;70(4):566–71. https://doi.org/10.1007/s12070-018-1371-y.

19 Meniere's Disease

Dimitrios Daskalakis and Peter Rea

Abstract

Meniere's disease (MD) is an idiopathic clinical illness which presents with acute attacks of vertigo lasting from 20 min to 24 h associated with nausea and sickness, along with a fluctuating low frequency sensorineural hearing loss that may become permanent. Tinnitus and aural fullness usually develop before or during the acute attack. Meniere's disease is classified as definite or probable by the American Academy of Otolaryngology—Head and Neck Surgery. Their recent Clinical Practice Guideline for Meniere's disease details the updated classification.

Case Presentation

You are called to see a 61-year-old male who has previously presented with recurrent right-sided hearing loss and fullness in the ear and now comes with a deterioration of his hearing on the right-hand side (Fig. 19.1). His initial audiogram had shown a mild right-sided low frequency sensorineural hearing loss which recovered on subsequent audiograms. He experienced further periods of up to a month of right-sided hearing loss and aural fullness followed by recovery. Several years later in the course of his illness, he developed bouts of right-sided low frequency tinnitus, aural fullness, and hearing loss followed by severe vertigo and vomiting lasting up to 2 h. There were no migrainous features, and there was no positional dizziness. His MRI of internal acoustic meatus (IAM) was normal. His audiogram on this last presentation is attached.

Questions

1. The differential diagnosis for patients presenting with episodic dizziness includes which of the following (more than one correct answer possible)?
   A. Vestibular migraine
   B. BPPV
   C. Persistent postural perceptual dizziness (PPPD)
   D. Hyperventilation
   E. Cardiac dysrhythmias
2. Which of the following conditions are more common in patients with Meniere's disease, than in the general population (more than one correct answer possible)?
   A. Migraine
   B. Otitis media with effusion
   C. BPPV

D. Daskalakis (✉)
ENT Head and Neck Surgery Department, 424 General Military Hospital, Thessaloniki, Greece

P. Rea
University Hospitals of Leicester NHS Trust, Leicester, UK

N. Tsetsos et al. (eds.), *Otolaryngology Study Guide*, https://doi.org/10.1007/978-3-031-77374-7_19

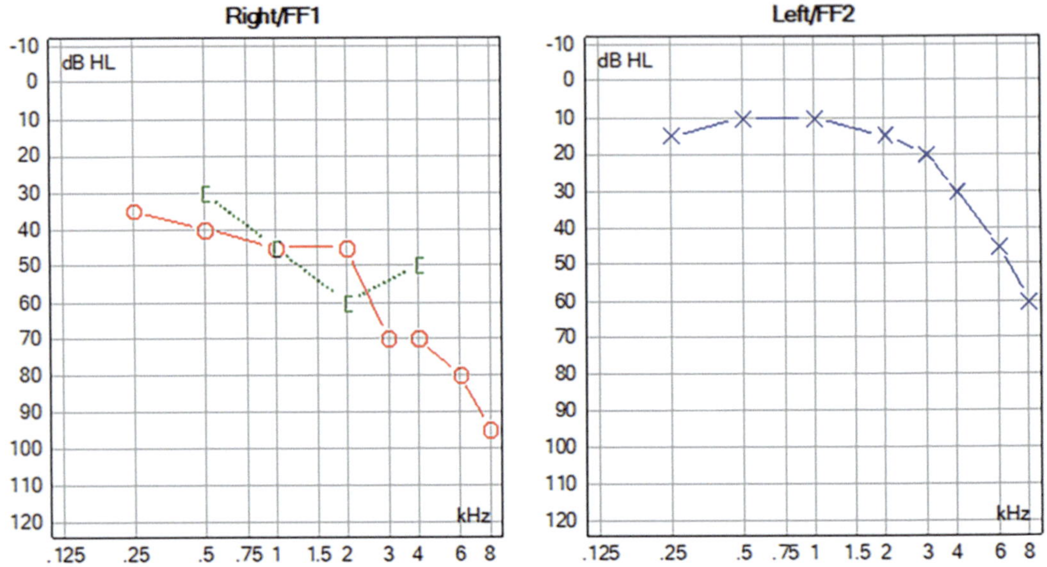

Fig. 19.1 Pure tone audiogram showing right-sided sensorineural hearing loss

   D. Otosclerosis
   E. Depression—Anxiety
3. Which of the following investigations should be considered in patients presenting with vertigo attacks consistent with Meniere's disease (more than one correct answer possible).
   A. EEG
   B. Audiogram
   C. Fluorescent treponemal antibody absorption
   D. MRI IAM
   E. Lying and standing BP
4. The likelihood of developing bilateral Meniere's disease is approximately:
   A. 1–10%
   B. 20–30%
   C. 40–50%
   D. 60–70%
   E. 80–90%
5. Regarding Tumarkin drop attacks (more than one correct answer possible).
   A. These are common events in patients with Meniere's disease
   B. They may lead to the withdrawal of a patient's driving licence, and the patient must be informed of this
   C. Patients have warning of when they may occur
   D. Patients are unlikely to injure themselves during a drop attack
   E. They tend to herald the late stages of Meniere's disease

Answers

1. **A, B, D, E**

   Common causes of episodic or recurrent vertigo include BPPV, vestibular migraine, and Meniere's disease. Rare vestibular causes of episodic vertigo include channelopathies (episodic ataxias) and vestibular paroxysmia. A wide range of non-vestibular causes should also be considered including posterior fossa transient ischaemic attacks, panic attacks, cardiac dysrhythmias, drug-induced dizziness, postural hypotension, and metabolic disorders among others [1, 2].

2. **A, C, E**

   There is significant evidence of increased rates of anxiety, depression, sleep-disorders, and migraine in patients diagnosed with Meniere's disease [3]. Migraine or a positive familial history of migraine has previously been associated with Meniere's disease [4]. Identifying and treating depression should allow for improvement of overall quality of life in patients with Meniere's disease [5].

BPPV is another condition that is seen more frequently in Meniere's disease [6]. Otolaryngologists should have a low threshold to screen and refer appropriately.

3. **B, C, D**

   When Meniere's disease is suspected, serial audiograms are the key diagnostic tests [1]. An MRI IAM is necessary to exclude retrocochlear pathology, and fluorescent treponemal antibody absorption is also often undertaken as syphilis can rarely manifest itself with symptoms identical to Meniere's disease [7].

4. **B**

   In most published studies, the frequency of bilateral Meniere's disease is between 20% and 30% [8–10].

5. **B, E**

   Tumarkin drop attacks [otherwise known as Vestibular Drop Attacks (VDA)] happen more frequently in Meniere's disease patients. The pooled frequency of VDA in Meniere's disease was 8% in hospital-based studies and often occurred in advanced stages of the disease [11]. In some studies, the VDA was defined as sudden imbalance without head movement occurring without warning or trigger [12–14]. This definition of VDA covers a wider spectrum of balance derangements compared to the original definition of "Tumarkin attacks" that refers to subjects who fall to the ground. Although VDA usually do not present with loss of consciousness, vestibular syncope has been described recently in VDA. VDA can develop with no warning, putting the patient at risk of developing injuries and decreasing their quality of life [11]. Patients with Meniere's disease and severe VDA were at a higher risk of experiencing a vertiginous attack while driving a car [15].

References

1. Basura GJ, Adams ME, Monfared A, Schwartz SR, Antonelli PJ, Burkard R, et al. Clinical practice guideline: Ménière's disease. Otolaryngol Head Neck Surg (United States). 2020;162(Suppl. 2):S1–55.
2. Bronstein A, Lempert T. Recurrent vertigo and dizziness. In: Dizziness. 2nd ed; 2017. p. 70–108.
3. Bruderer SG, Bodmer D, Stohler NA, Jick SS, Meier CR. Population-based study on the epidemiology of Ménière's disease. Audiol Neurotol. 2017;22(2):74–82.
4. Lempert T, Olesen J, Furman J, Waterston J, Seemungal B, Carey J, et al. Vestibular migraine: diagnostic criteria. J Vestib Res Equilib Orientat. 2022;32(1):1–6.
5. Patel JJ, Levy DA, Nguyen SA, Rizk HG, Meyer TA. Depression in Ménière's disease: a systematic review and meta-analysis. J Laryngol Otol. 2020;134(4):293–301.
6. Kutlubaev MA, Xu Y, Hornibrook J. Benign paroxysmal positional vertigo in Meniere's disease: systematic review and meta-analysis of frequency and clinical characteristics. J Neurol. 2021;268(5):1608–14. https://doi.org/10.1007/s00415-019-09502-x.
7. Johnson J, Lalwani A. Vestibular disorders. Meniere's disease. In: Current diagnosis & treatment in otolaryngology—head & neck surgery. 2nd ed; 2012.
8. Yazawa Y, Kitahara M. Bilateral endolymphatic hydrops in meniere's disease: review of temporal bone autopsies. Ann Otol Rhinol Laryngol. 1990;99(7):524–8.
9. Velázquez-Villaseñor L, Merchant SN, Tsuji K, Glynn RJ, Wall C, Rauch SD. Temporal bone studies of the human peripheral vestibular system. Normative Scarpa's ganglion cell data. Ann Otol Rhinol Laryngol Suppl. 2000;181:14–9.
10. Phillips J, Murdin L, Rea P, Harcourt J, Shepstone L, Sims E, et al. Development of a national Meniere's disease registry: a feasibility study. J Int Adv Otol. 2024;20(4):339.
11. Kutlubaev MA, Xu Y, Manchaiah V, Zou J, Pyykkö I. Vestibular drop attacks in Ménière's disease: a systematic review and meta-analysis of frequency, correlates and consequences. J Vestib Res Equilib Orientat. 2022;32(2):171–81.
12. Kentala E, Havia M, Pyykkö I. Short-lasting drop attacks in Meniere's disease. Otolaryngol Head Neck Surg. 2001;124(5):526–30.
13. Pyykkö I, Manchaiah V, Zou J, Levo H, Kentala E. Impact of Tumarkin attacks on complaints and work ability in Ménière's disease. J Vestib Res Equilib Orientat. 2018;28(3–4):319–30.
14. Pyykkö I, Manchaiah V, Zou J, Levo H, Kentala E. Vestibular syncope: a disorder associated with drop attack in Ménière's disease. Auris Nasus Larynx. 2018;45(2):234–41. https://doi.org/10.1016/j.anl.2017.03.023.
15. Pyykkö I, Manchaiah V. Driving habits and risk of traffic accidents among people with ménière's disease in Finland. J Int Adv Otol. 2019;15(2):289–95.

20 Vestibular Schwannoma

Konstantinos Geronatsios

Abstract

Vestibular schwannomas arise from Schwann cells, either from the vestibular or the cochlear nerve. They account for approximately 80% of cerebellopontine angle tumors, and their incidence is 0.7–1 per 100,000 population. They can remain asymptomatic for a long period of time, especially when they are small in size. The most common symptom is unilateral hearing loss, followed by unilateral tinnitus, imbalance, vertigo, headaches, facial weakness or numbness, swallowing difficulties, hoarseness of voice, palatal paresis, and hydrocephalus in large tumors. Most vestibular schwannomas have an intracanalicular component and can cause widening of the internal auditory meatus. Bilateral vestibular schwannomas can be related to neurofibromatosis type 2, a genetic condition characterized by the development of benign central nervous system tumors. Vestibular schwannomas can be managed by observation, surgical excision, and stereotactic radiotherapy.

K. Geronatsios (✉)
ENT Head and Neck Surgery Department,
424 General Military Hospital, Thessaloniki, Greece

Case Presentation

A 64-year-old male presented to the Otology clinic with moderate to severe hearing loss in his left ear, non-pulsatile tinnitus on the left, and mild difficulty swallowing. He also reported intermittent dizziness. These symptoms started 2 years ago with mild hearing loss and tinnitus in his left ear, but they have gradually worsened. His past medical history includes hypertension and dyslipidemia. There is no history of exposure to loud noises and no fluctuating hearing loss. Upon examination, both tympanic membranes appeared normal. The examination of the oral cavity and an endoscopy were unremarkable. There were no obvious signs of cranial nerve damage, and no automatic nystagmus was observed. The patient's pure tone audiogram (Fig. 20.1) and MRI scan of the Internal Auditory Meatus (IAM) (Fig. 20.2) are as follows.

Questions

1. Which of the following are possible symptoms of this tumor? (more than one correct answer possible)
   A. Right facial nerve palsy
   B. Left-sided hearing loss
   C. Bilateral tinnitus
   D. Imbalance and vertigo
   E. Dysphagia

N. Tsetsos et al. (eds.), *Otolaryngology Study Guide*, https://doi.org/10.1007/978-3-031-77374-7_20

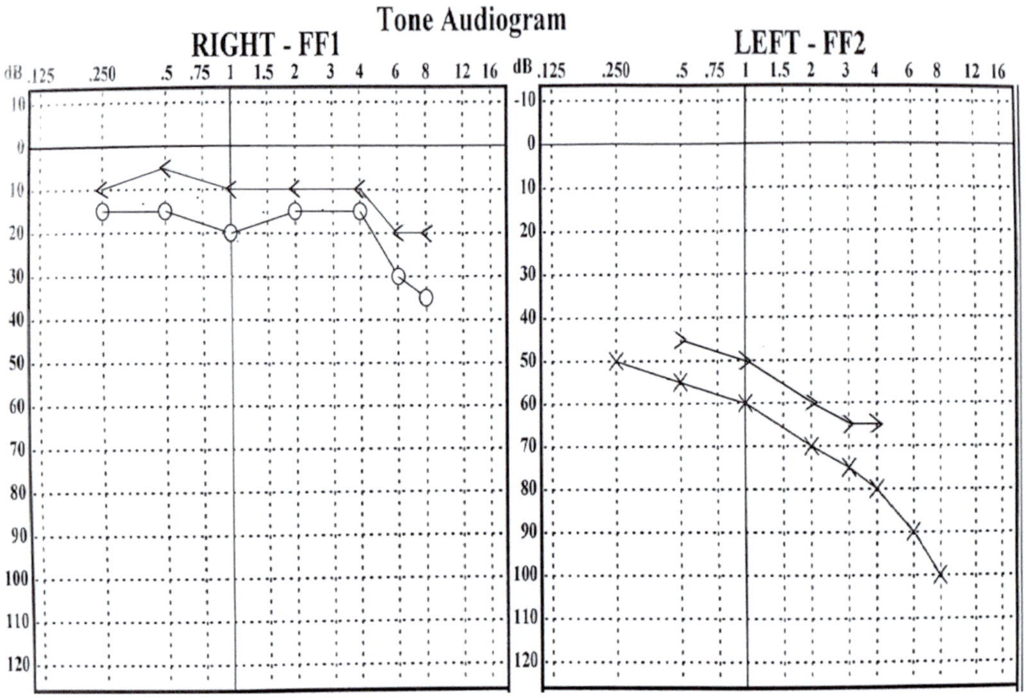

Fig. 20.1 Pure tone audiogram

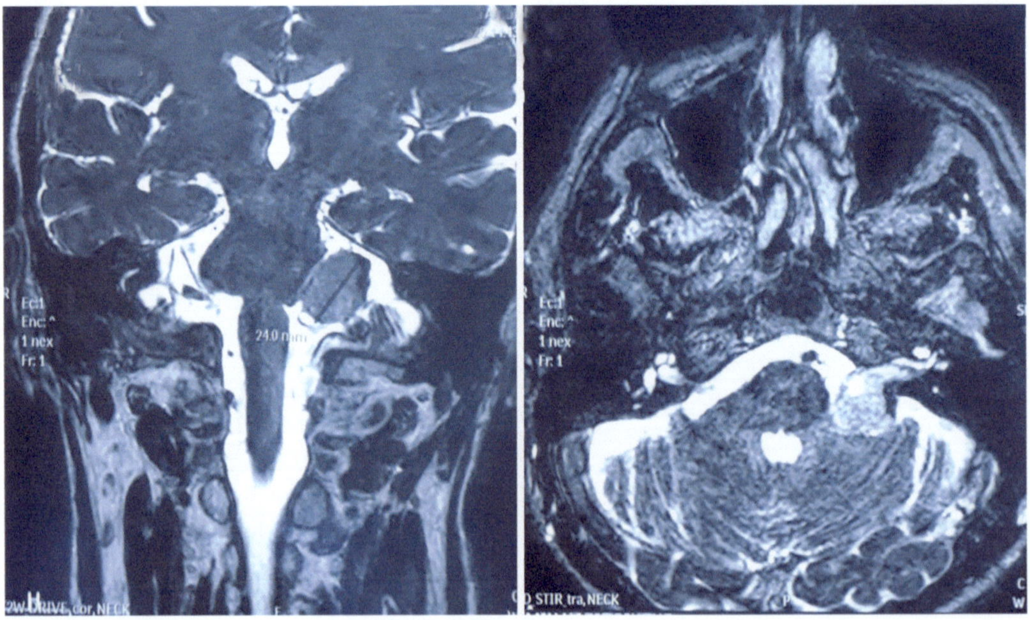

Fig. 20.2 MRI scan

2. Which of the following are true for the radiological findings of a vestibular schwannoma? (more than one correct answer possible)
   A. Most of these tumors do not have an intracanalicular component
   B. Intense contrast enhancement in T1 sequences is a common radiological finding
   C. CT scan of internal auditory meatus is the preferred examination for suspected vestibular schwannoma
   D. Large tumors may contain hypointense cystic areas
   E. On CT scan widening of the internal auditory canal may be noticed, but never evidence of bony erosion
3. In case of bilateral vestibular schwannomas, which systemic disorder is a possible diagnosis?
   A. Neurofibromatosis type 1
   B. Von Hippel-Lindau syndrome
   C. Neurofibromatosis type 2
   D. Li-Fraumeni syndrome
   E. Cowden syndrome
4. Which of the following statements are true? (more than one correct answer possible)
   A. For elderly patients with comorbidities, observation only is the proper management
   B. A vestibular schwannoma larger than 5 cm can metastasize to other sites of the body
   C. Radiation therapy increases mortality and morbidity
   D. Only a small percent of patients presenting with sudden unilateral sensorineural hearing loss are diagnosed with vestibular schwannoma
   E. People with small vestibular schwannomas, good hearing, and asymptomatic should be treated only surgically
5. Which is the treatment of Vestibular schwannoma? (more than one correct answer possible)
   A. Chemotherapy
   B. Observation
   C. Immunotherapy
   D. Surgical excision
   E. Stereotactic radiotherapy

Answers

1. **B, D, E**

   Vestibular schwannomas arise from Schwann cells, either from the vestibular or the cochlear nerve. They account for approximately 80% of cerebellopontine angle tumors, and their incidence is 0.7–1 per 100,000 population. They can remain asymptomatic for a long period of time, especially when they are small in size [1]. The most common symptom is unilateral hearing loss, followed by unilateral tinnitus, imbalance, vertigo, headaches, facial weakness or numbness, swallowing difficulties, hoarseness of voice, palatal paresis, and hydrocephalus in large tumors [1, 2].
2. **C, E**

   Most vestibular schwannomas have an intracanalicular component and can cause widening of the internal auditory meatus. An extracanalicular extension may cause an "ice cream cone" appearance. Only a small percentage of vestibular schwannomas have an extracanalicular component only. In MRI T1 images, most vestibular schwannomas are hypointense compared to the brain, and less commonly isointense. Cystic areas may also be noticed, especially in large tumors. In T1 images with contrast, the enhancement is intense. In MRI T2 images, the tumors appear heterogeneously hyperintense, compared to the brain [3, 4]. Cystic areas are presented with fluid intensity. The MRI scan of the internal auditory canals is the radiological examination of choice in suspected vestibular schwannomas [3, 5]. The temporal bone CT scan may reveal widening and possibly erosion of the internal auditory canal [5].
3. **C**

   Neurofibromatosis type 2 is a genetic condition, characterized by the development of benign central nervous system tumors, and it follows an autosomal inheritance pattern [6]. Most of these patients will present with bilateral vestibular schwannomas at a young age.

The average age of onset is 18–24 years. Approximately 50% of the patients may also develop meningiomas. The most common presentations are bilateral hearing loss, bilateral tinnitus, vertigo, and imbalance [7, 8]. Neurofibromatosis type 1 causes tumors along the nerves and changes in skin color. Von Hippel-Lindau syndrome is associated with brain hemangioblastomas. Cowden syndrome is related to the development of hamartomas, and Li-Fraumeni syndrome to the development of malignant tumors.

4. **A, D**

   Observation should only be recommended for elderly people, patients with comorbidities, in cases with small tumors and no hearing impairment, and when the tumor is on the side of the only hearing ear. MRI scans are recommended for surveillance follow-up [9]. Furthermore, patients with small and asymptomatic tumors can be observed only. Vestibular schwannoma is a benign tumor and cannot metastasize. Moreover, there is no chance of malignant transformation. Stereotactic radiotherapy is not related to increased morbidity and mortality. There are not enough data for secondary tumor induction by radiotherapy [10, 11]. Even though vestibular schwannoma can present with sudden hearing loss, only a small percentage of patients presenting with sudden unilateral sensorineural hearing loss are diagnosed with vestibular schwannoma.

5. **B, D, E**

   Chemotherapy and immunotherapy are not indicated as treatments for vestibular schwannoma. Observation should be recommended as above. Surgical treatment is indicated for symptomatic and growing tumors. Vestibular schwannomas are classified as large if the largest extracanalicular diameter is more than 2.5 cm. The three surgical approaches for vestibular schwannoma are the translabyrinthine approach, the retrosigmoid approach, and middle cranial fossa approach [12]. Stereotactic radiotherapy is an alternative to surgical therapy, with good results and fewer complications and morbidity. Patients receiving radiotherapy should remain in long-term follow-up with repetitive MRI scans, for the possibility of tumor re-growth [10, 11].

References

1. Greene J, Al-Dhahir MA. Acoustic neuroma [Updated 2022 Jun 4]. In: StatPearls. Treasure Island (FL): StatPearls Publishing; 2022.
2. Foley RW, Shirazi S, Maweni RM, et al. Signs and symptoms of acoustic neuroma at initial presentation: an exploratory analysis. Cureus. 2017;9(11):e1846.
3. Mulkens T, Parizel P, Martin J, et al. Acoustic schwannoma: MR findings in 84 tumors. AJR Am J Roentgenol. 1993;160(2):395–8.
4. Dunn IF, Bi WL, Mukundan S, et al. Congress of neurological surgeons systematic review and evidence-based guidelines on the role of imaging in the diagnosis and management of patients with vestibular schwannomas. Neurosurgery. 2018;82(2):E32–4.
5. Wu E, Tang Y, Zhang Y, Bai R. CT in diagnosis of acoustic neuromas. AJNR Am J Neuroradiol. 1986;7(4):645–50.
6. Tiwari R, Singh AK. Neurofibromatosis type 2. [Updated 2021 Oct 9]. In: StatPearls. Treasure Island (FL): StatPearls Publishing; 2022.
7. Evans DG. Neurofibromatosis 2. 1998 Oct 14 [Updated 2018 Mar 15]. In: Adam MP, Everman DB, Mirzaa GM, et al., editors. GeneReviews®. Seattle (WA): University of Washington, Seattle; 1998. 1993–2022.
8. Meola A, Chang SD. Bilateral vestibular schwannomas in neurofibromatosis type 2. N Engl J Med. 2018;379(15):1463. https://doi.org/10.1056/NEJMicm1804944.
9. Nellis JC, Sharon JD, Pross SE, et al. Multifactor influences of shared decision-making in acoustic neuroma treatment. Otol Neurotol. 2017;38(3):392–9.
10. Boari N, Bailo M, Gagliardi F, et al. Gamma Knife radiosurgery for vestibular schwannoma: clinical results at long-term follow-up in a series of 379 patients. J Neurosurg. 2014;121:123–42.
11. Powell C, Micallef C, Gonsalves A, Wharram B, Ashley S, Brada M. Fractionated stereotactic radiotherapy in the treatment of vestibular schwannoma (acoustic neuroma): predicting the risk of hydrocephalus. Int J Radiat Oncol Biol Phys. 2011;80(4):1143–50.
12. Silk P, Lane J, Driscoll C. Surgical approaches to vestibular schwannomas: what the radiologist needs to know. Radiographics. 2009;29(7):1955–70.

Presbycusis

21

Konstantinos Garefis

Abstract

Presbycusis or age-related hearing loss is a gradual, bilateral, and progressive type of sensorineural hearing loss associated with aging. The prevalence of presbycusis increases with age, affecting approximately 30–40% of individuals over 65 years old. The symptoms typically include difficulty hearing high-pitched sounds and difficulty understanding speech, particularly in noisy environments, and often tinnitus. The onset of symptoms may vary and can develop over many years or decades. Moreover, they tend to worsen over time, affecting communication abilities and significantly impacting quality of life. The exact pathophysiology of presbycusis is not fully understood but believed to involve a combination of genetic and environmental factors such as noise exposure, ototoxic medications, and vascular changes. Presbycusis can be classified into three main categories: sensory, neural, and metabolic. The diagnosis is made through a comprehensive audiological evaluation including a detailed medical history, physical exam, pure-tone audiometry which is the most common diagnostic test used, speech audiometry, and measures of speech understanding in noise. The management of presbycusis includes hearing aids, cochlear implants, auditory training as well as addressing any underlying medical conditions.

K. Garefis (✉)
2nd Academic ORL, Head and Neck Surgery Department, Aristotle University of Thessaloniki, Papageorgiou Hospital, Thessaloniki, Greece

Case Presentation

A 72-year-old man came to the audiology clinic complaining of hearing difficulty in both ears that had gradually worsened over several years. He reported difficulty understanding conversations, especially in noisy environments, and often had to ask people to repeat themselves. He also noticed he had to turn up the volume of the TV and phone. He denied any history of ear infections or exposure to loud noise. On examination, he had high-frequency hearing loss in both ears on audiometry testing while ear examination was normal (Fig. 21.1). Speech testing revealed difficulty understanding speech in noise. The patient was fitted with hearing aids, and he reported significant improvement in his ability to communicate and participate in social activities.

Questions

1. Which of the following is the most common type of presbycusis?
   A. Mechanical presbycusis
   B. Neural presbycusis

N. Tsetsos et al. (eds.), *Otolaryngology Study Guide*, https://doi.org/10.1007/978-3-031-77374-7_21

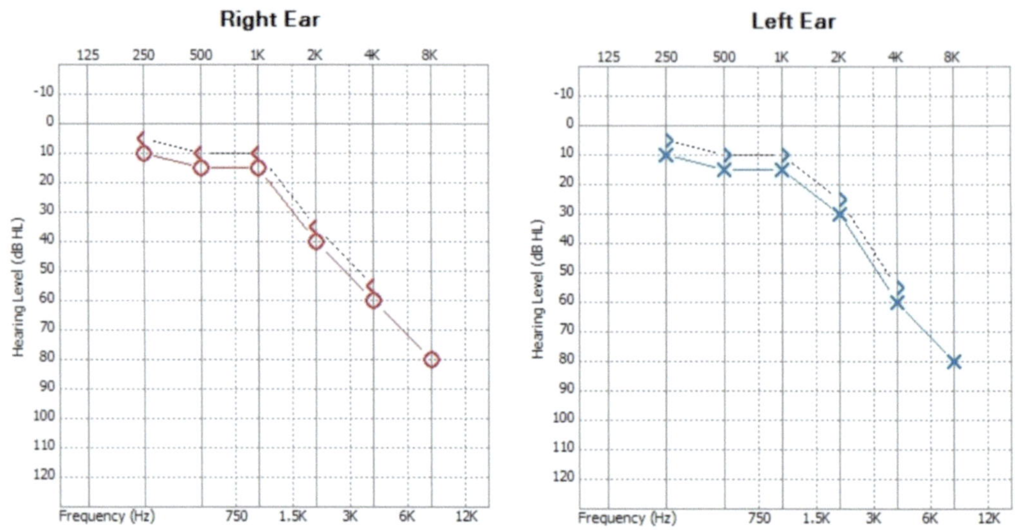

Fig. 21.1 Pure-tone audiogram showing bilateral symmetric sensorineural hearing loss indicating presbycusis

   C. Metabolic presbycusis
   D. Conductive presbycusis
   E. Sensory presbycusis
2. Which type of presbycusis is caused by a degeneration of the auditory nerve fibers that transmit sound signals from the cochlea to the brain?
   A. Metabolic presbycusis
   B. Neural presbycusis
   C. Conductive presbycusis
   D. Mechanical presbycusis
   E. None of the above
3. Which of the following are common symptoms of presbycusis? (more than one correct answer possible)
   A. Dizziness
   B. Tinnitus
   C. Ear discharge
   D. Difficulty hearing in noisy environments
   E. Nausea
4. What is the typical configuration of hearing loss observed in presbycusis?
   A. Flat
   B. Sloping
   C. Rising
   D. Inverted V
   E. None of the above
5. Which of the following surgical interventions may be considered for patients with severe presbycusis?
   A. Cochlear implant
   B. Stapedectomy
   C. Myringotomy
   D. Tympanoplasty
   E. None of the above

Answers

1. **E**

   Sensory presbycusis is the most common type, accounting for approximately 90% of cases of age-related hearing loss. It is caused by the degeneration of the sensory hair cells in the cochlea, which is associated with a decline in the number of inner and outer hair cells, as well as changes in the stria vascularis [1]. The hallmark of sensory presbycusis is a loss of sensitivity to high-frequency sounds, which often results in difficulty hearing and understanding speech, especially in noisy environments [2]. Several factors have been identified to contribute to the development of sensory presbycusis, including genetic susceptibility, environmental exposure to noise, and other health conditions, such as diabetes and cardiovascular disease [3, 4].

2. **B**

Neural presbycusis, caused by degeneration of the auditory nerve fibers that transmit sound signals from the cochlea to the brain, can affect both high- and low-frequency sounds [5]. In contrast, metabolic presbycusis is caused by changes in cochlear metabolic function leading to a decline in the production and regulation of proteins and enzymes necessary for normal hearing, often with reduced hearing sensitivity at high frequencies [6]. Conductive presbycusis is a loss of sound transmission through the outer or middle ear due to changes in the structure and function of the ossicles or ear canal, which can reduce overall hearing sensitivity, especially for low-frequency sounds [7]. Mechanical presbycusis results from age-related changes in the structure and function of the cochlea, including stiffening of the basilar membrane and loss of hair cell elasticity, which often reduces overall hearing sensitivity, especially for high-frequency sounds [8].

3. **B, D**

The gradual loss of hearing sensitivity, especially for high-frequency sounds, is the most common symptom of presbycusis, resulting in a reduced ability to hear and understand speech, particularly in noisy settings [1, 2]. Recent studies have shown reduced speech perception scores in individuals with presbycusis compared to controls, particularly in noisy environments [9, 10]. Tinnitus, which is a common accompanying symptom, may occur in up to 80% of cases, and is perceived as a high-pitched ringing, buzzing, or hissing sound that can be continuous or intermittent [7, 11]. Tinnitus can cause significant distress for patients with presbycusis and may require management in addition to the hearing loss itself.

4. **B**

Presbycusis is typically indicated by a specific pattern of hearing loss, known as sloping high-frequency hearing loss, which is reflected on a pure-tone audiogram. This configuration is characterized by elevated hearing thresholds at higher frequencies compared to lower frequencies [1, 7, 12]. While other audiogram configurations exist, including flat or rising patterns, they are not typically associated with presbycusis. Several studies have verified the predominance of the sloping configuration in pure-tone audiograms of presbycusis patients. For instance, a recent study revealed that 97.4% of presbycusis patients displayed a sloping configuration on their pure-tone audiogram [12]. These findings are consistent with the notion that (mainly sensory) presbycusis results from damage to the hair cells in the cochlea responsible for detecting high-frequency sounds [7].

5. **A**

Hearing aids are the most common treatment for presbycusis, as they can amplify sounds and improve speech understanding in noisy environments. According to the American Speech-Language-Hearing Association (ASHA) [13], hearing aids can also slow down the progression of presbycusis and reduce cognitive decline associated with hearing loss [2]. However, cochlear implants are a potential treatment option for patients with severe presbycusis who do not benefit from hearing aids or other interventions [14]. Cochlear implants bypass the damaged hair cells in the inner ear and stimulate the auditory nerve directly, allowing patients to perceive sound [15]. However, cochlear implants are not appropriate for all patients, and the decision to undergo surgery should be made in consultation with a healthcare provider [16].

References

1. Gates GA, Mills JH. Presbycusis. Lancet. 2005;366(9491):1111–20.
2. Lin FR, Yaffe K, Xia J, et al. Hearing loss and cognitive decline in older adults. JAMA Intern Med. 2013;173(4):293–9.
3. Frisina RD, Ding B, Zhu X, et al. Age-related hearing loss: prevention of threshold declines, cell loss and

apoptosis in spiral ganglion neurons. Aging (Albany NY). 2016;8(2):208–20.
4. Park SN, Back SA, Park KH, et al. Comparison of metabolic and inflammatory parameters in presbycusis and noise-induced hearing loss. Acta Otolaryngol. 2016;136(6):570–4.
5. Lin FR. Hearing loss and cognition among older adults in the United States. J Gerontol A Biol Sci Med Sci. 2011;66(7):815–20.
6. Jiang H, Sha SH, Schacht J. NF-κB pathway protects cochlear hair cells from aminoglycoside-induced ototoxicity. J Neurosci Res. 2005;82(4):525–32.
7. Sataloff RT, Sataloff J. Presbycusis: a review of clinical and histopathologic features. Ear Nose Throat J. 2011;90(5):E22–7.
8. Schuknecht HF, Gacek MR. Cochlear pathology in presbycusis. Ann Otol Rhinol Laryngol. 1993;102(7 Pt 2 Suppl. 159):1–16.
9. Wong LLN, Yu JKC, Chan SSM, Tong MCF, van Hasselt CA. Speech perception in noise: an exploration of presbycusis in Hong Kong. Clin Otolaryngol. 2021;46(1):40–8.
10. Vlaming MS, Koning RJ, Festen JM, Kramer SE. Age-related differences in auditory processing as assessed by speech-in-noise perception. Front Neurosci. 2019;13:910.
11. Spankovich C, Hood LJ, Silver H, et al. Prevalence and characteristics of tinnitus in individuals with audiometrically-defined hearing loss. Ear Hear. 2017;38(2):e69–75.
12. Jiang Y, Li X, Zhu Y, et al. Audiometric configurations of presbycusis. J Otol. 2017;12(1):7–12.
13. American Speech-Language-Hearing Association. Hearing aids. Available at: https://www.asha.org/public/hearing/hearing-aid/. Accessed on March 28, 2023.
14. Francis HW, Chee N, Yeagle JD, et al. Cochlear implantation in the very elderly. Otol Neurotol. 2013;34(6):1040–4.
15. Gaylor JM, Raman G, Chung M, et al. Cochlear implantation in adults: a systematic review and meta-analysis. JAMA Otolaryngol Head Neck Surg. 2013;139(3):265–72.
16. Kuthubutheen J, Sanli H, Rajan GP. Cochlear implantation in the elderly: outcomes and special considerations. J Laryngol Otol. 2013;127(Suppl. 2):S16–22.

22 Tinnitus

Konstantinos Geronatsios

Abstract

Tinnitus is one of the commonest ENT symptoms. The diagnostic process and management of the tinnitus is a challenge. Elderly people are more likely to suffer from tinnitus. We should ask the patient if they have bilateral or unilateral tinnitus, how loud are these, if the tinnitus is pulsatile or non-pulsatile, history of exposure to loud noises or working in a noisy environment, the impact of tinnitus in the quality of life, medication history, and if they have noticed what makes tinnitus worse. History of tinnitus accompanied by vertigo may raise concerns for Meniere's disease, intracranial lesions, and autoimmune ear disease. Visual problems (transient visual blurring, vertical diplopia-cranial nerve VI paresis, brief episodes of blindness, or seeing light flashes), combined with headaches and usually pulsatile tinnitus, are indicative of benign intracranial hypertension (Pseudotumor cerebri). Pulsatile tinnitus may be also related to vascular abnormalities, head and neck tumors, hypertension, atherosclerosis, paragangliomas, hyperthyroidism, and anemia. Non-synchronous pulsatile tinnitus may be related to palatal myoclonus.

K. Geronatsios (✉)
ENT Head and Neck Surgery Department,
424 General Military Hospital, Thessaloniki, Greece

Case Presentation

A 48-year-old lady presented to the clinic complaining of bilateral pulsatile tinnitus. The tinnitus started 6 months ago, and she mentioned that they have a severe impact on her quality of life, because of increased anxiety and sleep disturbance. Regarding her past medical history, she suffers from hypothyroidism, well controlled with medical treatment, she smokes occasionally, and she is overweight (BMI; 32). She also complains of sporadic headaches. She denies any family history of tinnitus or hearing impairment. Her blood pressure is 135/87 mmHg. Her tympanic membranes are bilateral normal. Neurological examination and carotid auscultation are normal. Tympanogram was type A bilaterally while audiogram was as follows (Fig. 22.1).

Questions

1. Which of the following is important to ask while taking the medical history from a patient who suffers from tinnitus?
   A. Visual problems, especially of recent onset
   B. Type of tinnitus (pulsatile or non-pulsatile)
   C. History of exposure to loud noises
   D. Vertigo symptoms combined with the tinnitus
   E. All the above

N. Tsetsos et al. (eds.), *Otolaryngology Study Guide*, https://doi.org/10.1007/978-3-031-77374-7_22

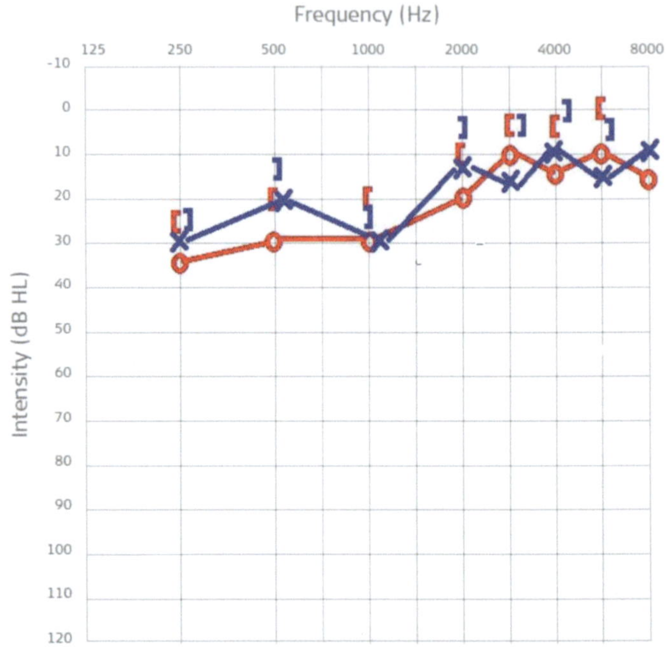

Fig. 22.1 Pure tone audiogram

2. Which of the following diagnostic imaging studies would be indicated for this patient? (more than one correct answer possible)
   A. Temporal bone CT scan with contrast
   B. MRI scan of the internal auditory meatus with contrast
   C. Head CT scan with contrast
   D. Head MRI scan with contrast
   E. Temporal bone CT scan without contrast
3. Which of the following is the commonest cause of tinnitus?
   A. Arteriovenous malformations
   B. Carotid stenosis
   C. Sensorineural hearing loss
   D. Hyperthyroidism
   E. Anemia
4. In cases in which tinnitus co-exists with autophony, which of the following would you suspect as a cause? (more than one correct answer possible)
   A. Patulous Eustachian tube
   B. Hyperthyroidism
   C. Noise-induced hearing loss
   D. Superior semicircular canal dehiscence syndrome
   E. Pseudotumor cerebri
5. In case that the investigations were negative for a specific clinical entity causing the symptoms, what would you recommend as treatment of tinnitus? (more than one correct answer possible)
   A. Inform the patient that tinnitus is a permanent problem, and she should learn to deal with this for her whole life
   B. Antidepressants
   C. Tinnitus masker
   D. Benzodiazepines
   E. Gingko Biloba tablets

Answers

1. **E**

All this information is critical for a detailed medical history of people who suffer from tinnitus. We should ask the patient if they have bilateral or unilateral tinnitus, how loud it is, whether the tinnitus is pulsatile or non-pulsatile, their history of exposure to loud noises or working in a noisy environment, the impact of tinnitus on their quality of life, their medication history, and if they have noticed what makes the tinnitus worse [1, 2]. A history of tinnitus accompanied by vertigo may raise concerns for Meniere's disease, intracranial lesions, and autoimmune ear disease. Visual problems (transient visual blurring, vertical diplopia-cranial nerve VI paresis, brief episodes of blindness, or seeing light flashes), combined with headaches and usually pulsatile tinnitus, are indicative of benign intracranial hypertension (Pseudotumor cerebri) [3]. Pulsatile tinnitus may also be related to vascular abnormalities, head and neck tumors, hypertension, atherosclerosis, paragangliomas, hyperthyroidism, and anemia [4, 5]. Non-synchronous pulsatile tinnitus may be related to palatal myoclonus.

2. **A, B, D**

   A temporal bone CT scan with contrast and an MRI of the internal auditory meatus may be the indicated diagnostic imaging studies in cases where we suspect a glomus tumor in the middle ear or another pathology of the middle and inner ear. MRA may also be helpful, if available, in order to exclude other vascular pathologies. An MRI scan of the head with contrast could provide more information in cases where we suspect benign intracranial hypertension. A temporal bone scan without contrast is not indicated. A CT scan of the head with contrast should be requested only in cases where we suspect intracranial pathology and an MRI is contraindicated (specific implants, severe claustrophobia) [6, 7].

3. **C**

   The most common cause of tinnitus is sensorineural hearing loss. This is why mostly elderly people, with age-related hearing loss, also complain about tinnitus. Additionally, people who have experienced sensorineural hearing loss suffer from unilateral tinnitus [1, 2, 8].

4. **A, D**

   Autophony is the perception that your own voice is echoing in your ears. Furthermore, it may be described as the ability to hear noises from distant parts of the body (arterial pulse, breathing). The coexistence of autophony is common in people who suffer from patulous Eustachian tube and superior semicircular canal dehiscence syndrome [9].

5. **B, C**

   Antidepressants, especially tricyclic antidepressants, have been used to treat the distress and anxiety symptoms associated with tinnitus. There are some studies that suggest tinnitus may worsen, especially with SSRIs [10]. Tinnitus maskers have been used successfully for several years, and some patients experience significant relief of their symptoms [11, 12]. We should never tell our patients that tinnitus is a permanent problem that will never improve, because this kind of advice can cause more distress and anxiety. Benzodiazepines have not been approved as a tinnitus treatment. There are not enough studies to prove the efficacy of Gingko Biloba for tinnitus [13].

References

1. Møller AR. Sensorineural tinnitus: its pathology and probable therapies. Int J Otolaryngol. 2016;2016:2830157. https://doi.org/10.1155/2016/2830157. Epub 2016 Feb 8
2. Biswas R, Lugo A, Akeroyd MA, Schlee W, Gallus S, Hall DA. Tinnitus prevalence in Europe: a multicountry cross-sectional population study. Lancet Reg Health Eur. 2021;
3. Mondragon J, Klovenski V. Pseudotumor cerebri. [Updated 2022 Sep 29]. In: StatPearls. Treasure Island (FL): StatPearls Publishing. p. 2022.
4. Hofmann E, Behr R, Neumann-Haefelin T, Schwager K. Pulsatile tinnitus: imaging and differential diagnosis. Dtsch Arztebl Int. 2013;110(26):451–8. https://doi.org/10.3238/arztebl.2013.0451.
5. Guo P, Sun W, Shi S, Wang W. Patients with pulse-synchronous tinnitus should be suspected to have elevated cerebrospinal fluid pressure. J Int Med Res. 2019;47(9):4104–13.
6. National Guideline Centre (UK). Evidence review for imaging to investigate the cause of pulsatile tinnitus: Tinnitus: assessment and management: Evidence review K. London: National Institute for Health and Care Excellence (NICE); 2020. (NICE Guideline, No. 155)
7. Cunnane MB. Imaging of Tinnitus. Neuroimaging Clin N Am. 2019;29(1):49–56. https://doi.org/10.1016/j.nic.2018.09.006.
8. Carolyn Crist. Nearly 15% of adults worldwide experience tinnitus symptoms— Medscape—Aug 17, 2022.
9. Palma Diaz M, Cisneros Lesser JC, Vega AA. Superior semicircular canal dehiscence syndrome—diagnosis and surgical management. Int Arch Otorhinolaryngol. 2017;21(2):195–8.

10. Baldo P, Doree C, Molin P, McFerran D, Cecco S. Antidepressants for patients with tinnitus. Cochrane Database Syst Rev. 2012;2012(9):CD003853.
11. Sandlin RE, Olsson RJ. Evaluation and selection of maskers and other devices used in the treatment of tinnitus and hyperacusis. Trends Amplif. 1999;4(1):6–26.
12. Attarha M, Bigelow J, Merzenich MM. Unintended consequences of white noise therapy for tinnitus—otolaryngology's Cobra effect: a review. JAMA Otolaryngol Head Neck Surg. 2018;144(10):938–43.
13. von Boetticher A. Ginkgo biloba extract in the treatment of tinnitus: a systematic review. Neuropsychiatr Dis Treat. 2011;7:441–7.

23 Otoacoustic Emissions

Manuela Cresswell and John Guy

Abstract

Otoacoustic emissions (OAE) tests are objective electrophysiologic tests that assess cochlear function in response to stimulus and are routinely used as a screening method for newborn hearing impairment. OAEs have high sensitivity but relatively low specificity.

A microphone in the ear canal records the sound produced by the outer hair cells in the cochlea, which can be spontaneous, or in response to a stimulus. The test is performed with a speaker and microphone probe in the ear canal.

The automated OAEs are used for screening purposes and remove the need for interpretation.

Transient-evoked OAEs measure the response to brief clicks at 80–86 decibels. Good responses are expected when hearing thresholds are above 20 dB. The responses are lost above 30 dB, independently of the aetiology of the hearing loss.

Distortion product OAEs are tested with two pure tones of different frequency presented simultaneously and for a longer period. The frequencies can be varied to estimate hearing thresholds across the frequencies.

One of the limitations of OAEs is that it can miss hearing impairment due to auditory neuropathy. In such patients, the OAEs can be present despite significant hearing impairment and absent or abnormal ABRs.

Case Presentation

A 2-day-old baby girl undergoes newborn hearing screening under the care of the health visitor at the child's home. She was born at 35 weeks of gestation via C-section due to maternal infection. The baby is currently being treated for mild neonatal jaundice but is otherwise well. She was fed shortly before the test was conducted.

Figure 23.1 shows the graph of failed OAEs.

Questions

1. If the OAEs show no response, what would be the next diagnostic step?
   A. Test ABR
   B. Repeat testing with OAEs in 2 months
   C. Perform a tympanogram to rule out middle ear effusion

M. Cresswell (✉)
Derriford Hospital, University Hospitals Plymouth NHS Trust, Plymouth, UK

J. Guy
University Hospitals Leicester NHS Trust, Leicester, UK

N. Tsetsos et al. (eds.), *Otolaryngology Study Guide*, https://doi.org/10.1007/978-3-031-77374-7_23

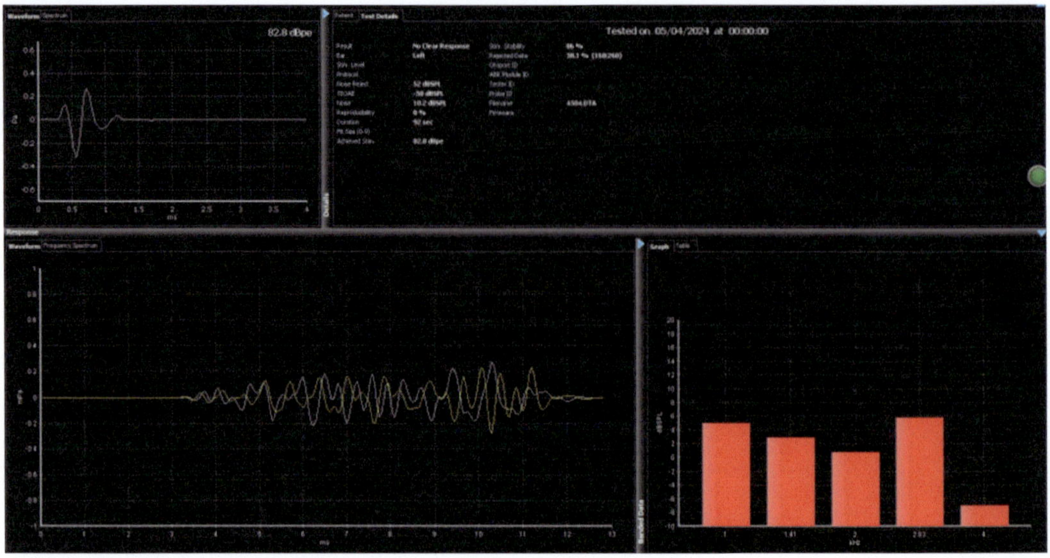

Fig. 23.1 GRAPH of failed OAEs

   D. Wait until the baby is old enough to perform pure-tone audiometry to ascertain true thresholds
   E. Advise parents to monitor the child's hearing as they mature
2. What tests would you expect the baby to routinely undergo as part of the newborn hearing screening programme? (Select one or more)
   A. Otoscopy
   B. Automated OAEs
   C. Automated ABR
   D. Play audiometry
   E. Visual reinforcement audiometry
3. If the baby had normal OAEs but absent ABRs, what would be the likely cause?
   A. Otitis media with effusion
   B. Auditory neuropathy
   C. Mild congenital sensorineural hearing loss
   D. Complete atresia of the ear canal
   E. Isolated congenital ossicular malformation
4. What proportion of newborn children are born with permanent hearing loss in one or both ears?
   A. 1 in 10
   B. 1 in 100
   C. 1 in 1000
   D. 1 in 10,000
   E. 1 in 100,000
5. Which of these conditions warrant audiological assessment (instead of the standard neonatal screening)?
   A. Microtia
   B. Bacterial meningitis
   C. Programmable shunt
   D. Confirmed congenital CMV
   E. Forceps delivery

Answers:

1. **A**

   If a baby fails OAEs, they should undergo full audiological assessment and have threshold assessment with ABRs. Delaying tests until the patient is older would delay appropriate and timely hearing rehabilitation with hearing aids or cochlear implantation. Although middle ear effusions are common in children, a tympanogram is not indicated until the patient has undergone ABR or if there is clinical appearance of middle ear effusion on examination.

2. **B and C**

   Although newborn hearing screening protocols vary across the world, automated OAEs and ABRs are the standard methods for screening [1].

Otoscopy would not assess hearing.

Visual reinforcement audiometry is indicated in babies between 6 months and 3 years old. The patient needs to be able to sit up unaided and turn the head to perform this test. It is a behavioural test where the child is seated, and there are loud speakers at 45 or 90° from the child. Sound stimuli are presented, and the child naturally turns to find the sound source and is rewarded with an animated toy.

3. **B**

   Patients with auditory neuropathy have normal OAE responses with absent or abnormal ABR [2]. Auditory neuropathy is associated with prematurity, cerebral palsy, severe neonatal jaundice, and mutations to the OTOF gene that interfere with inner hair cell synaptic transmission [1].

   Patients with mild hearing loss (conductive and sensorineural) would have ABR responses.

   Complete ear canal atresia is a contraindication for OAEs because the speaker/microphone probe needs to be inserted into the ear canal.

   Isolated congenital hearing loss is a rare disease unlikely to be the primary cause in this case.

4. **C**

   One to two babies in every 1000 are born with permanent hearing loss in 1 or both ears, increasing to 1 in 100 babies who have been in intensive care for over 48 h, and as such these patients are assessed [3]. Most of these babies are born into families with no history of permanent hearing loss.

5. **E**

   All of these except forceps delivery are contraindications to screening and should prompt immediate referral to an audiologist within 4 weeks of screen completion or by 44 weeks of gestational age [4].

References

1. Graham JM, Scadding JK, Bull PD. Pediatric ENT. 1st ed. Springer; 2007.
2. Flint P, Haughey B, Lund V, Robbins K, Thomas JR, Lesperance M, et al. Cummings otolaryngology: head and neck surgery, 7th ed. Elsevier; 2020.
3. NHS choices [Internet]. NHS; 2021 [cited 2024 Apr 2]. https://www.nhs.uk/conditions/baby/newborn-screening/hearing-test/.
4. England PH. Newborn hearing screening Programme (NHSP): care pathways for well babies [Internet]. Gov.uk; 2020 [cited 2024 Apr 2]. https://www.gov.uk/government/publications/newborn-hearing-screening-care-pathways/newborn-hearing-screening-programme-nhsp-care-pathways-for-well-babies.

Auditory Brainstem Responses (ABR)

24

Manuela Cresswell and John Guy

Abstract

ABR is an objective test of hearing that records the activity of both the vestibulocochlear cranial nerve and central nervous system in response to an auditory stimulus. It is often part of the evaluation in patients who are difficult to test (i.e. newborns, infants, and adults with suspected non-organic hearing loss) or as part of intraoperative monitoring of the cochlear nerve (i.e. hearing preservation surgery for vestibular schwannoma).

There is an automated ABR test which removes the need for interpretation by the tester. It is used mainly for screening purposes. Many healthcare systems around the world have set up a newborn hearing screening programme that includes ABR, first used for this purpose in 1979.

ABR can provide ear-specific and frequency-specific thresholds. The stimulus is called a click, and it consists of very short pulses presented at different frequencies. Electroencephalogram (EEG) activity is measured to see the corresponding waves generated after each click. The waveforms are known to change with the maturation of the auditory system; newborns tend to have more prominent waves I, III and V, while in adults the most prominent wave is V.

Case Presentation

A 4-month-old baby has failed the newborn hearing screening. The baby is assessed by the paediatric audiologists and paediatric ENT surgeon. The parents report that the baby was born at full term through normal vaginal delivery. The baby did not have any neonatal distress and did not require admission to the neonatal unit. They deny family history of hearing loss. The parents have noticed that the baby responds appropriately to loud sounds. The baby smiles and has a normal appearance with normal tympanic membranes on examination (Fig. 24.1).

Questions

1. Which of these tests would be appropriate for a 4-month-old baby who has failed the newborn hearing screening? (select one or more)
   A. Play audiometry
   B. Automated otoacoustic emissions

M. Cresswell (✉)
Derriford Hospital, University Hospitals Plymouth NHS Trust, Plymouth, UK

J. Guy
University Hospitals Leicester NHS Trust, Leicester, UK

N. Tsetsos et al. (eds.), *Otolaryngology Study Guide*, https://doi.org/10.1007/978-3-031-77374-7_24

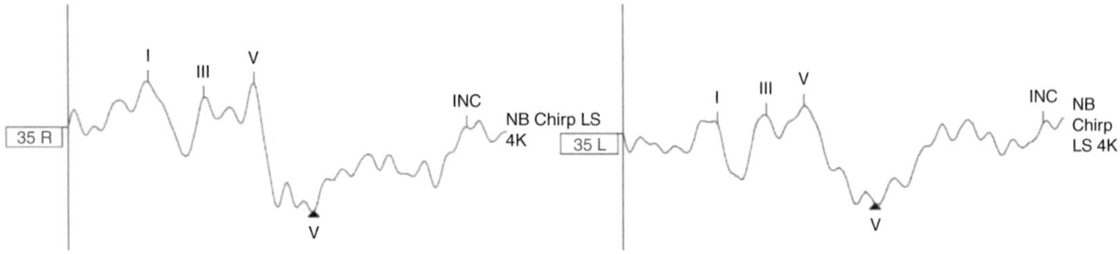

Fig. 24.1 Normal ABR on a newborn. Right ear in red. Left ear in blue

   C. Auditory brainstem responses
   D. Visual response audiometry
   E. Tympanometry
2. Which of the following are indications for ABR? (select one or more)
   A. Obtaining frequency-specific thresholds in infants
   B. Evaluating patients with suspected non-organic hearing loss
   C. First-line evaluation for adults with noise-induced hearing loss
   D. Newborn hearing screening
   E. Perioperative monitoring of cochlear nerve function in patients undergoing hearing preservation surgery for vestibular schwannoma
3. What are the known limitations to ABR testing? (select one or more)
   A. Noisy environment and electrical devices cause artefact and make the interpretation of ABR more difficult
   B. There is no correlation with audiometric testing
   C. Patients with vestibular schwannoma should not undergo ABR testing
   D. ABR cannot be performed if the patient is under general anaesthesia
   E. It requires a compliant patient, ideally asleep
4. What investigations are useful for investigating non-organic hearing loss?
   A. ABR
   B. CERA
   C. Stenger's test
   D. Serial audiograms
   E. Play audiogram
5. Through which of the following nuclei does electrical information NOT pass from the cochlear nerve to the auditory cortex?
   A. Cochlear nuclei
   B. Superior olivary complex
   C. Medial geniculate
   D. Inferior colliculi
   E. Broca's area

Answers

1. C

Newborn hearing screening using ABR, first described in 1979, has now become the standard in many countries [1, 2].

If a child fails the newborn hearing screening (generally includes automated OAE and automated ABR), they are referred for formal audiological assessment. ABR is useful to determine likely hearing thresholds and can be ear-specific [3].

Play audiometry is indicated in children between 2 and 5 years old. The child needs to be able to follow a 2-step command and have appropriate gross and fine motor skills. This test uses toys, and the child would be given a task to do (i.e. place toys in a bucket) every time they hear a sound stimulus.

Automated OAEs would already have been performed as part of the newborn hearing screening.

Visual reinforcement audiometry is indicated in babies between 7 months and 2.5 years old. The patient needs to be able to sit up unaided and turn the head to perform this test. It is a behavioural test where the child is seated, and there are loudspeakers at

45 or 90° from the child. Sound stimuli are presented, and the child naturally turns to find the sound source and is rewarded with an animated toy.

Tympanometry is an objective indirect measure of the middle ear pressure. It would not be indicated unless there is clinical suspicion of middle ear effusion.

2. A, B, D and E

   ABR is an essential part of the newborn hearing screening, and it is useful in evaluating infants, often providing ear-specific thresholds. Patients with suspected non-organic hearing loss can be assessed with ABR because the test results are not affected by the patient, although it does require the patient to be compliant with the test [4].

   The first-line test for noise-induced hearing loss is a pure tone audiogram.

   In hearing preservation surgery, the hearing thresholds are monitored using ABR.

3. A and E

   Interpretation is hampered by environmental noise and electrical devices but often this can be overcome by experienced ABR testers.

   The ideal testing conditions for ABR include an asleep or sedated patient with minimal or no movement.

   ABR results do correlate with audiometric testing within 10–15 dB [5].

   ABR was historically used as a diagnostic tool for vestibular schwannoma, but this has been largely replaced by cross-sectional imaging. ABR is used in patients with vestibular schwannoma who are undergoing hearing preservation surgery, which is performed under general anaesthesia.

4. A, B, C, D

   All answers except E are useful in non-organic hearing loss. ABR is automated and objective, as is Cortical Evoked Response Assessment. Stenger's test involves binaural testing of sounds of differing amplitude, exploiting the fact that when a sound is presented to both ears, the brain detects the sound only on the side with the higher amplitude [6]. Serial audiograms can also be used to assess for unexplained variance in results.

   Tympanometry is only useful in the sense that if abnormal it would imply an organic cause.

5. E

   The cochlear nucleus is the first nucleus on the auditory pathway. Found in the posterolateral portion of the brainstem, it relays low-frequency information through the ventral portion and high-frequency through its dorsal region.

   After the cochlear nucleus, fibres decussate into the superior olivary complex, then follow the ipsilateral inferior colliculus to the lateral lemniscus tract. The medial geniculate nucleus then transmits information to the auditory cortex [7].

   Broca's area is located in the dominant temporal lobe of the brain and is concerned with generating fluent speech. It is not involved in auditory processing.

References

1. Jacobson JT, Jacobson CA, Spahr RC. Automated and conventional ABR screening techniques in high-risk infants. J Am Acad Audiol. 1990;1(4):187–95. PMID: 2132603.
2. Schulman-Galambos C, Galambos R. Brain stem evoked response audiometry in newborn hearing screening. Arch Otolaryngol. 1979;105(2):86–90. https://doi.org/10.1001/archotol.1979.00790140032006.
3. Flint P, Haughey B, Lund V, Robbins K, Thomas JR, Lesperance M, et al. Cummings otolaryngology: head and neck surgery. 7th ed. Elsevier; 2020.
4. Joint Committee on Infant Hearing, American Academy of Pediatrics. Year 2007 position statement: principles and guidelines for early hearing detection and intervention programs. Pediatrics. 2007;120(4):898–921. https://doi.org/10.1542/peds.2007-2333.
5. Stapells DR, Oates P. Estimation of the pure-tone audiogram by the auditory brainstem response: a review. Audiol Neurootol. 1997;2(5):257–80. https://doi.org/10.1159/000259252.
6. Morita S, Suzuki M, Iizuka K. Non-organic hearing loss in childhood. Int J Pediatr Otorhinolaryngol. 2010;74(5):441–6.
7. Felix RA, Gourévitch B, Portfors CV. Subcortical pathways: towards a better understanding of auditory disorders. Hear Res. 2018;362:48–60.

25 Middle Ear Implants

Marios Stavrakas

Abstract

Active middle ear implants are devices aiming to transfer mechanical energy to the ossicular chain or directly to the inner ear fluids through the round or oval windows. They are an alternative to hearing aids, traditional reconstructive middle ear surgery, and bone conduction devices and are intended for people who cannot use these conventional solutions or who gain insufficient benefit from them. They are totally or partially implantable, and they comprise internal and external parts (microphone, audio processor, receiver unit, and transducer). The transducer can use piezoelectric, electromagnetic, or electromechanical energy. The main advantage of middle ear implants over conventional hearing aids is that they produce greater functional gain, with less distortion and feedback.

Case Presentation

A 42-year-old male patient who underwent combined approach tympanoplasty is struggling with his hearing and is unable to use his BTE hearing aid regularly due to recurrent infections. He's otherwise fir and well, and his audiogram is given below. He is keen to explore the possibility of having an active middle ear implant, and he has already excluded the option of a BAHA.

Questions

1. Which of the following are coupling options for the Vibrant Soundbridge (MED-EL)?
   A. Incus—long process
   B. Malleus handle
   C. Malleus neck
   D. Round window membrane
   E. A and D
2. Which of the following are indications for middle ear implants?
   A. B/L SNHL in whom ACHA have been used and found to be medically unsuitable due to conditions of the external ear
   B. Mixed hearing loss in whom ACHA have been used and found to be medically unsuitable due to conditions of the external ear [including microtia and other congenital conditions]
   C. And in whom a BAHA has been implanted and been associated with medical problems of the soft tissues or loss of fixture on more than one occasion
   D. A–C
   E. 80 dB HL at 2 or more frequencies (500 Hz, 1000 Hz, 2000 Hz, 3000 Hz, and 4000 Hz) bilaterally without acoustic hearing aids

M. Stavrakas (✉)
ENT Head and Neck Surgery Department,
University Hospitals Plymouth NHS Trust,
Plymouth, UK

N. Tsetsos et al. (eds.), *Otolaryngology Study Guide*, https://doi.org/10.1007/978-3-031-77374-7_25

3. What are the indications for vibroplasty in the round window?
   A. Failed stapedotomy
   B. Patient preference
   C. Open cavity following cholesteatoma surgery
   D. Ossicular chain discontinuity
   E. None of the above
4. Which of the following statements are true?
   A. The intrinsic dynamic range can be estimated as the difference between the maximum stable power or force output ('feedback free gain') and the noise floor
   B. The effective dynamic range can then be estimated by considering the sensorineural hearing loss (BC thresholds), a potential transmission loss (coupling deficit), and a worsening of bone conduction threshold due to an estimated natural or disease-related progression or the surgery itself as a safety margin
   C. The resulting effective dynamic range that determines the audiological result is—in the best case—just as large as the intrinsic dynamic range of the device, but rather almost always smaller
   D. All the above
   E. None of the above
5. Which of the following are not parts of the Vibrant Soundbridge?
   A. Abutment
   B. Microphone
   C. Magnet
   D. Receiving coil
   E. Floating mass transducer

Correct Answers

1. E

   The standard options for vibroplasty include coupling on the long or short process of incus, stapes suprastructure and round window membrane [1]. Other coupling solutions are directly to the stapes footplate, to the incus via a stapes prosthesis or through a stapedotomy [1]. The surgeon performing the vibroplasty has to take into consideration the intact structures and their mobility, the type of hearing loss, and possible underlying pathology (e.g. otosclerosis) and the audiological outcome we are aiming for.
2. D

   According to NICE commissioning policy (2013), the first three statements are correct. Statement E is relevant to cochlear implantation.
3. C

   One of the most frequent indications for vibroplasty in the round window is for patients with tympanoplasty cavities that are open due to cholesteatoma. In fact, the surgery can be combined with a subtotal petrosectomy and closure of the ear canal, to achieve better stability of the implant. This type of vibroplasty has also been reported for patients with conductive hearing loss as an alternative to hearing aids, or for patients with atresia of the external ear canal as an alternative to bone conduction implants [2].
4. D

   All the statements are correct [1].
5. A

   The Vibrant Soundbridge (MED-EL) is composed of both an internal implant and a wearable external component. The implanted portion of the device, also known as a vibrating ossicular replacement prosthesis (VORP), is composed of a receiving coil, a magnet, a demodulator, a conductor link, and a floating mass transducer (FMT). The external component, or audio processor, includes a microphone, an audio processor, a battery, a transmitter coil, and a retention magnet [3].

References

1. Rahne T, Plontke SK. Systematic and audiological indication criteria for bone conduction devices and active middle ear implants. Hear Res. 2022;421:108424.
2. Lassaletta L, Sánchez-Cuadrado I, Espinosa JM, Batuecas Á, Cenjor C, Lavilla MJ, Cavallé L, Huarte A, Nuñez F, Manrique M, Ramos Á. Active middle ear implants. Acta Otorrinolaringol Esp (Engl Ed). 2019;70(2):112–8.
3. Banakis Hartl RM, Jenkins HA. Implantable hearing aids: where are we in 2020? Laryngoscope Investig Otolaryngol. 2020;5(6):1184–91.

Bone-Anchored Hearing Aid (BAHA)

26

Konstantinos Garefis and Zoi Zachou

Abstract

A bone-anchored hearing aid (BAHA) is a hearing aid system comprising three main components: (1) a titanium screw implanted behind the ear, (2) an abutment fixed onto the screw and visible on the skin surface, and (3) an external sound processor. Its mechanism involves converting sound into vibrations that directly travel through the bone to stimulate the cochlea, bypassing the middle ear. Unlike traditional hearing aids, the BAHA is affixed to an abutment behind the ear and does not have any parts inside the external ear canal. BAHA was developed in the 1980s and is used by both adults and children. It is approved for treating conductive, mixed, and unilateral sensorineural hearing loss. The implantation procedure is straightforward and safe, characterized by a low incidence of osseointegration failure and minimal complications in soft tissue, with adverse skin reactions at the site of skin penetration being the most frequent. Patients fitted with BAHA typically experience enhanced hearing and improved quality of life.

Case Presentation

A 12-year-old girl attended the multidisciplinary Pediatric clinic. She was diagnosed with conductive hearing loss and outer/middle ear dysplasia in the context of Treacher Collins syndrome. She has been successfully using a bone conduction aid on a soft band for several years (Fig. 26.1). The patient and her parents are interested in a long-term solution and would like to discuss the available options.

Questions

1. Which of the following statements are true about BAHA? (more than one correct answer possible)
   A. A part of BAHA fits in the inner ear
   B. The minimum age of implantation is 2 years old
   C. Mandibulofacial dysostosis is commonly associated with BAHA implantation
   D. Children with Goldenhar syndrome are usually candidates

K. Garefis (✉)
2nd Academic ORL, Head and Neck Surgery Department, Aristotle University of Thessaloniki, Papageorgiou Hospital, Thessaloniki, Greece

Z. Zachou
1st ORL, Head and Neck Surgery Department, National & Kapodistrian University of Athens, Hippocration Hospital, Athens, Greece

N. Tsetsos et al. (eds.), *Otolaryngology Study Guide*, https://doi.org/10.1007/978-3-031-77374-7_26

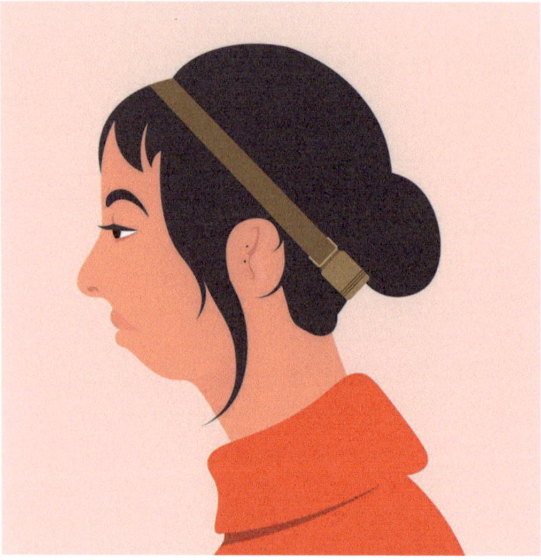

Fig. 26.1 Illustration of a patient with Treacher Collins syndrome, showing visible outer ear dysplasia and a BAHA on a soft band

   E. It provides better speech recognition compared to traditional hearing aids when the air-bone gap is greater than 35 dB
2. Which of the following is NOT an indication for placement of a BAHA?
   A. Congenital ossicular malformation
   B. Complete absence of the external ear (Grade III microtia)
   C. Chronically discharging ear
   D. Bilateral sensorineural hearing loss
   E. Learning difficulties and conductive hearing loss
3. Which of the following are complications of BAHA implantation: (more than one correct answer possible)
   A. CSF leak
   B. Peri-abutment skin problems
   C. Sigmoid sinus injury
   D. Loss of the osseointegrated fixture
   E. All of the above
4. Which of the following statements are NOT true about the percutaneous compared to transcutaneous BAHA? (more than one correct answer possible)
   A. They are prone to more infections
   B. They generate less gain
   C. Skin growth could be developed
   D. The quality of life is better in patients with transcutaneous devices
   E. All of the above are true
5. Which statements about osseointegration time in BAHA are true? (more than one correct answer possible)
   A. The usual osseointegration time is 9 months
   B. Inadequate bone thickness leads to a longer osseointegration period
   C. Failure of osseointegration could lead to loss of the fixture, more commonly in adults
   D. None of the above
   E. All of the above

Correct Answers

1. **C, D, E**

   In a BAHA system, a small titanium implant is surgically placed into the skull bone behind the ear, near the temporal line. This implant acts as a connection point for a sound processor, which sits on the outside of the head [1]. Thus, none of the BAHAs part fit in the outer, middle, or inner ear. It offers superior speech recognition compared to traditional hearing aids when the air-bone gap exceeds 35 dB. According to the medical product guidelines of the US FDA, the minimum age for a BAHA is 5 years old. This age recommendation generally corresponds to adequate bone thickness. A 4 mm length fixture is typically preferred, but a shorter 3 mm length fixture can be used when the calvarial bone thickness is reduced. In the UK, BAHA surgery is often performed before the age of 5, although it is acknowledged that complications may be more common in these cases [2]. Most children fitted with BAHA devices have conductive hearing loss due to craniofacial abnormalities, with the most common abnormality being mandibulofacial dysostosis (Treacher Collins syndrome). Other syndromes associated with BAHA use include hemifacial microsomia (Goldenhar syndrome), oculo-auriculo-vertebral dysplasia, Mobius syndrome, CATCH 22 syndrome,

Pfeiffer syndrome, Crouzon syndrome, and diabetic embryopathy [3]. Children with Down syndrome are considered good candidates for BAHA when conventional hearing aids have proven ineffective [4].

2. **D**

The current criteria for BAHA include various otological indications such as congenital malformations of the external and middle ear, like EAC atresia, chronic ear discharges such as chronic otitis externa or otitis media, and conductive hearing losses caused by ossicular disease. It is also considered when conventional air-conduction aids are not suitable for the patient. Another indication is unilateral profound sensorineural hearing loss, where the bone vibration from BAHA is transmitted to the cochlea of the opposite ear, allowing the perception of sound from the side of the head with the deaf ear [2, 5]. Additionally, BAHA serves as a third treatment option for otosclerosis in patients who cannot or opt out of stapedectomy and face problems with traditional hearing aids, as well as for patients with Paget's disease [5]. In general, for conductive or mixed hearing loss, the patient should demonstrate sufficient sensorineural reserve, with a bone conduction threshold of at least 45 dB HL and an unaided speech discrimination score (word recognition score) of 60% or higher [6]. Moreover, bilateral implantation seems superior to unilateral in selected cases, as subjective improvement has been seen in hearing thresholds, understanding speech in quiet, localization, and restoration of binaural hearing [7].

3. **E**

Dural exposure is a common intraoperative complication, particularly in children, potentially leading to cerebrospinal fluid (CSF) leakage. Another complication involves injury and bleeding of the sigmoid sinus. Loss of the osseointegrated fixture from the skull is a significant problem. Numerous cases of fixture loss have been documented, often due to direct trauma, especially in pediatric patients and individuals with poor hygiene. Percutaneous implants may be lost due to various factors, most commonly osseointegration failure, trauma, infection, bone disease, or radiation. This loss may occur in up to 10% of cases during long-term follow-up [5]. However, the most common complications involve the soft tissues around the abutment, such as erythema and tenderness of the skin, granulation tissue, cellulitis, abscess, skin overgrowth of the abutment, hypertrophic scars, and keloids. Some of these complications can be managed with topical steroids or, in severe cases, may require revision surgery [8].

4. **B, D**

The most commonly used bone conduction systems consist of an osseointegrated titanium fixture and an external unit that can be connected to this abutment. This procedure has been in use for over 30 years, and multiple studies have demonstrated the audiological benefit and improvement in quality of life with such percutaneous BAHA [9]. Although the overall complication rate for BAHAs is low and the required surgery is simple, the percutaneous approach may produce minor or major complications at the interface between the titanium screw and the surrounding skin [10]. The skin reactions to the BAHA site have been described according to Holger's classification:

Grade Description

0. Reaction-free skin around the abutment

1. Redness with slight swelling around the abutment

2. Redness, moistness, and moderate swelling

3. Redness, moistness, and moderate swelling with tissue granulation around the abutment

4. Overt signs of infection resulting in removal of the implant [11, 12]

To overcome these problems, transcutaneous bone conduction hearing aids have been developed. Passive magnetic implants stimulate an implanted magnet transcutaneously by an externally worn stimulator. These systems avoid the medical problems associated with the percutaneous screw but require significant contact forces and generate less gain than percutaneous devices. Published results of hearing performance and quality of life show similar functional results in appropriately selected subjects implanted with both types [13].

5. **B**

The ideal time between fixture implantation and placing the abutment (osseointegration time) continues to be a topic of debate. A 3-month period between surgeries has been common practice in the majority of pediatric BAHA centers. If difficulties are encountered at the first procedure, such as inadequate bone thickness, a longer osseointegration period is recommended [14]. Fixture loss due to osseointegration failure is significantly higher in younger children [15]. There is a general consensus that fixture failure is most common in the first postoperative year [16].

References

1. Powell R, Wearden A, Pardesi SM, Green K. Understanding the low uptake of bone-anchored hearing aids: a review. J Laryngol Otol. 2017;131(3):190–201.
2. Doshi J, McDermott AL. Bone anchored hearing aids in children. Expert Rev Med Devices. 2015;12(1):73–82.
3. Granström G. Osseointegrated implants in children. Acta Otolaryngol Suppl. 2000;543:118–21.
4. Sheehan PZ, Hans PS. UK and Ireland experience of bone anchored hearing aids (BAHA) in individuals with Down syndrome. Int J Pediatr Otorhinolaryngol. 2006;70(6):981–6.
5. Hagr A. BAHA: bone-anchored hearing aid. Int J Health Sci (Qassim). 2007;1(2):265–76.
6. Habal M, Frans N, Zelski R, Scheuerle J. Percutaneous bone-anchored hearing aid. J Craniofac Surg. 2003;14(5):637–42.
7. Heath E, Dawoud MM, Stavrakas M, Ray J. The outcomes of bilateral bone conduction hearing devices (BCHD) implantation in the treatment of hearing loss: a systematic review. Cochlear Implants Int. 2022;23(2):95–108.
8. Ghossaini SN, Roehm PC. Osseointegrated auditory devices: bone-anchored hearing aid and PONTO. Otolaryngol Clin North Am. 2019;52(2):243–51.
9. Gerdes T, Salcher RB, Schwab B, Lenarz T, Maier H. Comparison of audiological results between a transcutaneous and a percutaneous bone conduction instrument in conductive hearing loss. Otol Neurotol. 2016;37(6):685–91.
10. Verheij E, Bezdjian A, Grolman W, Thomeer HG. A systematic review on complications of tissue preservation surgical techniques in percutaneous bone conduction hearing devices. Otol Neurotol. 2016;37(7):829–37.
11. Holgers KM, Bjursten LM, Thomsen P, Ericson LE, Tjellström A. Experience with percutaneous titanium implants in the head and neck: a clinical and histological study. J Invest Surg. 1989;2(1):7–16.
12. Steehler MW, Larner SP, Mintz JS, Steehler MK, Lipman SP, Griffith S. A comparison of the operative techniques and the postoperative complications for bone-anchored hearing aid implantation. Int Arch Otorhinolaryngol. 2018;22(4):368–73.
13. Robinette K, Sims J, Pang B, Babu S. Transcutaneous versus percutaneous bone-anchored hearing aids: a quality of life comparison. Am J Otolaryngol. 2023;44(2):103758.
14. Tietze L, Papsin B. Utilization of bone-anchored hearing aids in children. Int J Pediatr Otorhinolaryngol. 2001;58(1):75–80.
15. de Wolf MJ, Hol MK, Huygen PL, Mylanus EA, Cremers CW. Nijmegen results with application of a bone-anchored hearing aid in children: simplified surgical technique. Ann Otol Rhinol Laryngol. 2008;117(11):805–14.
16. McDermott AL, Sheehan P. Paediatric Baha. Adv Otorhinolaryngol. 2011;71:56–62.

Cochlear Implants

27

Manuela Cresswell and John Guy

Abstract

Cochlear implants (CIs) are surgically implanted devices used to rehabilitate hearing in patients with severe to profound hearing loss. They have the potential to restore to near-normal hearing thresholds. Children born with profound hearing loss have much better outcomes in terms of speech and language development if they undergo cochlear implantation within the first year of life.

CIs devices are composed of three parts: a microphone and sound processor that are externally worn, which detect and process sound into electronic format; a transmitter coil, which sends information transcutaneously to the internal receiver; and an internal electrode array, which transmits electrical pulses to stimulate the cochlear nerve.

The candidacy for cochlear implantation varies internationally, and it has expanded in recent years. Children undergo a multidisciplinary assessment their speech, language, and listening skills according to their age, cognitive ability, and developmental stage.

Cochlear implantation surgery is carried out under general anaesthetic and in some cases, such as congenitally deaf children, simultaneous bilateral implants can be inserted. The surgical steps include a cortical mastoidectomy, posterior tympanotomy, identification of the round window and insertion of the electrode array. Audiological rehabilitation with regular audiology input starts weeks after surgery.

Case Presentation

A 2-year-old boy who is a refugee and missed his newborn hearing screening attends the paediatric otolaryngology clinic. The parents have noticed that he has a hearing impairment and although he makes some babbling noises, he has not developed speech. He communicates by signing with his hands. His other milestones are expected for his age. He was born at full term but developed severe jaundice at birth. There is no family history of hearing loss. On examination, there no syndromic features and his tympanic membranes are normal. He has absent otoacoustic emissions.

M. Cresswell (✉)
Derriford Hospital, University Hospitals Plymouth NHS Trust, Plymouth, UK

J. Guy
University Hospitals of Leicester NHS Trust, Leicester, UK

N. Tsetsos et al. (eds.), *Otolaryngology Study Guide*, https://doi.org/10.1007/978-3-031-77374-7_27

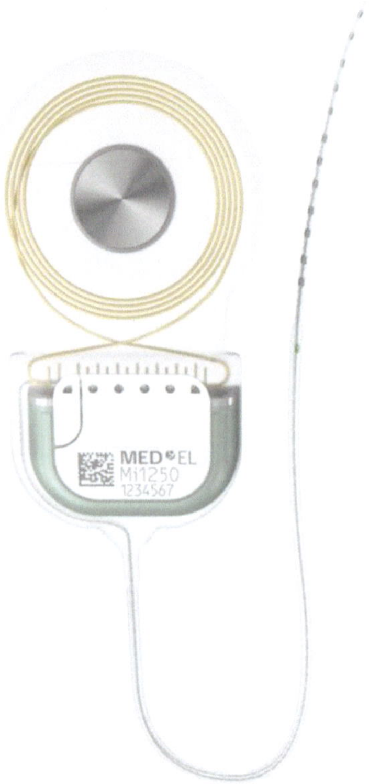

Fig. 27.1 Image provided by MED EL UK

The family have researched online and show you the picture of a cochlear implant device (Fig. 27.1).

Questions

1. What initial investigations would you order for this child? (more than one correct answer possible)
   A. Auditory brainstem responses
   B. Speech and language assessment
   C. Tympanogram
   D. Visual reinforcement audiometry
   E. CT and MRI scan of the temporal bones
2. The child undergoes full audiometric assessment and it is established that he has bilateral severe hearing loss (70 dB in the best hearing ear). He did not benefit from wearing conventional hearing aids. What tests would you request when assessing him for cochlear implantation?
   A. Pure tone audiogram
   B. Computerised tomography of the temporal bones
   C. Magnetic resonance imaging of the temporal bones
   D. Speech audiometry
   E. Formal speech and language assessment
3. What are the indications for cochlear implantation?
   A. Down's syndrome with moderate hearing loss
   B. Unilateral severe to profound hearing loss with inadequate benefit from hearing aid
   C. Bilateral severe to profound hearing loss with inadequate benefit from hearing aids
   D. Bilateral hearing loss secondary to congenital absence of cochlear nerves
   E. Moderate conductive hearing loss due to congenital stapes fixation
4. Which of the following is an indication for urgent cochlear implant insertion?
   A. Labyrinthitis ossificans
   B. Speech delay
   C. Otitis media with effusion
   D. Temporal bone fracture
   E. Sudden sensorineural hearing loss
5. Which three of the following are contraindications to CI insertion?
   A. Otitis media with effusion
   B. Ossicular discontinuity
   C. Tympanic membrane perforation
   D. Absent cochlear nerve
   E. Mastoiditis

Correct Answers

1. **A and D**

   In the first instance, it is important to ascertain the degree of hearing loss and ideally obtain ear-specific thresholds. This can be done with auditory brainstem responses and visual reinforcement audiometry which would be appropriate for the patient's age and development.

   The patient will require assessment by speech and language therapy after hearing thresholds have been established.

   Tympanogram is not indicated because there is no clinical suspicion of middle ear effusion or tympanic membrane perforation.

   CT and MRI scan are often performed as part of the work up for cochlear implantation but would only be indicated once it has been established that the patient has severe to profound hearing loss.

2. **B, C and E**

   Prior to cochlear implantation patients should undergo cross-sectional imaging to establish presence of cochlear nerves and identify any anatomical abnormalities prior to surgery [1].

   Speech discrimination tests are often used in the assessment of hearing loss for CI candidates. Sentence tests or word tests are speech discrimination tests. In the UK, the AB (Arthur-Boothroyd) word test is used for CI assessment. Words are played, and the patient is asked to repeat the words as accurately as possible. A percentage score is given for the correct responses. The NICE guidelines consider that a patient does not adequately benefit from hearing aids if they score less than 50% presented at 70 dB on the AB word test [2].

   However, in this case, speech discrimination in a patient that has not developed speech cannot be tested as the patient will not be able to repeat the words back. A patient that has not yet developed speech would need assessment by the speech and language therapy team. At this age, a pure tone audiogram would not be indicated.

3. **B and C**

   CIs are indicated for bilateral and unilateral (not in all countries) severe to profound hearing loss in patients who get inadequate benefit from conventional hearing loss.

   Absence of cochlear nerve is an absolute contraindication for cochlear implantation. Conductive hearing loss and moderate hearing loss in patient with Down's syndrome do not fulfil the criteria for CI.

   Criteria for CI vary between different countries. CIs have a significant cost to healthcare systems, thus cost-benefit analysis discussions help decide specific criteria. In the last few years, many healthcare systems have widened their CI criteria to include bilateral implantation and patients with single-sided deafness. In many countries such as Germany and Austria, the threshold criteria are 70 dB or worse [3].

   The NICE guidelines set out the eligibility criteria for CI in the United Kingdom [4]. The criteria are as follows:

   Unilateral CI is indicated for patients with bilateral severe to profound deafness (80 dB or worse at 2 or more frequencies 0.5, 1, 2, 3, and 4 kHz) who do not receive adequate benefit from hearing aids.

   Simultaneous bilateral CIs are indicated for children or adults with additional disability (i.e. blindness) with severe to profound deafness who do not receive adequate benefit from hearing aids.

4. **A**

   Labyrinthitis ossificans is the calcification of the inner ear following trauma or infection. As the membranous labyrinth ossifies, implantation of cochlear implants becomes more technically challenging, necessitating the need for prompt intervention, usually within a few months [5].

   Speech delay may indicate CI insertion but not on an urgent basis. Temporal bone fracture and SSNHL are not indications for CI insertion.

5. **D and E**

   These are contraindications to cochlear implant insertion. Absent cochlear nerve defeats the point of inserting a cochlear nerve stimulator. Active ear infection may cause colonisation of the implant and thus necessitate removal. In ossicular discontinuity, CI can only be considered once all other treatment options have been exhausted [6]. Otitis media with effusion is not a complete contraindication but can make it difficult to establish true hearing thresholds. In some centres, ventilation tubes are placed prior to CI assessment.

References

1. Graham JM, Scadding JK, Bull PD. Pediatric ENT, 1st ed. Springer; 2007.
2. Flint P, Haughey B, Lund V, Robbins K, Thomas JR, Lesperance M, et al. Cummings otolaryngology: head and neck surgery, 7th ed. Elsevier; 2020.
3. Van de Heyning P, Gavilán J, Godey B, et al. Worldwide variation in cochlear implant candidacy. J Int Adv Otol. 2022;18(3):196–202.

4. NICE. Cochlear Implants for children and adults with severe to profound deafness. 2017. https://www.nice.org.uk/guidance/ta566/chapter/1-Recommendations. Accessed 7 Mar 2023.
5. Taxak P, Ram C. Labyrinthitis and Labyrinthitis ossificans—A case report and review of the literature. J Radiol Case Rep. 2020;14(5):1.
6. Krogmann RJ, Al Khalili Y. Cochlear implants; 2019.

28 Bell's Palsy

Konstantinos Garefis and Nikolaos Tsetsos

Abstract

Bell's palsy (BP) is a condition affecting the facial nerve, leading to muscle weakness on one side of the face. It typically begins suddenly, usually within 72 h. Symptoms may include heightened sensitivity to sound, changes in facial sensation, pain around the neck or ear, or altered sense of taste. Bell's palsy is more commonly seen in individuals aged 15–45, with a slightly higher occurrence in middle and later life. It affects both genders equally, with an annual rate of 20–40 cases per 100,000 people. While the exact cause of Bell's palsy has traditionally been unknown, one potential factor is infection with herpes simplex virus type 1. Diagnosis is primarily based on clinical assessment and the exclusion of other possible causes. The severity of the condition is often evaluated using the House-Brackmann scale. Routine laboratory, imaging, or neurophysiological tests are generally not recommended at the initial presentation of typical Bell's palsy. Distinguishing Bell's palsy from other conditions involves considering factors such as congenital, cerebrovascular, infectious, neoplastic, inflammatory, autoimmune, and traumatic causes. Early treatment with corticosteroids has been found to improve facial function recovery, especially when administered within the first 72 h. Approximately 85% of patients experience some level of recovery within the first 3 weeks, with the remaining 15% recovering between 3 and 5 months. Ultimately, about 70% of all patients achieve full recovery.

Case Presentation

A 38-year-old man arrived at the emergency department with one-sided facial paralysis. He reported waking up with drooping on the left side of his face and an inability to close his left eye. He denied any prior injury, and his medical history showed no known underlying neurological conditions. Upon examination, there was noticeable weakness in the forehead, incomplete closure of the left eye, asymmetry of the mouth at rest (Fig. 28.1), and loss of taste sensation on the front two-thirds of the tongue.

Questions

1. Which of the following statements are true about BP? (more than one correct answer possible)

K. Garefis (✉)
2nd Academic ORL, Head and Neck Surgery Department, Aristotle University of Thessaloniki, Papageorgiou Hospital, Thessaloniki, Greece

N. Tsetsos
ENT Head and Neck Surgery Department, 424 General Military Hospital, Thessaloniki, Greece

N. Tsetsos et al. (eds.), *Otolaryngology Study Guide*, https://doi.org/10.1007/978-3-031-77374-7_28

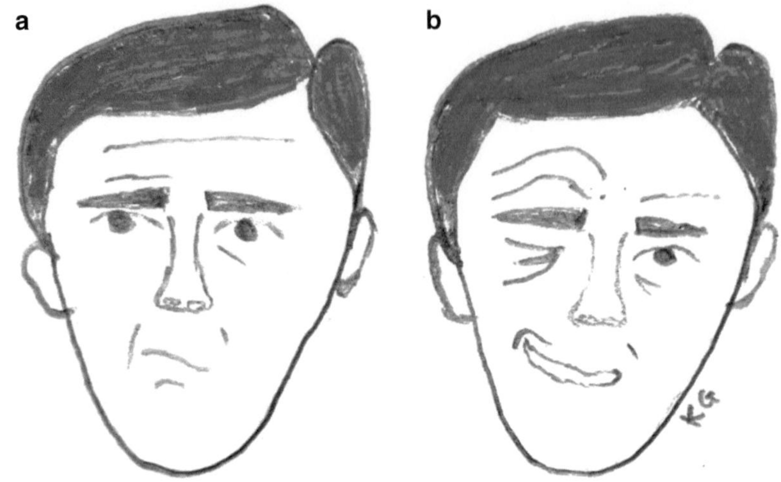

Fig. 28.1 Face of the patient at rest (**a**) and while moving (maximum effort) (**b**)

   A. The right sight of face is affected more often
   B. BP can be bilateral at about 12% of cases
   C. Most patients have spontaneous resolution
   D. It is more common in females
   E. Sternocleidomastoid can also be affected
2. Which level on House-Brackmann scale corresponds to the patient clinical appearance?
   A. Grade I
   B. Grade VII
   C. Grade III
   D. Grade IV
   E. Grade V
3. You examine a patient with left facial nerve palsy and observe that the forehead is unaffected, whereas the rest of the left side of the face is affected. Which of the following could be a potential diagnosis? (more than one correct answer possible)
   A. BP
   B. Stroke
   C. Brain tumor
   D. Lyme disease
   E. Sarcoidosis
4. Which of the following statements are true about BP diagnostic workup? (more than one correct answer possible)
   A. Laboratory testing to assess for specific diagnoses should be warranted only when sufficient clinical suspicion exists
   B. An MRI scan should always be performed at the time of initial presentation of BP
   C. MRI with gadolinium contrast often demonstrates enhancement of the intracanalicular and labyrinthine segments of the facial nerve
   D. If electroneuronography evaluation results are greater than 80% degeneration within the first 2 weeks, this tends to be a poor prognostic indicator
   E. Electromyography is most valuable in the time frame of 2–3 days to 3 weeks after the onset of BP
5. Which of the following statements are true about the management of BP? (more than one correct answer possible)
   A. The use of oral steroids is strongly recommended
   B. Oral antiviral monotherapy is not recommended in patients with new onset BP
   C. The role of physical therapy in Bell's palsy has been well established
   D. Ocular protection is essential to protecting vision
   E. Surgical decompression should be exclusively considered in patients with incomplete paralysis

Correct Answers

1. **C**

BP presents with a sudden onset of one-sided facial paralysis, with bilateral paralysis affecting only 0.3% of patients [1]. There is no specific preference for which side of the face is affected, and there is no apparent sea-

Table 28.1 The House-Brackmann grading system

GRADE I. Normal Normal facial function in all areas
GRADE II. Mild dysfunction Slight weakness noticeable on close inspection. No synkinesis, contracture, or hemifacial spasm. Normal symmetry and tone at rest. Moderate to good forehead function. Complete eye closure with minimal effort. Slight asymmetry of mouth
GRADE III. Moderate dysfunction Obvious, but not disfiguring difference between the sides. Noticeable, but not severe, synkinesis, contracture, or hemifacial spasm. Normal symmetry and tone at rest. Slight to moderate movement of forehead. Complete but asymmetric eye closure with effort. Slightly weak mouth movements with maximum effort
GRADE IV. Moderately severe dysfunction Obvious weakness or disfiguring asymmetry. Normal symmetry and tone at rest. No forehead movement. Incomplete eye closure. Asymmetry of mouth with maximum effort
GRADE V. Severe dysfunction Only barely perceptible motion. Asymmetry at rest. No forehead movement. Incomplete eye closure with only slight movement of lid with maximal effort. Slight movement of corner of mouth
GRADE VI. Total paralysis No movement

sonal pattern [1, 2]. BP affects both males and females relatively equally, although it is slightly more common in men over 40, women under 20 years of age, and women in pregnancy [1, 3]. Individuals with BP commonly experience weakness or complete paralysis of all the facial muscles on one side, while sternocleidomastoid remains unaffected [2]. The vast majority of patients undergo spontaneous recovery. Approximately 84% of them regain near-normal facial function, and 71% achieve complete resolution. In cases of incomplete paralysis, 94% of patients make a full recovery within 4 months from the onset [1].

2. **D**

   The House-Brackmann facial nerve grading system is the established approach for assessing facial nerve function. This scale is highly practical for clinical purposes as it swiftly evaluates eye closure, mouth, and forehead movement to estimate functionality. It ranges from Grade I (100% function) to Grade VI (0% function) (Table 28.1) [4].

3. **B, C**

   Central nervous system damage, which can result from various sources such as multiple sclerosis, stroke, or tumors, may also lead to facial nerve paralysis [2]. In cases of central paralysis, the muscles responsible for raising the eyebrows are often left unaffected, resulting in a balanced forehead appearance when raised. Conversely, in peripheral paralysis, these forehead muscles are typically affected, leading to an uneven or incomplete raising of the forehead on the affected side. It's worth noting that some nerve fibers responsible for forehead movement cross over at the brainstem level, originating from both sides of the cerebral hemispheres [2, 5]. Consequently, supranuclear (central) lesions affecting the facial nerve will not cause paralysis in the forehead on the affected side. BP often appears suddenly, whereas central paralysis may exhibit a gradual or abrupt onset. Furthermore, central paralysis can be accompanied by other neurological symptoms such as speech difficulties, limb weakness, or balance issues, depending on the underlying cause [2]. Individuals with Lyme disease often have a medical history that includes previous encounters with ticks, skin rashes, or joint discomfort [2]. For those living in regions where the disease is prevalent, a diagnosis becomes more likely, particularly when facial paralysis affects both sides of the face or when it occurs in a pediatric patient [6]. The most common neurological symptom of sarcoidosis is peripheral facial nerve palsy, which is usually bilateral and accompanied by additional symptoms [2, 7].

4. **A, C**

While laboratory tests themselves pose minimal risk to patients, the expenses associated with many tests conducted to identify uncommon causes can be significant. It is justified to test for these conditions when there is enough clinical suspicion. The routine use of diagnostic imaging is not recommended during the initial presentation of these patients. However, there is a specific role for imaging in cases of suggestive history or physical findings (such as temporal bone trauma or a history of tumors), or if the paralysis does not recover within the expected timeframe or worsens [8]. In BP, MRI with gadolinium contrast often reveals enhancement of the intracanalicular and labyrinthine segments of the facial nerve, as well as more pronounced enhancement of the geniculate ganglion, tympanic, and mastoid segments [9]. If the results of electroneuronography show over 90% degeneration within the first 2 weeks, this tends to indicate a poor prognosis and is associated with incomplete recovery [1]. Electromyography is most useful within the 2–3 week to 3-month timeframe following the onset of BP. It is beneficial for monitoring regeneration if reinnervation occurs and should be used and interpreted in conjunction with clinical examinations [10].

5. **A, B, D**

The primary proposed cause of BP is believed to be inflammation and swelling resulting from the compression of the facial nerve as it passes through the fallopian (facial) canal. Medications that target the inflammatory process, such as oral corticosteroids, may reduce nerve swelling and aid in the restoration of facial nerve function. Since the pathophysiology of BP involves the activation of HSV-1, healthcare providers have included antiviral therapy in the acute treatment of BP. However, the use of antiviral therapy has been a topic of controversy. While oral antiviral treatment alone is not recommended for patients with new onset Bell's palsy, it is suggested to administer oral antiviral therapy along with oral steroids within 72 h of symptom onset [8]. Various treatment approaches have been studied, including thermal treatment, electrotherapy, massage, facial exercise, and biofeedback, but there is insufficient evidence to support the effectiveness or harm of physical therapy as a treatment for BP [8]. To prevent corneal exposure and dryness, it is recommended to regularly apply artificial tears and lubrication, and to tape the eyelid shut at night. Healthcare providers should consider early implantation of eyelid weights to help patients maximize eye protection [1]. Patients with complete paralysis, more than 90% reduction in amplitude on electroneurography testing compared to the unaffected side of the face, and no voluntary nerve activity on electromyography are less likely to recover spontaneously or with medical treatment alone. In this specific patient group, early intervention could lead to improved recovery rates. Therefore, considering the significant impact of permanent facial paralysis, more proactive intervention could be warranted [8].

References

1. Vakharia K, Vakharia K. Bell's palsy. Facial Plast Surg Clin North Am. 2016;24(1):1–10.
2. Tiemstra JD, Khatkhate N. Bell's palsy: diagnosis and management. Am Fam Physician. 2007;76(7):997–1002.
3. Holland NJ, Bernstein JM. Bell's palsy. BMJ Clin Evid. 2014;2014:1204.
4. House JW. Facial nerve grading systems. Laryngoscope. 1983;93(8):1056–69. https://doi.org/10.1288/00005537-198308000-00016.
5. Eviston TJ, Croxson GR, Kennedy PG, Hadlock T, Krishnan AV. Bell's palsy: aetiology, clinical features and multidisciplinary care. J Neurol Neurosurg Psychiatry. 2015;86(12):1356–61.
6. Reich SG. Bell's palsy. Continuum (Minneap Minn). 2017;23(2, Selected Topics in Outpatient Neurology):447–466.
7. Said G. Sarcoidosis of the peripheral nervous system. Handb Clin Neurol. 2013;115:485–95.
8. Baugh RF, Basura GJ, Ishii LE, et al. Clinical practice guideline: Bell's palsy. Otolaryngol Head Neck Surg. 2013;149(3 Suppl):S1–S27.
9. Gupta S, Mends F, Hagiwara M, Fatterpekar G, Roehm PC. Imaging the facial nerve: a contemporary review. Radiol Res Pract. 2013;2013:248039.
10. Guntinas-Lichius O, Volk GF, Olsen KD, et al. Facial nerve electrodiagnostics for patients with facial palsy: a clinical practice guideline. Eur Arch Otorrinolaringol. 2020;277(7):1855–74.

Part III

Rhinology

29 Nasal Septum Deviation

Alexandros Poutoglidis
and Christodoulos Dimakis

Abstract

Nasal septum deviation is a common deformity that can significantly impact a patient's quality of life. The most common symptom is nasal obstruction, which can vary in severity among individuals. The extent to which nasal septum deviation contributes to overall obstruction can be assessed during a physical examination with vasoconstriction. It's common to find mucosal hypertrophy of the inferior turbinate on the non-deviated side due to compensatory mechanisms. The most common surgical approaches in septoplasty are hemi-transfixion and Killian incisions. In cases where bilateral mucosa tearing occurs during mucoperichondrial flap elevation, an interposition graft should always be considered. To achieve a good cosmetic and functional outcome, it's crucial to conservatively resect only deviated spurs and open the nasal valve. However, septoplasty can have complications. Persistent, subjective, postoperative obstruction is not uncommon among patients and is often due to inappropriate surgical indications. The percentage of dissatisfied patients can be reduced with optimal techniques and accurate preoperative diagnosis. Inferior turbinate hypertrophy due to allergic rhinitis or other factors can significantly affect the normal airflow of inspired air, and septoplasty alone may not provide a satisfactory outcome. Objective measurements like acoustic rhinometry or airflow rhinometry can objectively assess the need for surgical management.

Case Presentation

A 34-year-old man presented to the outpatient clinic with the chief complaints of nasal obstruction and snoring in the last 5 years following a car accident. He also reported mild episodes of epistaxis and facial pain. His medical history was significant for a nasal fracture after the aforementioned accident. The fracture was conservatively treated without surgical intervention. It should be stated that the patient had no aesthetic deformity. On physical examination, anterior rhinoscopy revealed a right-sided septal deviation mainly in the anterior part. Flexible nasendoscopy confirmed the findings of the rhinoscopy and ruled out any other pathologies (Fig. 29.1). Anterior airflow rhinomanometry indicated high resistant values on the right side. A septoplasty was rec-

A. Poutoglidis
ENT Department, Lister Hospital, East and North Hertfordshire NHS Trust, Stevenage, UK

C. Dimakis (✉)
ENT Head and Neck Surgery Department, Athens Naval Hospital, Athens, Greece

N. Tsetsos et al. (eds.), *Otolaryngology Study Guide*, https://doi.org/10.1007/978-3-031-77374-7_29

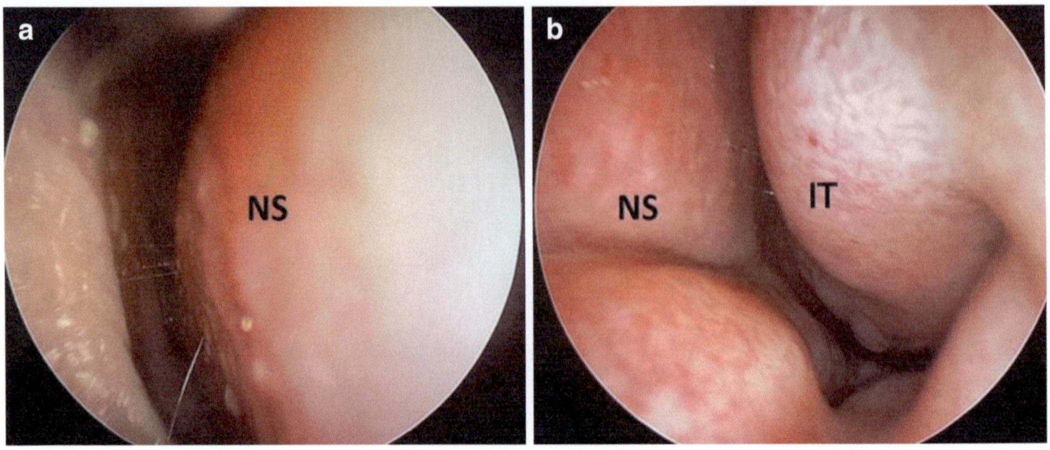

Fig. 29.1 Endoscopic view of the nasal cavity. An anterior deviation of the nasal septum is noted on the right side. Left inferior turbinate demonstrates hypertrophy. *NS* nasal septum, *IT* inferior turbinate, (**a**) right side, (**b**) left side

ommended to correct the deviation and relieve the patient of nasal obstruction and snoring. Two months later, the patient underwent an uneventful septoplasty and he was discharged the following day. Five months later, the patient reported significant improvement in his nasal breathing with no nasal obstruction and snoring.

Questions

1. Septal hematoma is a complication of septoplasty and should be treated:
   A. Oral antibiotics and corticosteroids
   B. Nasal irrigations
   C. Incision, drainage, and antibiotics
   D. Watchful waiting
   E. Incision and drainage are indicated only when it is further complicated by an abscess
2. Which of the following structures belong to the nasal septum?
   A. Perpendicular plate of the ethmoid bone
   B. Vomer
   C. Quadrangular cartilage
   D. Maxillary crest
   E. Inferior turbinate
3. The internal nasal valve consists of:
   A. Vomer
   B. Upper lateral cartilage
   C. Pyriform aperture
   D. Nasal septum
   E. Inferior turbinate
4. Which of the following belongs to the postoperative complications of septoplasty?
   A. Perforation of the nasal septum
   B. Nasal septum hematoma
   C. "Saddle" nose deformity
   D. Cerebrospinal fluid rhinorrhea
   E. Epistaxis
5. Which of the following belongs to the objective measurements of nasal obstruction?
   A. X-ray
   B. Acoustic rhinometry
   C. Nasal endoscopy
   D. Airflow rhinometry
   E. Magnetic resonance imaging (MRI)

Correct Answers

1. **C**

   Nasal hematoma is typically a result of nasal trauma or a post-surgery complication following septoplasty. It involves the accumulation of blood between the nasal septum cartilage and the mucoperichondrium that covers it. If not treated promptly, it can cause irreversible necrosis of the nasal septum within 72–96 h [1]. This can lead to nasal collapse and significant cosmetic deformity, known as "saddle" nose deformity. Bacterial infection of the hematoma can lead to abscess formation, particularly in cases with delayed presentation. To prevent severe complications, nasal hematoma and abscesses should be treated aggressively. Initial treatment involves wide incision and drainage. A corrugator can be sutured into the hematoma cavity to prevent re-accumulation. Antibiotics for a minimum of one week and nasal packs for 48 h can help control infection and bleeding, respectively [2].

2. **A, B, C, D**

   The nasal septum framework includes both cartilaginous and bony components. The bony structures include the maxillary crest of the maxillary and palatine bone, which forms the nasal spine, the perpendicular plate of the ethmoid bone, and the vomer. The quadrangular cartilage forms the cartilaginous component. The inferior turbinate, a separate bone of the lateral nasal wall, does not contribute to the formation of the nasal septum [3].

3. **B, C, D, E**

   Nasal blockage results from obstructions in the external and internal nasal valves. The former is made up of the nasal septum and lower lateral cartilage, while the latter consists of the upper lateral cartilage, pyriform aperture, inferior turbinate, and nasal septum. The resistance to airflow depends on the orientation of the nasal bones, the position of the nasal septum, and the size of the turbinates, particularly the inferior one. The internal nasal valve is the narrowest part of the nasal passage. Even a slight increase in its axial diameter can significantly improve overall airflow. This is based on Poiseuille's law, which describes the relationship between resistance and radius. Therefore, restoring the internal valve is crucial for relieving nasal obstruction [3].

4. **A, B, C, D, E**

   Nasal septum surgery can have complications. Mild nosebleeds in the first few days after surgery are common. Persistent and severe nosebleeds may occur when the surgery involves interventions on the inferior turbinate [1]. Septal perforation, often due to poor surgical technique, can occur in the hands of inexperienced surgeons. If bilateral fenestrations during the elevation of mucoperichondrial flaps are left unrepaired and an interposition graft is not used, postoperative perforation is almost inevitable. The health of the cartilage depends on the blood supply from the overlying perichondrium. Therefore, a bilateral deficit can lead to necrosis and permanent perforation. Repairing a nasal septum perforation with a second operation is challenging and often unsuccessful [4]. Overly aggressive resection of the upper bony segment of the nasal septum can result in a deficit in the skull base and postoperative cerebrospinal fluid rhinorrhea or changes in nasal shape with ptosis of the tip, "saddle" nose deformity, and devastating cosmetic and functional outcomes. Lastly, the formation of synechiae between the inferior turbinate and nasal septum is usually due to trauma [5].

5. **B, D**

   The dimensions of the nasal airway are measured using acoustic rhinometry. This non-invasive and accurate method evaluates nasal geometry [6]. Sound waves are sent into the nasal cavity, and their reflections are recorded on a chart known as a rhinogram. This can assess both nasal resistance and the areas with the smallest axial dimensions. The rhinogram typically shows two dips, the first due to the nasal valves and the second due to the size of the inferior and middle turbinates. Therefore, the decision to perform septoplasty can be guided by the rhinogram, and postoperative acoustic rhinometry can be used to evaluate the outcome. Airflow rhinometry can be used to assess the resistance of airflow through the nasal cavity [7]. The process can be repeated after vasoconstriction to document the results of medical management and to determine if surgical intervention would benefit the patient. It's important to remember that nasal obstruction is often not due to nasal septum spurs but rather inferior turbinate hypertrophy. Despite the sensitivity and objectivity of both methods, their time-consuming nature and the need for specialized and expensive equipment limit their widespread use.

References

1. Flint PW, Haughey BH, Lund VJ, Niparko JK, Richardson MA, Robbins KT, et al. Cummings otolaryngology—head and neck surgery, 5th ed. Mosby; 2010.
2. Hong CX, Husain S, Wan Hamizan AK, Zahedi FD. Recurrent nasal septal hematoma and abscess: a rare manifestation of leukemia. Clin Med Res. 2021;19(1):35–8.
3. Hsu DW, Suh JD. Anatomy and physiology of nasal obstruction. Otolaryngol Clin North Am. 2018;51(5):853–65.
4. Rajzer I, Stręk P, Wiatr M, Skladzien J, Kurowska A, Kopeć J, Swiezy K, Wiatr A. Biomaterials in the reconstruction of nasal septum perforation. Ann Otol Rhinol Laryngol. 2021;130(7):731–7.
5. Kim SJ, Chang DS, Choi MS, Lee HY, Pyo JS. Efficacy of nasal septal splints for preventing complications after septoplasty: a meta-analysis. Am J Otolaryngol. 2021;42(3):102389.
6. Edizer DT, Erisir F, Alimoglu Y, Gokce S. Nasal obstruction following septorhinoplasty: how well does acoustic rhinometry work? Eur Arch Otorrinolaringol. 2013;270(2):609–13.
7. Tan MFM, Whitcroft KL, Mehta N, Schilder A, Leung TS, Andrews PJ. Investigating the nasal cycle using unilateral peak nasal inspiratory flow and acoustic rhinometry minimal cross-sectional area measurements. Clin Otolaryngol. 2019;44(4):518–24.

30 Hereditary Haemorrhagic Telangiectasia

Harry Carter

Abstract

Hereditary Haemorrhagic Telangiectasia (HHT), also known as Osler-Weber-Rendu Syndrome, causes Arteriovenous Malformations (AVM), increasing the risk of haemorrhage. It is inherited in an autosomal dominant fashion and has high penetrance, estimated around 95% by late adulthood. Prevalence is approximately 1:10,000 in North America. The condition commonly presents with recurrent epistaxis in teenage years, followed by the presence of telangiectasia (small AVMs) on the lips, tongue and gastrointestinal tract mucosa in adulthood. Larger AVMs can occur in the brain, lungs and liver, occasionally causing life-threatening complications. Gastrointestinal involvement may lead to occult or overt bleeding per rectum and iron deficiency anaemia. The management of HHT largely depends on the site and symptoms of the AVMs. Although an awareness of the multi-organ pathology HHT can cause is important, epistaxis management is the challenge that ENT practitioners face. Simple measures such as regular humidification or moisturisers are followed by medical treatments, including oral antifibrinolytic or systemic antiangiogenic agents. Finally, there are a range of surgical approaches to control epistaxis, depending on the severity of symptoms.

Case Presentation

A 34-year-old man with a background of HHT presents to the ENT outpatient department with a history of recurrent epistaxis (at least one epistaxis per day) (Fig. 30.1). He uses humidification and nasal moisturisers regularly at home, but the episodes seem to be worsening. He wants to discuss different approaches to preventing nosebleeds.

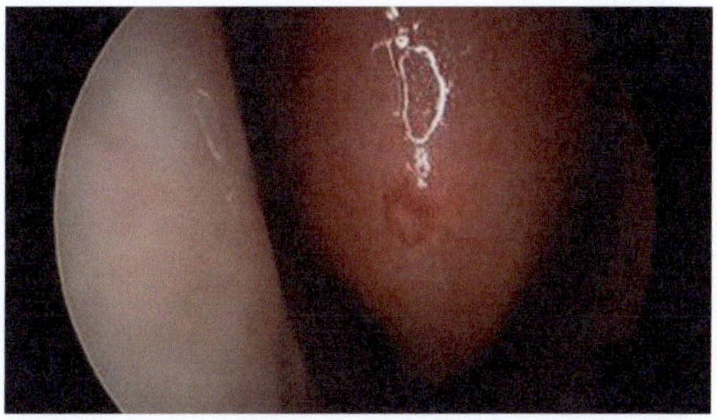

Fig. 30.1 An endoscopic view of nasal telangiectasia in HHT. (Image used with permission from Dr. Brian Rotenberg, Otolaryngology—Head and Neck Surgery Department, Schulich School of Medicine and Dentistry)

H. Carter (✉)
ENT Head and Neck Surgery Department,
Morriston Hospital, Swansea, UK

N. Tsetsos et al. (eds.), *Otolaryngology Study Guide*, https://doi.org/10.1007/978-3-031-77374-7_30

Questions

1. A patient with known HTT presents to the emergency department with epistaxis which has not resolved with 30 min of nasal pressure. Which method to arrest the bleeding should be avoided?
   A. High-pressure rapid rhino
   B. Nasopore
   C. Tranexamic acid
   D. Floseal
   E. Merocel
2. Which medication is not a recognised medical therapy for HHT?
   A. Bevacizumab (Avastin)
   B. Oestrogen
   C. Tranexamic acid
   D. Saline
   E. Vitamin K
3. What procedure is the last line of treatment in recurrent epistaxis with HHT?
   A. Septodermoplasty
   B. Sclerotherapy
   C. Laser photocoagulation
   D. Young's procedure
   E. Coblation
4. A patient with HHT walks from the waiting room into your clinic room. You notice that they are cyanosed and dyspnoeic. What is the likely pathophysiology of this?
   A. Emphysematous bullae reducing gas exchange
   B. Acute respiratory distress syndrome
   C. COVID-19
   D. Systemic arteriovenous shunting
   E. Portal hypertension
5. Which of the options is not one of the diagnostic criteria?
   A. Multiple telangiectasia at classical sites
   B. Bleeding per rectum
   C. Spontaneous and recurrent epistaxis
   D. Visceral AVMs
   E. First-degree relative with HHT

Answers

1. A

   Active epistaxis in the context of HHT should be managed similarly to standard cases with a few exceptions. First-aid measures should always be used initially, as this is non-invasive and often effective. Silver nitrate cautery should be avoided in HHT as it often worsens the severity of epistaxis and is relatively imprecise [1]. If used repeatedly or broadly, it is high risk for septal perforation [2]. Nasal packing should be considered next, however, pneumatic, high-pressure devices such as a Rapid Rhino should also be avoided as this may worsen bleeding [1]. Either absorbable (such as Naspore) or low-pressure, non-absorbable packs (such as Merocel) are preferable as they are less likely to traumatise non-bleeding telangiectasia [3]. Haemostatic agents or tranexamic acid would also be appropriate options [1, 4].
2. E

   Vitamin K can be used as a warfarin reversal agent, but is not a recognised therapy for HHT [5]. Topical agents are used as first-line treatments for HHT, including saline sprays, beta-blockers, and oestrogens [6]. Oral tranexamic acid may be considered next, as trials demonstrate reduction in frequency and duration of epistaxis [7, 8]. If surgical ablative therapy does not improve epistaxis, systemic antiangiogenic therapy (Bevacizumab), which inhibits vascular endothelial growth factor (VEGF), can be used. Case series have demonstrated reduced epistaxis with improved anaemia and quality of life. However, effects may be transient and the treatment carries risks [9, 10]. There is some evidence that oral oestrogens reduce the need transfusion from gastrointestinal bleeding and epistaxis, but are not tolerated by males and increase venous thromboembolism risk [11, 12].
3. D

   Young's procedure is surgical closure of the nostrils and is reserved as a last line of treatment for epistaxis with HHT [6]. The procedure has a reported 94% cessation of epistaxis but the effects of anosmia and permanent mouth breathing can be poorly tolerated [13], and reversal is sometimes required [14]. Various ablative therapies are available. Laser therapy is a popular option but can be difficult to reach posterior telangiectasia if flexible fibres are not available [3]. Coblation is an alternative to laser therapy, using radiofrequency energy to break molecular bonds at low temperatures, reducing risk to surrounding mucosa [15]. Sclerotherapy also reports good efficacy for reduction in epistaxis but carries a risk of tissue necrosis, cellulitis, and visual loss [16, 17].

4. D

   HHT is associated with the development of pulmonary AVMs. In most patients, these are asymptomatic but can manifest with dyspnoea, cyanosis, haemoptysis, polycythaemia, or clubbing [18]. The AVM creates a direct communication between arteries and veins called a shunt [19]. This results in poorly oxygenated blood entering pulmonary veins and cyanosis. The larger the AVM or shunt fraction, often the worse the symptoms [20]. In HHT patients, screening for pulmonary AVMs should take place as treatment may be indicated to reduce complications of emboli, haemorrhage, and shunting [19].

5. B—Bleeding per rectum

   The Curaçao Diagnostic Criteria is the internationally accepted framework for the diagnosis of HHT. There are four criteria:
   - Spontaneous and recurrent epistaxis
   - Multiple mucocutaneous telangiectasia
   - Visceral involvement (e.g. pulmonary/hepatic/cerebral AVMs, gastrointestinal telangiectasia)
   - A first-degree relative with HHT

   A patient with three criteria would be 'definite', two 'suspected' and one 'unlikely' [21]. The diagnosis can be confirmed with genetic testing; however, this is not required [6]. Bleeding per rectum alone is not a diagnostic criterion as telangiectasia affecting the gastrointestinal mucosa would need to be visualised.

References

1. Sautter NB, Smith TL. Treatment of hereditary hemorrhagic telangiectasia-related epistaxis [Internet]. Vol. 49, Otolaryngologic Clinics of North America. W.B. Saunders; 2016 [cited 2022 Sep 1]. p. 639–654. https://pubmed.ncbi.nlm.nih.gov/27267016/.
2. Raghavan U. Septal perforation. In: Symptom oriented otolaryngology—head and neck surgery: rhinology and facial plastics (Volume 2) [Internet]. Jaypee Brothers Medical Publishers (P) Ltd.; 2017 [cited 2022 Sep 5]. p. 191–191. https://www.ncbi.nlm.nih.gov/books/NBK537208/.
3. Chin CJ, Rotenberg BW, Witterick IJ. Epistaxis in hereditary hemorrhagic telangiectasia: an evidence based review of surgical management. J Otolaryngol—Head Neck Surg [Internet]. 2016 [cited 2022 Sep 1];45(1):3. http://www.journalotohns.com/content/45/1/3.
4. Lee JM, Wu V, Faughnan ME, Lasso A, Figol A, Kilty SJ. Prospective pilot study of Floseal® for the treatment of anterior epistaxis in patients with hereditary hemorrhagic telangiectasia (HHT). J Otolaryngol—Head Neck Surg [Internet]. 2019 [cited 2022 Sep 1];48(1):48. https://journalotohns.biomedcentral.com/articles/10.1186/s40463-019-0379-y.
5. Crowther MA, Julian J, McCarty D, Douketis J, Kovacs M, Biagoni L, et al. Treatment of warfarin-associated coagulopathy with oral vitamin K: a randomised controlled trial. Lancet [Internet]. 2000 [cited 2022 Sep 1];356(9241):1551–3. https://linkinghub.elsevier.com/retrieve/pii/S0140673600031251.
6. Faughnan ME, Mager JJ, Hetts SW, Palda VA, Lang-Robertson K, Buscarini E, et al. Second international guidelines for the diagnosis and management of hereditary hemorrhagic telangiectasia [Internet]. Vol. 173, Annals of Internal Medicine. American College of Physicians; 2020 [cited 2022 Sep 1]. p. 989–1001. https://pubmed.ncbi.nlm.nih.gov/32894695/.
7. Geisthoff UW, Seyfert UT, Kübler M, Bieg B, Plinkert PK, König J. Treatment of epistaxis in hereditary hemorrhagic telangiectasia with tranexamic acid—A double-blind placebo-controlled cross-over phase IIIB study. Thromb Res [Internet]. 2014 [cited 2022 Sep 1];134(3):565–71. https://pubmed.ncbi.nlm.nih.gov/25005464/.
8. Gaillard S, Dupuis-Girod S, Boutitie F, Rivière S, Morinière S, Hatron PY, et al. Tranexamic acid for epistaxis in hereditary hemorrhagic telangiectasia patients: a European cross-over controlled trial in a rare disease. J Thromb Haemost [Internet]. 2014 [cited 2022 Sep 1];12(9):1494–502. https://pubmed.ncbi.nlm.nih.gov/25040799/.
9. Rosenberg T, Fialla AD, Kjeldsen J, Kjeldsen AD. Does severe bleeding in hht patients respond to intravenous bevacizumab? Review of the literature and case series [Internet]. Vol. 57, Rhinology. International Rhinologic Society; 2019 [cited 2022 Sep 1]. p. 242–51. https://pubmed.ncbi.nlm.nih.gov/30907391/.
10. Guilhem A, Fargeton AE, Simon AC, Duffau P, Harle JR, Lavigne C, et al. Intra-venous bevacizumab in hereditary hemorrhagic telangiectasia (HHT): a retrospective study of 46 patients. PLoS One [Internet]. 2017 Nov 1 [cited 2022 Sep 1];12(11). https://pubmed.ncbi.nlm.nih.gov/29190827/.

11. van Cutsem E, Rutgeerts P, Vantrappen G. Treatment of bleeding gastrointestinal vascular malformations with oestrogen-progesterone. Lancet [Internet]. 1990 [cited 2022 Sep 1];335(8695):953–5. https://pubmed.ncbi.nlm.nih.gov/1970032/.
12. Jameson JJ, Cave DR. Hormonal and Antihormonal therapy for epistaxis in hereditary hemorrhagic telangiectasia [Internet]. Vol. 114, Laryngoscope; 2004 [cited 2022 Sep 1]. p. 705–9. https://pubmed.ncbi.nlm.nih.gov/15064628/.
13. Lund VJ, Darby Y, Rimmer J, Amin M, Husain S. Nasal closure for severe hereditary haemorrhagic telangiectasia in 100 patients. The Lund modification of the Young's procedure: a 22-year experience. Rhinol J [Internet]. 2017 [cited 2022 Sep 1];55(2):135–41. https://pubmed.ncbi.nlm.nih.gov/28064338/.
14. Oozeer NB, Bingham BJ. Reversal of Young's procedure in hereditary haemorrhagic telangiectasia. J Laryngol Otol [Internet]. 2012 [cited 2022 Sep 1];126(11):1169–71. https://pubmed.ncbi.nlm.nih.gov/22932648/.
15. Luk L, Mace JC, Bhandarkar ND, Sautter NB. Comparison of electrosurgical plasma coagulation and potassium-titanyl-phosphate laser photocoagulation for treatment of hereditary hemorrhagic telangiectasia-related epistaxis. Int Forum Allergy Rhinol [Internet]. 2014 [cited 2022 Sep 1];4(8):640–5. https://pubmed.ncbi.nlm.nih.gov/24719397/.
16. Boyer H, Fernandes P, Le C, Yueh B. Prospective randomized trial of sclerotherapy vs standard treatment for epistaxis due to hereditary hemorrhagic telangiectasia. Int Forum Allergy Rhinol [Internet]. 2015 [cited 2022 Sep 1];5(5):435–40. https://pubmed.ncbi.nlm.nih.gov/25643928/.
17. Boyer H, Fernandes P, Duran O, Hunter D, Goding G. Office-based sclerotherapy for recurrent epistaxis due to hereditary hemorrhagic telangiectasia: a pilot study. Int Forum Allergy Rhinol [Internet]. 2011 [cited 2022 Sep 1];1(4):319–23. https://pubmed.ncbi.nlm.nih.gov/22287439/.
18. Gefen AM, White AJ. Asymptomatic pulmonary arteriovenous malformations in children with hereditary hemorrhagic telangiectasia. Pediatr Pulmonol [Internet]. 2017 [cited 2022 Sep 1];52(9):1194–7. https://pubmed.ncbi.nlm.nih.gov/28608633/.
19. Meier NM, Foster ML, Battaile JT. Hereditary hemorrhagic telangiectasia and pulmonary arteriovenous malformations: clinical aspects [Internet]. Vol. 8, Cardiovascular Diagnosis and Therapy. AME Publishing Company; 2018 [cited 2022 Sep 1]. p. 316–24. /pmc/articles/PMC6039799/.
20. Faughnan ME, Lui YW, Wirth JA, Pugash RA, Redelmeier DA, Hyland RH, et al. Diffuse pulmonary arteriovenous malformations: characteristics and prognosis. Chest [Internet]. 2000 [cited 2022 Sep 1];117(1):31–8. https://pubmed.ncbi.nlm.nih.gov/10631195/.
21. Shovlin CL, Guttmacher AE, Buscarini E, Faughnan ME, Hyland RH, Westermann CJJ, et al. Diagnostic criteria for hereditary hemorrhagic telangiectasia (Rendu-Osler-Weber syndrome). Am J Med Genet [Internet]. 2000 [cited 2022 Sep 1];91(1):66–7. https://pubmed.ncbi.nlm.nih.gov/10751092/.

Allergic Rhinitis

31

Alexandros Poutoglidis, Despoina Beka, and Christodoulos Dimakis

Abstract

The aerodigestive tract is susceptible to Th2-related immune response, with allergic rhinitis and asthma being the most common manifestations. Allergic rhinitis has a significant socioeconomic impact, affecting both the quality of life of patients and the cost of national healthcare systems. Specifically, allergens trigger an IgE-dependent reaction in sensitized patients, leading to the release of mast cells and subsequent inflammation. Eosinophils and basophils play a crucial role in nasal mucosa hypersensitivity, becoming irritated by specific allergens. Common symptoms include pruritus, nasal congestion, nasal secretions, sneezing, and lacrimation following antigen exposure. Currently, allergic rhinitis is categorized as mild, moderate, or severe based on symptom severity, and as intermittent or persistent based on symptom duration. H1-antihistamines and leukotriene antagonists can partially control symptoms but do not fully alleviate nasal congestion. Intranasal steroids are often the first-line treatment as they improve quality of life and can be used alongside antihistamines for enhanced results. However, the only definitive solution is immunotherapy (sublingual and subcutaneous), due to its ability to modify the natural progression of the disease, often leading to permanent relief.

Case Presentation

A 32-year-old woman presented to the outpatient department, primarily complaining of persistent nasal congestion. Her medical history revealed severe allergic asthma. She also mentioned frequent bouts of sneezing and watery eyes, which had significantly worsened after she adopted a stray cat. The nasal congestion was causing her considerable discomfort, affecting her sleep, leisure activities, and work performance. A nasal rhinoscopy showed that her inferior turbinates were pale and swollen, with clear secretions visible in the inferior and middle meatus (Fig. 31.1). Allergic skin prick tests confirmed an allergy to cats, with a wheal >4 mm, and identified three other allergens (Fig. 31.1). The patient was diagnosed with severe persistent allergic rhinitis and was advised to avoid the allergens that triggered her symptoms. Intranasal steroids were pre-

A. Poutoglidis
ENT Department, Lister Hospital, East and North Hertfordshire NHS Trust, Stevenage, UK

D. Beka
ENT Head and Neck Surgery Department, General Hospital of Athens "Laiko", Athens, Greece

C. Dimakis (✉)
ENT Head and Neck Surgery Department, Athens Naval Hospital, Athens, Greece

N. Tsetsos et al. (eds.), *Otolaryngology Study Guide*, https://doi.org/10.1007/978-3-031-77374-7_31

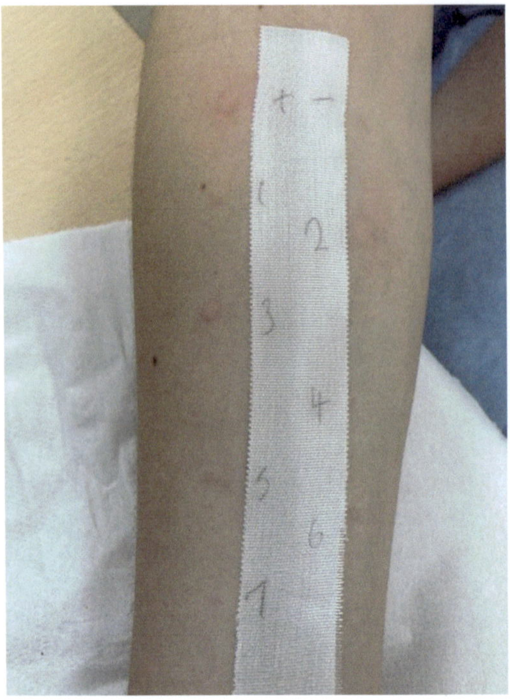

Fig. 31.1 Skin prick tests

scribed as the primary treatment for 3 months to manage her symptoms. At the three-month follow-up, her symptoms had significantly improved, indicating effective control of her allergic rhinitis.

Questions

1. Which of the following factors are associated with the development of allergic rhinitis?
   A. Genetics
   B. Geography
   C. Hygiene
   D. Socioeconomic factors
   E. Animal dander exposure
2. Which of the following tests aid in the diagnosis of allergic rhinitis?
   A. Coagulation tests
   B. Skin prick test
   C. Serum total IgE
   D. Specific IgE for serum antigen
   E. Allergen challenge testing
3. Immunotherapy for allergic rhinitis:
   A. Can be administrated both subcutaneous and sublingual
   B. Achieves a long-term control of allergic rhinitis
   C. Has a similar mechanism action with the intranasal steroids
   D. Is the first-line treatment for patients with moderate intermittent allergic rhinitis
   E. Sublingual immunotherapy can be performed only in a special clinic
4. Which of the following drugs are considered effective medications for allergic rhinitis?
   A. Intranasal steroids
   B. H_1-antihistamines
   C. Decongestants
   D. Anticholinergics
   E. Omalizumab
5. Non-allergic rhinitis includes:
   A. Rhinitis medicamentosa
   B. Occupational rhinitis
   C. Gustatory rhinitis
   D. Infectious rhinitis
   E. Granulomatous rhinitis

Answers

1. **A, B, C, D, E**

   Allergic rhinitis has a strong connection to genetics and epigenetics, with genes encoding subtypes of human leukocyte antigen (HLA) and cytokines associated with the condition. Other factors like air pollution and parental smoking can lead to DNA methylation, a crucial step in the disease's pathogenesis [1]. The decline in infectious diseases due to antibiotics, vaccinations, and improved hygiene has been linked to an increase in allergic rhinitis. This theory is based on the protective effect of environmental microflora on the nasal mucosa [2]. As a result, developed countries have a higher incidence of allergic rhinitis. Current research indicates that allergic rhinitis is more prevalent in people living in Northern Europe and America, likely due to differences in climate (temperature) and economy [3].
2. **B, C, D, E**

   The skin prick test is widely regarded as the most method reliable for diagnosing the cause of allergic rhinitis [4]. It involves applying common allergens to the skin and observing for a local reaction. While total serum IgE levels can indicate atopy, they cannot identify the specific allergen. However, the specific-serum IgE test can detect the allergen in vitro. A detailed medical history is essential to guide the selection of testing antigens. The ratio of total IgE to specific IgE can serve as an index for the effectiveness of immunotherapy. If all these tests fail to diagnose allergic rhinitis, an allergen challenge may be performed as a last resort [5].

3. **A, B**

   Allergen immunotherapy is seen as a long-term solution for allergic rhinitis as it targets the disease's cause rather than the symptoms In. contrast, steroids and antihistamines only control the symptoms and not the underlying cause of allergic rhinitis. Immunotherapy can be administered either subcutaneously or sublingually. While the subcutaneous route is commonly used in modern immunotherapy, there is growing interest in sublingual administration due to its safety. Sublingual immunotherapy can be self-administered, while subcutaneous administration requires a clinic visit [6]. Both routes of administration (subcutaneous and sublingual) should be continued for a minimum of 3 years [7].

4. **A, B, D**

   H1-antihistamines can be administered orally or intranasally. They work by binding to H1 receptors to antagonize histamine. First-generation antihistamines had significant side effects, with sedation being the most common. Second-generation antihistamines, however, do not cross the blood–brain barrier in high concentrations and have significantly fewer side effects [8]. Intranasal corticosteroids are recommended as the first-line treatment. If they fail to provide satisfactory results, an antihistamine may be added. Decongestants work by stimulating adrenergic receptors, providing rapid symptom relief through vascular constriction. However, their prolonged use can lead to reduced effectiveness and eventually to rhinitis medicamentosa. Therefore, decongestants are strongly contraindicated for treating allergic rhinitis. Intranasal anticholinergics, particularly ipratropium bromide, control clear anterior nasal discharge and may be used in patients where rhinorrhea is the primary symptom. Omalizumab is a monoclonal anti-IgE antibody that prevents mast cell activation. It is an approved treatment for severe asthma and chronic rhinosinusitis with nasal polyps. While it is beneficial for controlling allergic rhinitis, it is not yet an approved treatment modality [9].

5. **A, B, C, D, E**

   Rhinitis is traditionally divided into allergic and non-allergic types. Allergic rhinitis is diagnosed with positive skin tests, IgE tests, or allergic challenge tests if the first two are negative. Any type of rhinitis not linked to exposure to a specific agent or allergen is simply referred to as non-allergic rhinitis. Non-allergic rhinitis with eosinophilia is a type where eosinophils are detected in nasal smears but all allergic tests are negative. Infectious rhinitis can be bacterial, viral, or fungal. Autoimmune diseases like granulomatosis with polyangiitis can initially present with nasal mucosa inflammation. Sarcoidosis can also have similar nasal cavity symptoms. Gustatory odors and occupational irritants can lead to gustatory and occupational rhinitis, respectively. Neoplasms, unilateral choana atresia, adenoid hypertrophy, and other obstructive lesions often cause nasal obstruction and may be misdiagnosed as rhinitis. Finally, any type of rhinitis not linked to exposure to a specific agent or allergen was previously known as vasomotor rhinitis. Today, it is simply referred to as non-allergic rhinitis [10].

References

1. Choi BY, Han M, Kwak JW, Kim TH. Genetics and epigenetics in allergic rhinitis. Genes (Basel). 2021;12(12):2004.
2. Lambrecht BN, Hammad H. The immunology of the allergy epidemic and the hygiene hypothesis. Nat Immunol. 2017;18(10):1076–83.
3. Katelaris CH, Lee BW, Potter PC, Maspero JF, Cingi C, Lopatin A, Saffer M, Xu G, Walters RD. Prevalence and diversity of allergic rhinitis in regions of the world beyond Europe and North America. Clin Exp Allergy. 2012;42(2):186–207.
4. Tatar EC, Sürenoğlu UA, Saylam G, Işık E, Ozdek A, Korkmaz H. Is there any correlation between the results of skin-prick test and the severity of symp-

toms in allergic rhinitis? Am J Rhinol Allergy. 2012;26(1):e37–9.

5. Beken B, Eguiluz-Gracia I, Yazıcıoğlu M, Campo P. Local allergic rhinitis: a pediatric perspective. Turk J Pediatr. 2020;62(5):701–10.
6. Durham SR, Penagos M. Sublingual or subcutaneous immunotherapy for allergic rhinitis? J Allergy Clin Immunol. 2016;137(2):339–49.
7. Penagos M, Eifan AO, Durham SR, Scadding GW. Duration of allergen immunotherapy for long-term efficacy in allergic rhinoconjunctivitis. Curr Treat Options Allergy. 2018;5(3):275–90. https://doi.org/10.1007/s40521-018-0176-2.
8. Kawauchi H, Yanai K, Wang DY, Itahashi K, Okubo K. Antihistamines for allergic rhinitis treatment from the viewpoint of nonsedative properties. Int J Mol Sci. 2019;20(1):213.
9. Oba Y, Salzman GA. Cost-effectiveness analysis of omalizumab in adults and adolescents with moderate-to-severe allergic asthma. J Allergy Clin Immunol. 2004;114:265–9.
10. Wilson KF, Spector ME, Orlandi RR. Types of rhinitis. Otolaryngol Clin North Am. 2011;44(3):549–59.

Chronic Rhinosinusitis 32

Nikolaos Tsetsos

Abstract

Chronic rhinosinusitis (CRS) is characterized by inflammation in the nose and paranasal sinuses lasting a minimum of 12 weeks. Depending on whether nasal polyps are present, CRS can be categorized into two types: CRS with nasal polyps (CRSwNP) and CRS without nasal polyps (CRSsNP). CRSwNP is marked by high tissue eosinophilia and an increase in T helper (Th)-2 cytokine expression. In contrast, CRSsNP is typified by Th-1 polarization and less eosinophilic infiltration. The EPOS2020 steering has decided to examine CRS from the perspective of primary and secondary classifications, further subdividing each based on the anatomical spread of the disease into localized and diffuse categories. In the case of primary CRS, the disease is categorized based on the predominance of endotypes, specifically type 2 or non-type 2. Key symptoms of CRS encompass anterior and/or posterior mucopurulent nasal discharge, nasal blockage, facial discomfort/pressure/fullness, and a diminished sense of smell (hyposmia or anosmia). Certain alarming symptoms, such as unilateral symptoms, blood-tinged rhinorrhea, orbital symptoms, swelling of the forehead, and specific neurological signs, call for immediate medical attention. As per prevailing clinical guidelines, the primary treatment for CRS involves intranasal corticosteroids. For patients who do not respond adequately to conservative treatment, endoscopic sinus surgery is suggested. Lately, biologics have emerged as a potential treatment option for CRSwNP patients who have a recalcitrant disease.

Case Presentation

A 29-year-old man visited the rhinology clinic, troubled by a constant nasal blockage that had lasted for the past 9 months. He also reported symptoms of runny nose, postnasal drip, and a loss of smell and taste. Despite having taken two separate rounds of antibiotics over a span of three months as prescribed by his general practitioner, he saw no significant improvement. The patient had a history of allergic rhinitis and severe asthma. Upon examination through nasal endoscopy, bilateral, mobile, smooth, grey, and semi-translucent growths were observed, originating and extending beyond the middle meatus (Fig. 32.1). His nasal turbinates were swollen and exhibited a pale, bluish-grey hue. The patient was then asked to undergo high-resolution computed tomography (CT) and was prescribed intranasal corticosteroids and nasal saline irrigations for a three-month period as an initial treatment plan.

N. Tsetsos (✉)
ENT Head and Neck Surgery Department,
424 General Military Hospital, Thessaloniki, Greece

N. Tsetsos et al. (eds.), *Otolaryngology Study Guide*, https://doi.org/10.1007/978-3-031-77374-7_32

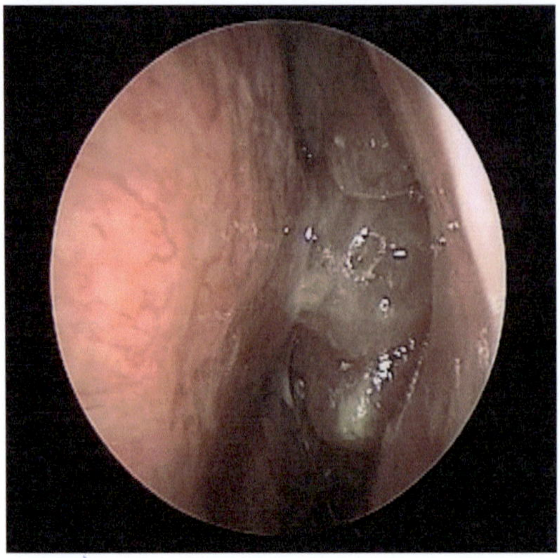

Fig. 32.1 Endoscopic view of the left nasal cavity showing nasal polys originating and extending beyond the middle meatus

Questions

1. Which of the following statements accurately define chronic rhinosinusitis (CRS)? (multiple correct answers possible)
   A. The symptoms should persist for a minimum of 12 weeks in both adults and children
   B. Nasal blockage/obstruction/congestion or nasal discharge should always be present in adults, but not necessarily in children with CRS
   C. It is defined by the occurrence of two or more symptoms in both adults and children, one of which must be facial pain/pressure
   D. In adults, a decrease in or complete loss of smell must always be a symptom
   E. In children, cough can be one of the two symptoms used to diagnose CRS
2. Which statements are accurate regarding CRS? (multiple correct answers possible)
   A. CRSwNP is linked to increased T helper (Th)-1 cytokine expression
   B. The presence of *Staphylococcus aureus* on the sinonasal mucosa has been connected to chronic rhinosinusitis with nasal polyps (CRSwNP)
   C. Biofilms are believed to cause persistent, hard-to-treat disease
   D. Fungi have been exclusively associated with allergic fungal rhinosinusitis
   E. Nearly all individuals with cystic fibrosis experience CRS symptoms
3. Which of the following are warning signs and symptoms that need immediate referral ENT doctor? (multiple correct answers possible)
   A. Bilateral symptoms
   B. Blood-stained rhinorrhea, bleeding
   C. Facial pressure
   D. Reduced or double vision
   E. Frontal swelling
4. What types of medical treatments are recommended in adult CRS? (multiple correct answers possible)
   A. Nasal irrigation with saline
   B. Nasal corticosteroids
   C. Systemic corticosteroids
   D. Antihistamines
   E. Topical antibiotics
5. Which of the following are true about surgical management of CRS (multiple correct answers possible)
   A. Functional Endoscopic Sinus Surgery (FESS) can be used as the first treatment prior to medical therapy
   B. The aim of surgery is to restore sinus aeration and drainage by enlarging sinus ostia while destroying the sinus mucosa.
   C. CRSwNP patients have a higher risk for revision sinus surgery.
   D. CRSwNP patients with concomitant asthma have a higher risk for revision sinus surgery
   E. Dupilumab is a monoclonal antibody indicated for patients with bilateral polyps who had had sinus surgery.

Correct Answers

1. A, B, E

   CRS (with or without nasal polyps) in adults is the inflammation of the nose and paranasal sinuses characterized by the presence of two or more symptoms for ≥12 weeks.

One of which should be nasal blockage/obstruction/congestion or nasal discharge (anterior/posterior nasal drip):

- ± facial pain/pressure
- ± reduction in or loss of smell

with validation by telephone or interview [1].

CRS (with or without nasal polyps) in children is the inflammation of the nose and paranasal sinuses characterized by the presence of two or more symptoms for ≥12 weeks.

One of which should be nasal blockage / obstruction / congestion or nasal discharge (anterior / posterior nasal drip):

- ± facial pain/pressure
- ± cough

with validation by telephone or interview [1].

2. B, C

Chronic rhinosinusitis with nasal polyps (CRSwNP) is associated with high tissue eosinophilia and an increase in T helper (Th)-2 cytokine expression, specifically interleukin (IL)-5 and IL-13. In contrast, chronic rhinosinusitis without polyps (CRSsNP) typically exhibits Th-1 polarization and less eosinophilic infiltration [2]. Over half of CRSwNP patients have been found to have *Staphylococcus aureus* colonization in the sinonasal mucosa. The exotoxins produced by this bacterium, which act as superantigens, can trigger T cell activation and massive proliferation, leading to the formation of polyps [3]. Biofilms, which provide bacteria with a protective barrier against both host defense mechanisms and antibiotics, are believed to contribute to recurrent, stubborn disease. Various bacterial species, including *Haemophilus influenzae*, *Staphylococcus aureus*, *Streptococcus pneumoniae*, and *Moraxella catarrhalis*, have been identified in CRS biofilms [4]. Interestingly, fungi have been detected in the sinonasal mucosa of nearly all CRS patients and controls in several studies. The "Fungal Hypothesis of CRS" suggests that an overactive, non-IgE-mediated response to common airborne fungi could be the underlying cause of both CRSwNP and CRSsNP [4, 5]. In the context of cystic fibrosis, up to 100% of patients exhibit radiologic and endoscopic signs of sinonasal pathology, and two-thirds have nasal polyposis. However, less than 20% of cystic fibrosis patients report symptoms of CRS [6].

3. B, D, E

Cardinal symptoms of CRS consist of ongoing persistent nasal obstruction, postnasal drip, complete (anosmia), or reduced (hyposmia) loss of smell, facial pain, headache, facial pressure, and purulent nasal discharge. Both allergic and non-allergic rhinitis, nasal turbinate enlargement, septal deviation, and vasculitis should be considered in the differential diagnosis of CRS. Furthermore, benign growths like inverted papilloma, antrochoanal polyp, angiofibroma, and encephalocele, as well as malignant tumors such as squamous cell carcinoma (SCC), esthesioneuroblastoma, nasal lymphoma, and rhabdomyosarcoma should always be taken into account. Red flag signs and symptoms that require immediate referral to an ENT specialist include: one-sided symptoms (e.g., unilateral nasal obstruction), blood-tinged rhinorrhea, bleeding, crusting, cacosmia, orbital symptoms, periorbital swelling, displaced eye globe, reduced or double vision, ophthalmoplegia, intense unilateral or bilateral frontal headache, frontal swelling, and indications of meningitis or focal neurological signs [7, 8].

4. A, B, C

Several studies have thoroughly assessed the effectiveness of nasal irrigation, and the application of nasal saline irrigation using isotonic saline or Ringer's lactate is advised. A substantial amount of evidence suggests that the long-term use of intranasal corticosteroids is both safe and effective in treating patients with Chronic Rhinosinusitis (CRS), enhancing nasal symptoms and overall quality of life. A short course of systemic corticosteroids, whether combined with local corticosteroid treatment or not, has proven effective in reducing nasal symptoms and shrinking polyp size. Short courses of oral steroid treatment, administered once or twice annually, can improve the management of chronic rhinosinusitis with nasal polyps. While oral steroids can be safely taken for short durations, they are typically not continued over the long term due to their potential side effects. However, there is a lack of sufficient data to support the regular use of antihistamines in treating patients with CRS; hence, their use is not recommended. Additionally, topical antibiotics have not demonstrated any significant advantage over a placebo in patients with CRS [1].

5. C, D, E

   Surgery is typically only recommended for both CRSwNP and CRSsNP patients who who have failed adequate control with medical treatment [1]. FESS aims to open up the sinus openings, improve sinus ventilation and mucus drainage, and provide better access for medication administration while respecting sinonasal mucosa [1, 9]. Patients with chronic rhinosinusitis with nasal polyps and asthma are at higher risk of needing repeat surgery [1, 10]. New monoclonal antibody treatments, which target type 2 inflammation, are now available for severe chronic rhinosinusitis with nasal polyps that does not improve with other treatments. Three monoclonal antibodies approved for chronic rhinosinusitis with nasal polyps in the United States are dupilumab, omalizumab, and mepolizumab. Specifically, dupilumab is a fully human monoclonal antibody that blocks interleukin-4 and interleukin-13, which are key drivers of type 2 inflammation. It is approved for patients with nasal polyps on both sides of the nose who have already had sinus surgery [1, 11].

References

1. Fokkens WJ, Lund VJ, Hopkins C, et al. European position paper on rhinosinusitis and nasal polyps 2020. Rhinology. 2020;58(Suppl S29):1–464. Published 2020 Feb 20.
2. Van Zele T, Claeys S, Gevaert P, et al. Differentiation of chronic sinus diseases by measurement of inflammatory mediators. Allergy. 2006;61(1): 1280–9.
3. Chegini Z, Didehdar M, Khoshbayan A, Karami J, Yousefimashouf M, Shariati A. The role of Staphylococcus aureus enterotoxin B in chronic rhinosinusitis with nasal polyposis. Cell Commun Signal. 2022;20(1):29.
4. Bachert C, Pawankar R, Zhang L, Bunnag C, Fokkens WJ, Hamilos DL, Jirapongsananuruk O, Kern R, Meltzer EO, Mullol J, Naclerio R, Pilan R, Rhee CS, Suzaki H, Voegels R, Blaiss M. ICON: chronic rhinosinusitis. World Allergy Organ J. 2014;7(1):25.
5. Ponikau JU, Sherris DA, Kern EB, et al. The diagnosis and incidence of allergic fungal sinusitis. Mayo Clin Proc. 1999;74(9):877–84.
6. Tipirneni KE, Woodworth BA. Medical and surgical advancements in the management of cystic fibrosis chronic rhinosinusitis. Curr Otorhinolaryngol Rep. 2017;5(1):24–34.
7. Al-Ahmad M, Alsaleh S, Al-Reefy H, et al. Expert opinion on biological treatment of chronic rhinosinusitis with nasal polyps in the Gulf region. J Asthma Allergy. 2022;15:1–12. Published 2022 Jan 4.
8. London NR Jr, Reh DD. Differential diagnosis of chronic rhinosinusitis with nasal polyps. Adv Otorhinolaryngol. 2016;79:1–12.
9. Bachert C, Zhang L, Gevaert P. Current and future treatment options for adult chronic rhinosinusitis: focus on nasal polyposis. J Allergy Clin Immunol. 2015;136(6):1431–40.
10. Gill AS, Smith KA, Meeks H, et al. Asthma increases long-term revision rates of endoscopic sinus surgery in chronic rhinosinusitis with and without nasal polyposis. Int Forum Allergy Rhinol. 2021;11(8):1197–206.
11. Book R, Eligal S, Tal Y, Eliashar R. Biological treatment for uncontrolled chronic rhinosinusitis with nasal polyps: preliminary real-world results from a Tertiary Medical Center. J Clin Med. 2023;12(11):3671. Published 2023 May 25.

Olfactory Disorders

33

Konstantinos Garefis and Nikolaos Tsetsos

Abstract

Olfactory disorders are frequently reported by adults and can significantly affect their overall quality of life. These problems can manifest in both quantitative and qualitative ways. The incidence of olfactory disorders exceeds 20%, with 15% experiencing hyposmia (reduced sense of smell) and 5% experiencing anosmia (complete loss of smell). Various factors contribute to these disturbances, including inflammatory conditions in the sinonasal region, viral upper respiratory tract infections, head trauma, aging, neurodegenerative diseases, and exposure to toxic substances. A comprehensive approach is essential for accurately diagnosing and managing olfactory disorders. This includes a thorough assessment of medical history, nasal examination with endoscopy, psychophysical olfaction testing (the most common diagnostic method), subjective evaluation, and, in some cases, imaging studies. The choice of therapy for olfactory disorders depends on the underlying cause. Treatment options may include pharmaceutical agents, such as corticosteroids, and olfactory training, which has been shown to be effective in addressing many causative factors.

K. Garefis
2nd Academic ORL, Head and Neck Surgery Department, Aristotle University of Thessaloniki, Papageorgiou Hospital, Thessaloniki, Greece

N. Tsetsos (✉)
ENT Head and Neck Surgery Department, 424 General Military Hospital, Thessaloniki, Greece

Case Presentation

A 45-year-old female visited the Ear, Nose, and Throat (ENT) Department due to a five-month period of anosmia (loss of smell). She also mentioned that certain odors were perceived as unpleasant. The onset of these symptoms was sudden, and the patient linked them to a COVID-19 infection she had experienced five months earlier. Nasoendoscopy and the rest of the ENT examination showed normal results. Olfactory function was evaluated using the Sniffin' Sticks test (Fig. 33.2), which indicated hyposmia (Fig. 33.1).

Questions

1. Which of the following are the most common causes of olfactory disorders?
   A. Chronic rhinosinusitis, allergic rhinitis, viral infection
   B. Head trauma, chronic rhinosinusitis, idiopathic
   C. Allergic rhinitis, congenital, aging
   D. Covid-19 infection, chronic rhinosinusitis, head trauma
   E. Infections, iatrogenic, tumors

N. Tsetsos et al. (eds.), *Otolaryngology Study Guide*, https://doi.org/10.1007/978-3-031-77374-7_33

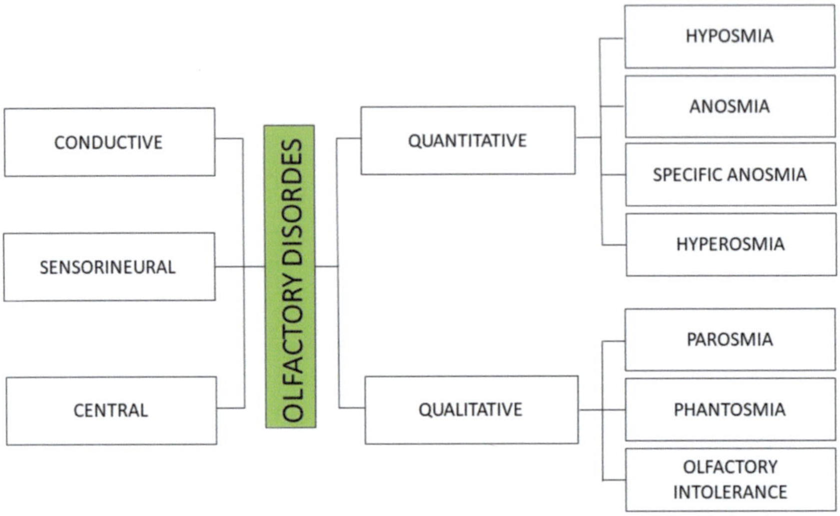

Fig. 33.1 Classification of olfactory disorders—dysfunction

2. The olfactory system is closely related to which cranial nerve? (more than one correct answer possible)
   A. Cranial nerve V (Trigeminal)
   B. Cranial nerve VII (Facial)
   C. Cranial nerve IX (Glossopharyngeal)
   D. Cranial nerve I (Olfactory)
   E. Cranial nerve X (Vagus)
3. Which of the following methods is appropriate for assessing olfactory disorders? (more than one correct answer possible)
   A. Nasoendoscopy
   B. Brain magnetic resonance imaging
   C. Sniffin' Sticks battery test
   D. UPSIT test
   E. All of the above
4. According to the Sniffin' Sticks battery test, the patient has a TDI score of 18. What is the diagnosis for the patient described above? (more than one correct answer possible)
   A. Post-viral hyposmia
   B. Congenital anosmia
   C. Parosmia
   D. Presbyosmia
   E. Phantosmia
5. Which of the following therapies would you recommend for the patient? (more than one correct answer possible)
   A. Corticosteroids
   B. Monoclonal antibodies
   C. Olfactory training
   D. Doxycycline
   E. All of the above

Correct Answers

1. D

   The most common causes of olfactory disorders are post-infectious olfactory dysfunction (OD) (COVID-19-associated and non-COVID-19-associated, due to rhinoviruses, parainfluenza, etc.), OD secondary to sinonasal disease (mainly rhinosinusitis), and post-traumatic OD. However, there are several etiologies for olfactory disorders including: OD associated with neurological disease, OD associated with exposure to drugs/toxins, congenital OD, OD associated with aging (presbyosmia), other possible causes such as iatrogenic complications (e.g., sinonasal and skull base surgery), tumors, multiple systemic co-morbidities, and idiopathic OD [1, 2].

2. A, D

   The olfactory system consists of two main components essential for perceiving odors: the peripheral and central divisions [1, 3]. The peripheral olfactory system comprises the olfactory epithelium and nerve fascicles, while the central olfactory system encompasses the olfactory bulb and its central connections. Olfactory perception relies on approximately 6–30 million neurosensory cells located within the olfactory neuroepithelium in the posterosuperior region of each nasal cavity. Unlike other nerves, the olfactory nerve does not form a single bundle; instead, olfactory axons join with other axons to create small bundles known as fila olfactoria. These bundles exit the nasal cavity, traverse the ethmoid bone's lamina cribrosa, and enter the brain. Collectively, these fascicles constitute the olfactory nerve. Notably, olfactory sensory neurons, whose axons comprise the olfactory nerve, establish a direct connection between the nasal cavity and the brain, without any intermediary relay. Inside the brain, the olfactory nerve terminates in the olfactory bulb, where its neurons receive synaptic connections from the terminals of the olfactory axon [4]. Numerous odors can simultaneously activate the olfactory and trigeminal nerves, especially when they are present in high concentrations [5]. For example, the sensation of cooling produced by menthol and the tingling sensation induced by carbon dioxide in carbonated drinks are both perceived through the trigeminal nerve in the nasal region [1, 5]. These two systems closely interact at both central and peripheral levels of neural processing, indicating a potential interdependence [5]. As a result, the trigeminal nerve plays multiple roles, contributing to functions such as olfaction, nasal airflow, and nasal defense mechanisms [5, 6]. It provides innervation to both nasal cavities, with the anterior section receiving branches from the anterior ethmoidal and infraorbital nerves, and the posterior part being innervated by fibers from the posterior superior medial nasal nerve and nasopalatine nerve [5].

3. E

   The evaluation of the sense of smell involves a comprehensive assessment, including the patient's medical history, clinical examination, chemosensory testing, and potentially structural imaging. Patients should undergo a thorough examination by an ENT specialist, which should include nasal endoscopy to carefully inspect the olfactory cleft. Subjective evaluations are crucial to fully understand their quality of life and the impact of the condition. These assessments can be facilitated through the use of validated questionnaires or recognized evaluation methods, such as a visual analogue scale, when questionnaires are not feasible. The most commonly employed approach to evaluate OD involves psychophysical assessments. These evaluations typically consist of tests measuring odor threshold and/or one of odor identification or discrimination. A wide range of validated psychophysical olfactory tests are available, with the Sniffin Sticks, University of Pennsylvania Smell Identification Test (UPSIT), and Connecticut Chemosensory Clinical Research Center (CCCRC) test being among the most widely accepted and validated [1]. Electrophysiological tests, like olfactory-evoked potentials and electroencephalography, provide an objective assessment of olfactory function. However, these tests necessitate specialized and costly equipment, as well as high levels of expertise [1, 7]. When it comes to structural imaging, the choice of imaging method depends on the suspected underlying cause. Computed Tomography (CT) is the initial choice for imaging the paranasal sinuses when there are suspicions of sinonasal inflammation or bony abnormalities. Magnetic Resonance Imaging (MRI) should be the first choice when intracranial abnormalities are suspected, or when measuring the size of the olfactory bulbs is necessary. Notably, MRI can provide valuable insights in cases of congenital anosmia or post-traumatic olfactory dysfunction, revealing characteristic patterns that confirm the suspected cause, such as aplastic or hypoplastic olfactory bulbs and olfactory sulcus in congenital anosmia, or specific post-traumatic lesions [1, 7, 8].

4. A, C

   Olfactory disorders can be classified into two main types: quantitative and qualitative. Quantitative smell disorders encompass conditions such as anosmia (total loss of smell), specific anosmia (difficulty smelling a particular odor while maintaining the ability to

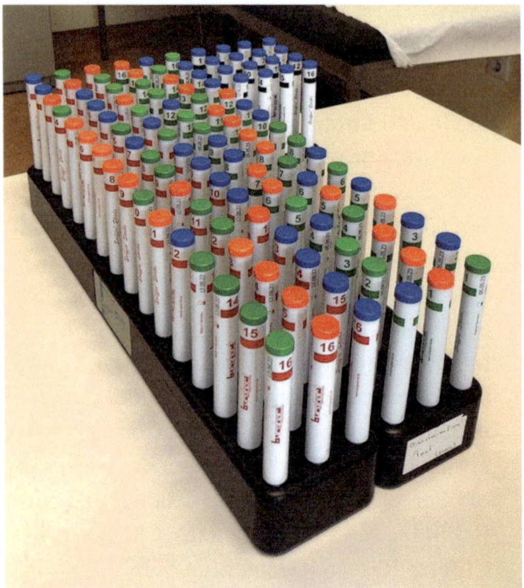

Fig. 33.2 The Sniffin' Stick battery test

detect most other odors), hyposmia (reduced sense of smell), and hyperosmia (heightened sensitivity to odors). On the other hand, qualitative smell disorders consist of olfactory intolerance (an increased sensitivity to everyday smells without distortion), parosmia (perception of odors as distorted in the presence of a smell source), and phantosmia (perceiving odors when there are no actual stimuli) [1, 7]. Parosmia and phantosmia often co-occur, typically following post-viral or post-traumatic disorders. Qualitative OD usually accompanies quantitative smell disorders like hyposmia and anosmia [1, 9]. OD can also be categorized based on the location of the lesion: conductive dysfunction occurs due to a blockage that hinders the transmission of odors to the olfactory neuroepithelium, sensorineural dysfunction results from damage or loss of the olfactory neuroepithelium or nerve, and central dysfunction arises from damage or loss of the olfactory processing pathways in the central nervous system [1] (Fig. 33.1). Regarding the TDI score, this is a measure that combines scores from Threshold, Discrimination, and Identification subtests, ranging from 1 to 48 points (Fig. 33.2). Anosmia is defined as a TDI score of ≤16.5, normosmia as a TDI score of >30.5, and hyposmia as a score falling between these two values [10].

5. C

   The existing body of evidence does not definitively endorse any particular pharmaceutical agent for the treatment of post-viral olfactory dysfunction. The efficacy of pharmacological interventions appears to be contingent upon the underlying cause of olfactory impairment. In cases of acute and chronic rhinosinusitis, where initial medical management with corticosteroids is advised, both topical and systemic steroids are commonly employed [11]. Limited supporting evidence exists for the use of steroids in addressing OD stemming from other causes [1]. Oral and topical steroids may still find utility as a short course in specific patients with olfactory dysfunction after viral infection, serving as a diagnostic tool [2]. Conversely, antibiotics do not play a role in managing post-viral olfactory dysfunction [1, 2]. For patients experiencing olfactory loss across various etiologies, olfactory training can be a beneficial approach [1]. Notably, olfactory training has demonstrated significant clinical improvements in patients with post-viral OD [11]. Additionally, monoclonal antibody therapies represent a promising and secure alternative treatment option for patients with chronic rhinosinusitis with nasal polyps [12].

References

1. Whitcroft KL, Altundag A, Balungwe P, Boscolo-Rizzo P, Douglas R, Enecilla MLB, Fjaeldstad AW, Fornazieri MA, Frasnelli J, Gane S, Gudziol H, Gupta N, Haehner A, Hernandez AK, Holbrook EH, Hopkins C, Hsieh JW, Huart C, Husain S, Kamel R, Kim JK, Kobayashi M, Konstantinidis I, Landis BN, Lechner M, Macchi A, Mazal PP, Miri I, Miwa T, Mori E, Mullol J, Mueller CA, Ottaviano G, Patel ZM, Philpott C, Pinto JM, Ramakrishnan VR, Roth Y, Schlosser RJ, Stjärne P, Van Gerven L, Vodicka J, Welge-Luessen A, Wormald PJ, Hummel T. Position paper on olfactory dysfunction: 2023. Rhinology. 2023;61(33):1–108.
2. Addison AB, Wong B, Ahmed T, Macchi A, Konstantinidis I, Huart C, Frasnelli J, Fjaeldstad AW, Ramakrishnan VR, Rombaux P, Whitcroft KL, Holbrook EH, Poletti SC, Hsieh JW, Landis BN,

Boardman J, Welge-Lüssen A, Maru D, Hummel T, Philpott CM. Clinical Olfactory Working Group consensus statement on the treatment of postinfectious olfactory dysfunction. J Allergy Clin Immunol. 2021;147(5):1704–19.
3. Smith TD, Bhatnagar KP. Anatomy of the olfactory system. Handb Clin Neurol. 2019;164:17–28.
4. Crespo C, Liberia T, Blasco-Ibáñez JM, Nácher J, Varea E. Cranial pair I: the olfactory nerve. Anat Rec (Hoboken). 2019;302(3):405–27.
5. Hummel T, Frasnelli J. The intranasal trigeminal system. Handb Clin Neurol. 2019;164:119–34.
6. Garefis K, Konstantinidis I. The human perception of breathing: how do we perceive breathing and why surgery cannot always resolve nasal congestion. Curr Otorhinolaryngol Rep. 2023;11:245–51. https://doi.org/10.1007/s40136-023-00476-z.
7. Luke L, Lee L, Jegatheeswaran L, Philpott C. Investigations and outcomes for olfactory disorders. Curr Otorhinolaryngol Rep. 2022;10(4):377–84.
8. Van Regemorter V, Rombaux P, Dricot L, Kupers R, Grégoire A, Hox V, Huart C. Functional imaging in olfactory disorders. Curr Otorhinolaryngol Rep. 2022;10(4):421–6.
9. Landis BN, Konnerth CG, Hummel T. A study on the frequency of olfactory dysfunction. Laryngoscope. 2004;114(10):1764–9.
10. Rumeau C, Nguyen DT, Jankowski R. How to assess olfactory performance with the Sniffin' Sticks test(®). Eur Ann Otorhinolaryngol Head Neck Dis. 2016;133(3):203–6.
11. Kattar N, Do TM, Unis GD, Migneron MR, Thomas AJ, McCoul ED. Olfactory training for postviral olfactory dysfunction: systematic review and meta-analysis. Otolaryngol Head Neck Surg. 2021;164(2):244–54.
12. Tsetsos N, Markou K, Konstantinidis I. Effect of monoclonal antibodies on olfactory dysfunction caused by chronic rhinosinusitis with nasal polyps: a systematic review and meta-analysis. Int Forum Allergy Rhinol. 2020;10:893–900.

34 Mucocele of Paranasal Sinuses

Yazan Kanaan

Abstract

Paranasal sinus mucocele is a benign disease resulting from obstruction of paranasal sinus ostia, leading to the paranasal sinuses' mucus filling. This can lead to expansion and pressure on surrounding structures. The most commonly involved sinuses are the frontal and ethmoid.

Paranasal sinus mucoceles are usually caused by obstruction of the sinus ostia, which leads to mucus filling of the sinuses. They can result from chronic inflammation and obstruction of sinus ostia; they can also result from previous endoscopic sinus surgery or facial trauma resulting in sinus flow tract obstruction. Paranasal sinus mucoceles are rare in children, but cystic fibrosis should be considered, especially in the paediatric population.

Clinically, besides the usual symptoms of sinusitis, patients with mucoceles usually present specifically with headache or facial pain. However, patients can have an intracranial or orbital extension and may report visual changes or proptosis. Histologically, they are usually lined by pseudostratified columnar epithelium but, in some cases, may be associated with areas of squamous epithelium, inflammatory cell infiltration, bone resorption, and new bone formation. Surgery is the only curative treatment; endoscopic marsupialization has proven an effective therapeutic modality. Some patients with frontal mucocele will require combined access, especially when the lesion is located more laterally.

Y. Kanaan (✉)
University Hospitals Plymouth NHS Trust, Plymouth, UK

Case Presentation

A 73-year-old gentleman presented with a 2-week history of progressively worsening diplopia. He denied any nasal symptoms or recent history of sinus infection. He did not report headaches or other neurological symptoms. Neurological and eye examinations were normal. Flexible nasal endoscopy showed patent nasal cavities with no signs of infection, tumours, or nasal polyps. CT and MRI scans were requested and showed a mucocele of the right sphenoid sinus (Figs. 34.1 and 34.2).

Questions

1. Paranasal sinus mucoceles most frequently affect. (more than one correct answer possible)
   A. Frontal sinus
   B. Ethmoid sinus

N. Tsetsos et al. (eds.), *Otolaryngology Study Guide*, https://doi.org/10.1007/978-3-031-77374-7_34

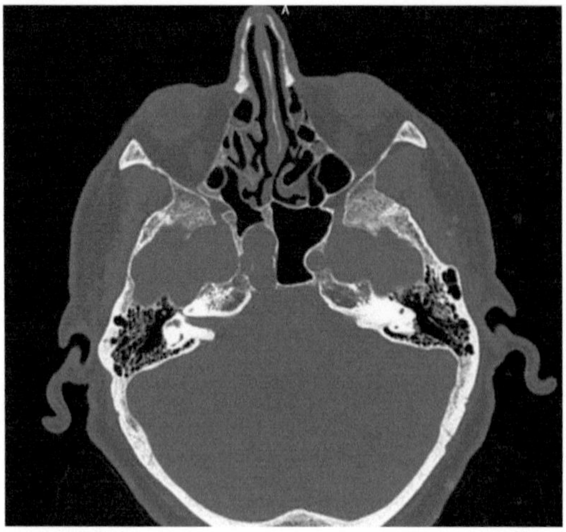

Fig. 34.1 Mucocele of the right sphenoid sinus—CT scan, axial plane

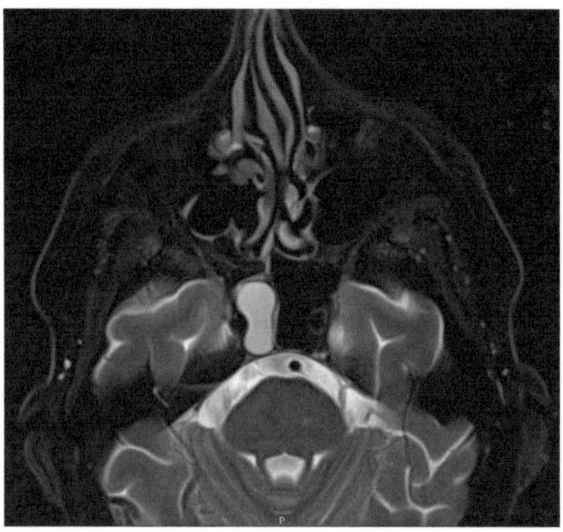

Fig. 34.2 Mucocele of the right sphenoid sinus—MRI scan, axial plane

   C. Maxillary sinus
   D. Sphenoid sinus
   E. Middle turbinate

2. Which of the following are associated with paranasal sinus mucoceles?
   A. Cystic fibrosis
   B. Previous functional endoscopic sinus surgery
   C. Trauma
   D. Sinonasal tumours
   E. All the above
3. Which of the following is not true about paranasal sinus mucoceles?
   A. The most common presenting symptoms are seizures and other neurological symptoms
   B. They are usually lines by pseudostratified columnar epithelium
   C. In the paediatric population, patients should be investigated for cystic fibrosis
   D. Surgery is the only curative treatment
   E. Patient may present with visual disturbances and proptosis
4. What is the most effective treatment modality for paranasal sinus mucoceles?
   A. Surgical drainage (endoscopic marsupialization)
   B. Steroid nasal sprays
   C. Systemic steroids
   D. Long-term intravenous antibiotics
   E. Watchful waiting
5. What are the possible complications of mucoceles? (more than one correct answer possible).
   A. Intraorbital extension
   B. Intracranial extension
   C. Epistaxis
   D. Mucopyocele
   E. TIA

Answers

1. **A and B**

   Paranasal sinus mucocele is a benign disease resulting from obstruction of paranasal sinus ostia, leading to the paranasal sinuses' mucus filling [1]. This can lead to expansion and pressure on surrounding structures. The most commonly involved sinuses are the frontal and ethmoid [1, 2].

2. **E**

   Paranasal sinus mucoceles are usually caused by obstruction of the sinus ostia, which leads to mucus filling of the sinuses. They can result from chronic inflammation and obstruction of sinus ostia; they can also result from previous endoscopic sinus surgery or facial trauma resulting in sinus flow tract obstruction [1, 3]. Paranasal sinus mucoceles are rare in children, but cystic fibrosis should be considered, especially in the paediatric population [4, 5].

3. **A**

   Clinically, besides the usual symptoms of sinusitis, patients with mucoceles usually present specifically with headache or facial pain. However, patients can have an intracranial orbital extension and may report visual changes or proptosis [1]. Histologically, they are usually lined by pseudostratified columnar epithelium but, in some cases, may be associated with areas of squamous epithelium, inflammatory cell infiltration, bone resorption, and new bone formation [6]. Surgery is the only curative treatment. Endoscopic marsupialization has proven to be an effective therapeutic modality. Some patients with frontal mucocele will require combined access, especially when the lesion is located more laterally [1].

4. **A**

   Surgery is the only curative treatment. Endoscopic marsupialization has proven to be an effective therapeutic modality. Some patients with frontal mucocele will require combined access, especially when the lesion is located more laterally [1].

5. **A, B, and D**

   If left untreated, the natural progression of the pathology may result in complications. Mucus production within the obstructed sinus leads to accumulation of secretions which may become infected, creating a mucopyocele, or they may result in expansion of the bony structures. Mucocele expansion leads to remodelling and erosion of surrounding bone, which may provide routes for intracranial or intraorbital extension. The pathophysiological mechanism of this process is rather complex. The increased pressure within the mucocele cavity causes a stress-induced bony remodelling, while chronic inflammation within the obstructed sinus leads to the release of cytokines, collagenases, and prostaglandins, which stimulate osteoclastic bone resorption [7].

References

1. Plantier DB, Neto DB, Pinna FR, Voegels RL. Mucocele: clinical characteristics and outcomes in 46 operated patients. Int Arch Otorhinolaryngol. 2019;23(1):88–91. https://doi.org/10.1055/s--0038-1668126. Epub 2018 Oct 24
2. Har-El G. Endoscopic management of 108 sinus mucoceles. Laryngoscope. 2001;111(12):2131–4. https://doi.org/10.1097/00005537-200112000-00009.
3. Obeso S, Llorente JL, Pablo Rodrigo J, Sánchez R, Mancebo G, Suárez C. Mucoceles de senos paranasales. Nuestra experiencia en 72 pacientes [Paranasal sinuses mucoceles. Our experience in 72 patients]. Acta Otorrinolaringol Esp. 2009;60(5):332–9. Spanish. https://doi.org/10.1016/j.otorri.2009.05.006. Epub 2009 Sep 5.
4. Di Cicco M, Costantini D, Padoan R, Colombo C. Paranasal mucoceles in children with cystic fibrosis. Int J Pediatr Otorhinolaryngol. 2005;69(10):1407–13. https://doi.org/10.1016/j.ijporl.2005.03.037.
5. Nicollas R, Facon F, Sudre-Levillain I, Forman C, Roman S, Triglia JM. Pediatric paranasal sinus mucoceles: etiologic factors, management and outcome. Int J Pediatr Otorhinolaryngol. 2006;70(5):905–8. https://doi.org/10.1016/j.ijporl.2005.10.002. Epub 2005 Nov 15
6. Lund VJ, Milroy CM. Fronto-ethmoidal mucocoeles: a histopathological analysis. J Laryngol Otol. 1991;105(11):921–3. https://doi.org/10.1017/s0022215100117827.
7. Scangas GA, Gudis DA, Kennedy DW. The natural history and clinical characteristics of paranasal sinus mucoceles: a clinical review. Int Forum Allergy Rhinol. 2013;3(9):712–7.

35 Cerebrospinal Fluid Leak

Yazan Kanaan and Marios Stavrakas

Abstract

Cerebrospinal fluid leak (CSF leak) is typically classified into spontaneous/idiopathic, traumatic, and iatrogenic. The most common cause of cerebrospinal fluid leak is a craniofacial trauma, making up 80% of CSF leaks in some reviews. During endoscopic sinus surgery, the most common site of injury is the cribriform plate/fovea ethmoidalis (80%) followed by the frontal and sphenoid sinuses. During neurosurgical procedures, the sphenoid sinus is the most common site of injury; this is related to the advances and frequency of transnasal endoscopic approaches to pituitary tumors. Following history taking and clinical examination, if a CSF leak is suspected, confirmation with beta-2 transferrin and/or beta-trace protein is essential. Site identification can be aided by HRCT, MRI, and CT cisternogram. Intraoperative identification of the CSF leak site can be achieved by intrathecal fluorescein or topical fluorescein application. Treatment varies depending on the cause, site, and size of defect.

Y. Kanaan
University Hospitals Plymouth NHS Trust, Plymouth, UK

M. Stavrakas (✉)
ENT Head and Neck Surgery Department, University Hospitals Plymouth NHS Trust, Plymouth, UK

Case Presentation

A 34-year-old lady was referred to the ENT clinic with a left clear nasal discharge that occurs spontaneously, worse with leaning forward. She had previous history of head trauma without any significant findings. There were no history of sinus surgery and no headache or other neurological symptoms. Nasal endoscopy was unremarkable. Sample of the fluid was sent for analysis. CT scan of the sinuses was requested followed by CT cisternogram (Fig. 35.1).

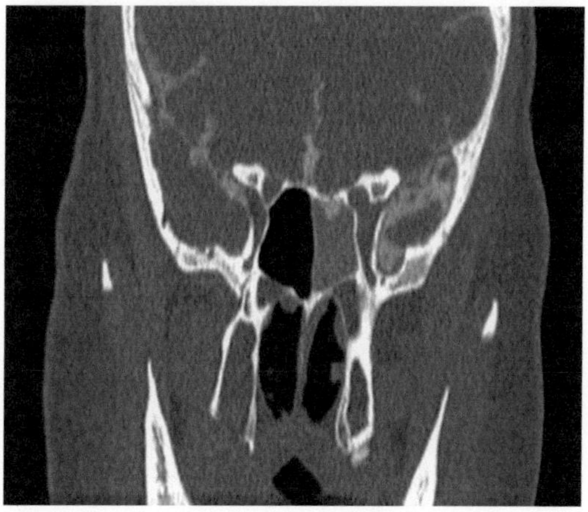

Fig. 35.1 CT cisternogram depicting a CSF leak associated with a defect at the left sphenoid sinus

N. Tsetsos et al. (eds.), *Otolaryngology Study Guide*, https://doi.org/10.1007/978-3-031-77374-7_35

Questions

1. What is the most common cause of CSF leak?
   A. Endoscopic sinus surgery
   B. Craniofacial trauma
   C. Hydrocephalus
   D. Benign intracranial hypertension
   E. Sinonasal cancer
2. The most common site of injury leading to CSF leak during neurosurgical procedures is:
   A. Cribriform plate
   B. Frontal sinus
   C. Sphenoid sinus
   D. Posterior ethmoid sinus
   E. Fovea ethmoidalis
3. Which of the following are useful in identifying the site when a CSF leak is suspected?
   A. MRV
   B. HRCT
   C. MRI FLAIR/CISS
   D. B and C
   E. Lumbar puncture
4. Which of the following statements are true about beta-2 transferrin and beta-trace protein?
   A. Beta-2 transferrin is found in CSF, perilymph, aqueous humor, and vitreous humor
   B. The sample for beta-2 transferrin testing can be stored for up to 14 days
   C. Beta-trace protein is made by the meninges
   D. None of the above
   E. All of the above
5. Which of the statements below represent diagnostic criteria for idiopathic intracranial hypertension (IIH)?
   A. Papilledema
   B. Normal neurological examination and normal CSF constituents
   C. Elevated lumbar puncture pressure ≥25 cm CSF
   D. Neuroimaging—normal brain parenchyma, venous thrombosis excluded
   E. All of the above

Answers

1. **B**

   The most common cause of cerebrospinal fluid leak is a craniofacial trauma, making up 80% of CSF leaks in some reviews. Iatrogenic causes comprise 16% of CSF leaks, with the last 4% due to varied etiologies. CSF leak is typically classified into spontaneous/idiopathic, traumatic, and iatrogenic [1–3].
2. **C**

   Around 16% of CSF leaks are a result of iatrogenic injury. During endoscopic sinus surgery, the most common site of injury is the cribriform plate/fovea ethmoidalis (80%) followed by the frontal and sphenoid sinuses. During neurosurgical procedures, the sphenoid sinus is the most common site of injury; this is related to the advances and frequency of transnasal endoscopic approaches to pituitary tumors [1, 2].
3. **D**

   Radiologically, CSF leaks can be investigated with a high-resolution CT scan (HRCT), which can demonstrate a skull base defect. It is very helpful in trauma cases, where the surgeon needs to know about other fractures or impinged bone fragments. A heavy T2 MRI can also pick up skull base CSF leaks, especially when FLAIR and CISS sequences are included. More specifically, the signal in FLAIR and CISS can help differentiate between CSF (bright in CISS, dark in FLAIR) and inflammation/edema (bright in CISS, bright in FLAIR). A CT cisternogram is also an alternative. Intraoperative intrathecal fluorescein can identify the site of leak and is extremely helpful in cases of multiple CSF leak sites and also allows control of the repair integrity [4].
4. **E**

   Beta-2 transferrin is almost exclusively found in CSF, which makes this test highly sensitive. It can also be detected in the perilymph, aqueous humor, and vitreous humor. Its sensitivity and specificity vary in the literature between 87–100% and 97–100%, respectively. Testing is most commonly performed using immunofixation electrophoresis, and a minimum of 2–5 mL of the suspected fluid is required. Beta-2 transferrin samples can be kept refrigerated or in room temperature up to 14 days until processed in the laboratory. Beta-trace protein is made by the meninges and the choroid plexus and acts as a prostaglandin D synthetase. It is found in high concentrations in the CSF, which makes it a specific marker. It is tested through nephelometric assay; it is cheaper and faster to process and has a high CSF/serum ratio. Its sensitivity is reported between 80 and 100%, and its specificity is around 100%. The test should be avoided in patients with renal insufficiency and active bacterial meningitis, as the serum or CSF levels are altered [4, 5]. There are various approaches, but the algorithm we follow in our institution is the following:

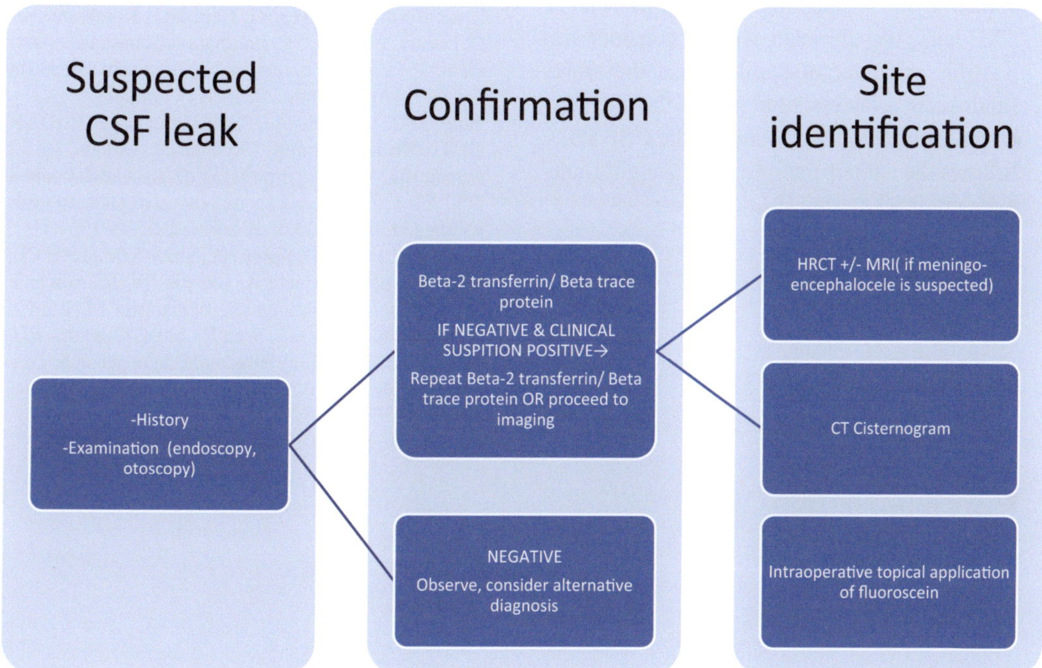

5. **E**

According to the 2018 consensus guidelines for IIH, all the statements are correct [6]. IIH can present with a variety of symptoms, with the most common being headache of increased severity and frequency, visual changes, dizziness, pulsatile tinnitus, and back pain. Less common symptoms are neck pain, blurred vision, and cognitive disturbance. Imaging findings suggestive of IIH include empty sella, flattening of the posterior aspect of the globe, distention of the perioptic subarachnoid space +/− tortuous optic nerve, and also transverse sinus stenosis [6]. When it comes to the management of IIH-associated CSF leak, the clinician should consider the possible existence of papilledema; therefore, fundoscopy is an essential part of the diagnostic pathway. Surgical closure of the CSF leaks follows the same principles, but weight management is a key step [6].

References

1. Le C, Strong EB, Luu Q. Management of anterior skull base cerebrospinal fluid leaks. J Neurol Surg B Skull Base. 2016;77(5):404–11. https://doi.org/10.1055/s--0036-1584229. Epub 2016 Jun 2.
2. Banks CA, Palmer JN, Chiu AG, O'Malley BW Jr, Woodworth BA, Kennedy DW. Endoscopic closure of CSF rhinorrhea: 193 cases over 21 years. Otolaryngol Head Neck Surg. 2009;140(6):826–33. https://doi.org/10.1016/j.otohns.2008.12.060. Epub 2009 Feb 28.
3. Ziu M, Savage JG, Jimenez DF. Diagnosis and treatment of cerebrospinal fluid rhinorrhea following accidental traumatic anterior skull base fractures. Neurosurg Focus. 2012;32(6):E3. https://doi.org/10.3171/2012.4.FOCUS1244.
4. Georgalas C, Oostra A, Ahmed S, Castelnuovo P, Dallan I, van Furth W, Harvey RJ, Herman P, Kombogiorgas D, Locatelli D, Meco C. International consensus statement: spontaneous cerebrospinal fluid rhinorrhea. Int Forum Allergy Rhinol. 2021;11(4):794–803.
5. Tang DM, Bastien AJ, Sindwani R. CHAPTER OUTLINE introduction, 19 chemical markers, 19 B2 transferrin, 19 B-trace protein, 20. In: Cerebrospinal fluid rhinorrhea-e-book: comprehensive guide to evaluation and management. Elsevier; 2023. p. 19.
6. Mollan SP, Davies B, Silver NC, Shaw S, Mallucci CL, Wakerley BR, Krishnan A, Chavda SV, Ramalingam S, Edwards J, Hemmings K, Williamson M, Burdon MA, Hassan-Smith G, Digre K, Liu GT, Jensen RH, Sinclair AJ. Idiopathic intracranial hypertension: consensus guidelines on management. J Neurol Neurosurg Psychiatry. 2018;89(10):1088–100. https://doi.org/10.1136/jnnp-2017-317440. Epub 2018 Jun 14.

36 Sinonasal Inverted Papilloma

Konstantinos Garefis and John Goudakos

Abstract

Sinonasal inverted papilloma (SNIP) is a rare benign epithelial lesion of the epithelial tissue found in the sinonasal region, accounting for 0.4–7% of tumors in this area. It is more common in men, with a male-to-female ratio ranging from 2:1 to 5:1, and typically affects adults in their fifth to sixth decades of life. While the exact cause of inverted papilloma is not fully understood, viral infections, particularly human papilloma virus (HPV), are considered a major contributing factor. Other factors that may play a role include abnormalities in cell cycle regulation, angiogenic factors, environmental and occupational exposures, and chronic inflammation. SNIP usually originates from the Schneiderian sinonasal epithelium in the lateral nasal wall. Patients with inverted papilloma often experience nonspecific symptoms such as one-sided nasal blockage, nasal polyps, nosebleeds, excessive nasal discharge, and reduced sense of smell. SNIP is clinically significant due to its tendency to grow aggressively, high likelihood of recurrence, and potential to become cancerous. Diagnosis is based on the patient's medical history, physical examination, and imaging studies, with confirmation achieved through biopsy and histological examination of the lesion. Currently, endoscopic treatment methods are considered the preferred approach, as they have shown lower recurrence rates compared to external approaches.

Case Presentation

A 58-year-old man was sent to the Ear, Nose, and Throat (ENT) Department due to ongoing issues with blockage in his right nostril and repeated nosebleeds over the last 6 months. The patient did not have any significant medical history or exposure to occupational hazards. During a nasal endoscopy, a lumpy reddish-gray growth was seen, taking up nearly the entire right nasal cavity (Fig. 36.1). The opposite nasal cavity looked normal, and no irregularities were found during a neck examination. A computed tomography (CT) scan showed a soft tissue growth coming from the side of the nasal wall, along with signs of inflammation in the bone near the growth. To investigate further, a sample of tissue was taken for examination under local anesthesia.

K. Garefis (✉)
2nd Academic ORL, Head and Neck Surgery Department, Aristotle University of Thessaloniki, Papageorgiou Hospital, Thessaloniki, Greece

J. Goudakos
ENT Head and Neck Surgery Department, 424 General Military Hospital, Thessaloniki, Greece

N. Tsetsos et al. (eds.), *Otolaryngology Study Guide*, https://doi.org/10.1007/978-3-031-77374-7_36

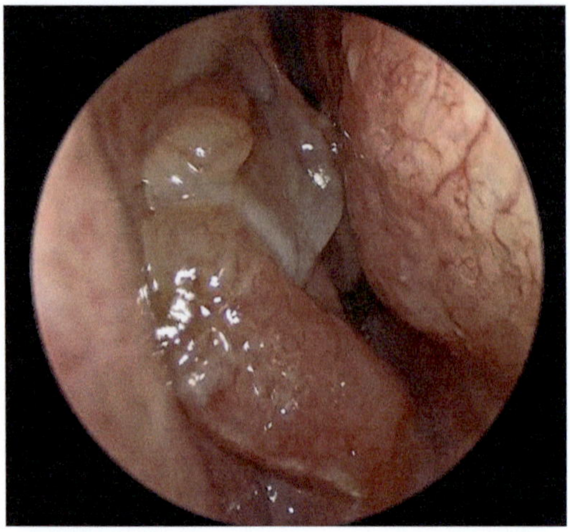

Fig. 36.1 Endoscopic image showing the mass into the right nasal cavity

Questions

1. Which of the following statements are true about SNIP (more than one correct answer possible)?
   A. It predominantly occurs in children
   B. Women affected more often
   C. The most frequent risk factor is Epstein-Barr virus (EBV)
   D. It is a malignant tumor
   E. It arises from the Schneiderian epithelium
2. Which nasal site is most commonly involved by SNIP?
   A. Olfactory cleft
   B. Lateral nasal wall
   C. Frontal sinus
   D. Sphenoid sinus
   E. Nasal septum
3. Which of the following is NOT a CT finding for SNIP?
   A. Unilateral opacification of nasal cavity
   B. Sclerotic or eroded adjacent bone
   C. Plaque-like bone thickening
   D. Lobulated soft tissue density mass
   E. Cystic mass of middle turbinate or maxillary sinus
4. What is currently the preferred treatment approach for the patient described above?
   A. Endoscopic approach
   B. Radiation therapy
   C. External paralateronasal approach with medial maxillectomy
   D. Antibiotics and corticosteroids
   E. Combination of endoscopic and external approach
5. Which of the following statements regarding the recurrence and malignant transformation of SNIP are true (more than one correct answer possible)?
   A. HPV subtypes are associated with increased risk of malignant SNIP
   B. HPV infection is not associated with the recurrence of SNIP
   C. Adenocarcinoma is the most common type of malignant SNIP
   D. The incidence of malignant SNIP is less than 30%
   E. A minimum follow-up of 2 years after treatment is required

Answers

1. **E**

The majority of SNIPs occur in individuals aged between their fifth and sixth decades, with an average age of 53 years [1, 2]. The age range of patients affected spans from 6 to 89 years, although SNIP is generally uncommon in children [2]. The behavior of the lesion in children appears to be similar to that in adults. The male-to-female ratio ranges from 3:1 to 5:1 [1, 2]. The exact etiology of inverted papilloma remains unclear. Many factors have been associated with its occurrence, including chronic inflammation, viral infections, smoking, occupational and environmental exposures, cell cycle-related proteins, and angiogenic factors. HPV is considered a significant contributing factor, while EBV has not shown a significant association [1, 3]. SNIP is a benign epithelial tumor that belongs to the sinonasal Schneiderian papilloma category. It originates from the sinonasal Schneiderian membrane, which is derived from both the neuroectoderm of the olfactory placode and the nasopharyngeal mucosa of endodermal origin. Among sinonasal papillomas, inverted, oncocytic, and exophytic papillomas account for approximately 62%, 6%, and 32%, respectively, according to the World Health Organization 2005 classification. The term "inverted papilloma" describes the histological appearance of the epithelium, with its inward growth into the stroma, while a distinct and intact basement membrane separates the epithelial component from the underlying connective tissue stroma [1, 2, 4, 5].

2. **B**

Inverted papillomas commonly originate with greater frequency from the lateral aspects, such as the lateral nasal wall and the sinuses, compared to the medial areas, including the turbinates or septum [1, 2]. The lateral nasal wall, particularly in proximity to the middle turbinate and behind the uncinate process, is the primary site of development [1]. Extension of these papillomas often involves the paranasal sinuses. Among these sinuses, the ethmoidal and maxillary sinuses are the most frequently affected sites. The prevalence of inverted papillomas involving different nasal sites, in descending order, is as follows: lateral nasal wall, ethmoid cells, maxillary sinus, and, less commonly, frontal and sphenoid sinuses, as well as the nasal septum [2].

3. **E**

The CT scan remains the preferred imaging modality for assessing SNIP, despite its limitations [1]. It can reveal specific characteristics, such as the opacification of a single nasal cavity and sinus mass [2]. Another notable finding is the presence of a lobulated mass of soft tissue density in the middle meatus region, with or without calcification, as well as lobulated margins [2, 6]. Bone remodeling is observed in a significant percentage of cases [1]. As the tumor grows, adjacent bone structures may show thinning, bowing, erosion, or sclerotic changes. Two distinct patterns of localized bone thickening can be observed on CT scans: "plaque-like bone thickening," primarily involving the lateral wall of the nasal cavity, and "cone-shaped bone thickening," which is limited to the walls of the paranasal sinuses or the bony septum. Importantly, the presence of focal hyperostosis on preoperative CT scans is strongly correlated with the origin of the inverted papilloma, providing valuable information for predicting tumor origin before surgery [1, 2, 6]. Nevertheless, magnetic resonance imaging (MRI) proves to be a highly effective method for outlining the centrifugal extent of SNIP. This is attributed to its capacity to differentiate between the tumor and inflammatory changes. MRI is particularly useful in the context of unilateral masses. An acknowledged MRI characteristic, observed in 80% of IPs, is the "convoluted cerebriform pattern" [6].

4. **C**

Surgical resection is considered the primary treatment option for SNIP, aiming to achieve complete eradication of the disease in the first attempt. A crucial principle during surgery is the removal of both the tumor and the mucoperiosteum from which the tumor originates [1]. Traditionally, external approaches such as the Caldwell-Luc procedure, lateral rhinotomy, medial maxillectomy, frontal trephination, and osteoplastic flap have commonly been used due to their extensive surgical access [1, 2]. However, the current gold standard treatment is endoscopic approaches. These endoscopic techniques offer numerous advantages, including significantly lower recurrence rates compared to open approaches, lower complication rates, shorter hospital stays, absence of external scars, and superior visualization [1, 2, 7, 8]. While combined and external approaches may still be appropriate for specific complex SNIP presentations, preoperative medical treatment often involves the administration of antibiotics and corticosteroids to reduce inflammation and intraoperative bleeding, thereby improving surgical conditions [1, 2, 5]. In some case reports, radiotherapy has been described as a treatment option when the tumor is inoperable, complete resection is impossible, or when SNIP is associated with malignancy [5]. Moreover, as an adjuvant therapy in the postoperative management of challenging SNIP, topical 5-fluorouracil, a chemotherapeutic drug, seems promising [9].

5. **A, D, E**

HPV plays a significant role in SNIP, not only as a risk factor but also in the malignant transformation and recurrence of the disease. In particular, patients infected with HPV types 16, 11/16, 18, and 16/18 are associated with an increased risk of malignant SNIP [10]. HPV infection is also significantly linked to the recurrence of SNIP, indicating its pathological involvement in the disease [11]. The reported incidence of metachronous or synchronous malignancies with SIP varies, ranging from 2 to 27%, with the most common estimation being between 5 and 10%, and a median rate of 9%. Squamous cell carcinoma is the most common malignancy observed in inverted papillomas, although other types such as adenocarcinoma, mucoepidermoid carcinoma, sinonasal undifferentiated carcinoma, and small cell carcinoma have also been reported [1, 12, 13]. Recurrence and metachronous carcinoma can develop after a prolonged period, emphasizing the importance of long-term follow-up. Incomplete resection is often implicated in recurrence, which frequently occurs at the initial inverted papilloma site, usually within 2 years of surgery [5, 12]. To mitigate these risks, recent publications suggest lifelong follow-up, particularly for advanced tumors, HPV-positive tumors, and cases of incomplete tumor resection [11, 12, 14, 15].

References

1. Upadhya IB, Rao K. Sinonasal inverted papilloma: a narrative review. Indian J Otolaryngol Head Neck Surg. 2022;74(Suppl 2):1017–22.
2. Anari S, Carrie S. Sinonasal inverted papilloma: narrative review. J Laryngol Otol. 2010;124(7):705–15.
3. Wang MJ, Noel JE. Etiology of sinonasal inverted papilloma: a narrative review. World J Otorhinolaryngol Head Neck Surg. 2016;3(1):54–8.
4. Barnes L, Eveson J, Reichart P, Sidransky D. World Health Organization classification of tumours. Pathology and genetics of head and neck tumours. Lyon: IARC Press; 2005.
5. Lisan Q, Laccourreye O, Bonfils P. Sinonasal inverted papilloma: from diagnosis to treatment. Eur Ann Otorhinolaryngol Head Neck Dis. 2016;133(5):337–41.
6. Chawla A, Shenoy J, Chokkappan K, Chung R. Imaging features of Sinonasal inverted papilloma: a pictorial review. Curr Probl Diagn Radiol. 2016;45(5):347–53. https://doi.org/10.1067/j.cpradiol.2015.10.004.
7. Peng R, Thamboo A, Choby G, Ma Y, Zhou B, Hwang PH. Outcomes of sinonasal inverted papilloma resection by surgical approach: an updated systematic review and meta-analysis. Int Forum Allergy Rhinol. 2019;9(6):573–81.
8. Goudakos JK, Blioskas S, Nikolaou A, Vlachtsis K, Karkos P, Markou KD. Endoscopic resection of Sinonasal inverted papilloma: systematic review and meta-analysis. Am J Rhinol Allergy. 2018;32(3):167–74.
9. Adriaensen GF, Lim KH, Georgalas C, Reinartz SM, Fokkens WJ. Challenges in the management of inverted papilloma: a review of 72 revision cases. Laryngoscope. 2016;126(2):322–8.
10. Ding R, Sun Q, Wang Y. Association between human papilloma virus infection and malignant Sinonasal inverted papilloma. Laryngoscope. 2021;131(6):1200–5.
11. Rha MS, Kim CH, Yoon JH, Cho HJ. Association of the human papillomavirus infection with the recurrence of sinonasal inverted papilloma: a systematic review and meta-analysis. Rhinology. 2022;60(1):2–10.
12. Suh JD, Chiu AG. What are the surveillance recommendations following resection of sinonasal inverted papilloma? Laryngoscope. 2014;124(9):1981–2.
13. Re M, Gioacchini FM, Bajraktari A, Tomasetti M, Kaleci S, Rubini C, Bertini A, Magliulo G, Pasquini E. Malignant transformation of sinonasal inverted papilloma and related genetic alterations: a systematic review. Eur Arch Otorrinolaringol. 2017;274(8):2991–3000.
14. Jiang XD, Dong QZ, Li SL, Huang TQ, Zhang NK. Endoscopic surgery of a sinonasal inverted papilloma: surgical strategy, follow-up, and recurrence rate. Am J Rhinol Allergy. 2017;31(1):51–5.
15. Binz GHA, Soyka MB, Holzmann D, Meerwein CM. Need for long-term follow-up in sinonasal inverted papilloma: a single-institution experience. Head Neck. 2021;43(2):630–8.

Nasopharyngeal Carcinoma 37

Konstantinos Garefis and Yazan Kanaan

Abstract

Nasopharyngeal carcinoma (NPC) is a relatively uncommon malignancy originating from the epithelial lining of the nasopharynx. Its global distribution shows a significant geographical imbalance, with over 70% of new cases occurring in East and Southeast Asia. The occurrence of NPC is more prevalent among males compared to females. Several risk factors contribute to its development, including Epstein-Barr virus (EBV) infection, which is a primary causal agent, as well as host genetics, ethnic, a family history of NPC, smoking, consumption of preserved foods and alcohol, and poor oral hygiene. Clinical presentation of NPC varies depending on the affected anatomical structures, and common symptoms include epistaxis, unilateral nasal obstruction, serous otitis media, cervical lymphadenopathy, and cranial nerve palsies. Approximately three-quarters of patients experience nodal metastasis in the neck. Diagnosis of NPC involves a combination of nasendoscopy, nasopharyngeal biopsy, and imaging studies such as magnetic resonance imaging (MRI), computed tomography (CT), and ^{18}F-fluorodeoxyglucose (^{18}F-FDG)-PET/CT, which are commonly used for staging and treatment planning. Radiotherapy, either as monotherapy or in combination with chemotherapy, remains the primary treatment modality for NPC. However, advances in treatment approaches, including targeted therapies and immunotherapy, are being explored and show promise in recurrent or metastatic cases.

Case Presentation

A 57-year-old male, heavy smoker for several years, presented to the ENT department with a 4-month history of progressive nasal obstruction, a sense of auditory fullness, and decreased hearing on the left side. Nasoendoscopy revealed a mass originating from the left nasopharynx (Fig. 37.1). During neck palpation, a palpable left level II cervical lymph node was detected, while otoscopy revealed left serous otitis. Further investigations included an MRI of the nasopharynx and cervical region, which confirmed the presence of a tumor involving the left nasopharyngeal wall and a pathological node in the left level II measuring approximately 3 cm (Fig. 37.2). To establish a definitive diagnosis, biopsies were performed on the nasopharyngeal tumor under local anesthesia.

K. Garefis
2nd Academic ORL, Head and Neck Surgery Department, Aristotle University of Thessaloniki, Papageorgiou Hospital, Thessaloniki, Greece

Y. Kanaan (✉)
University Hospitals Plymouth NHS Trust, Plymouth, UK

N. Tsetsos et al. (eds.), *Otolaryngology Study Guide*, https://doi.org/10.1007/978-3-031-77374-7_37

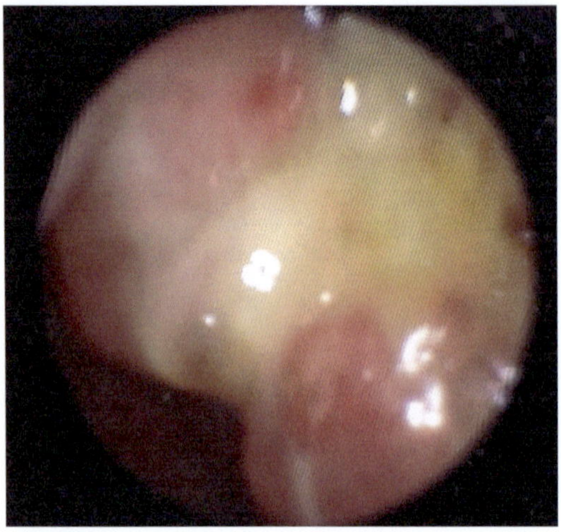

Fig. 37.1 Endoscopy image showing the mass in the nasopharynx

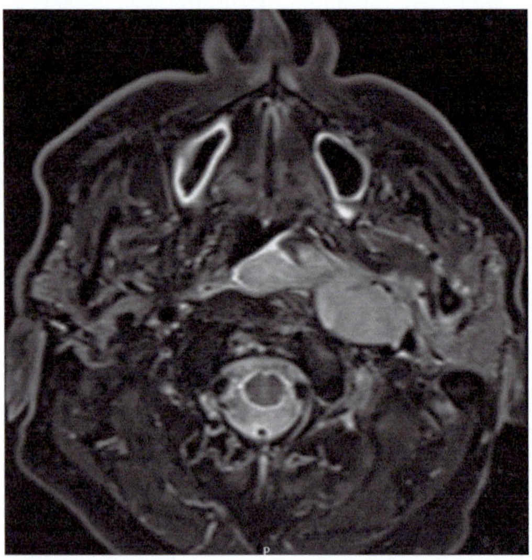

Fig. 37.2 MRI showing the tumor in the left nasopharyngeal area

Questions

1. Which of the following statements are true about nasopharyngeal carcinoma (NPC) (more than one correct answer possible)?
   A. The Asian population has a higher risk compared to Europeans.
   B. It is more frequent in females.
   C. The peak age of disease occurrence is 50–60 years.
   D. Human papilloma virus is a major risk factor.
   E. Consumption of Chinese-style salted fish is associated with the disease.
2. What is the most common site from which NPC arises?
   A. Roof of nasopharynx
   B. Fossa of Rosenmüller
   C. Torus tubarius
   D. Posterior pharyngeal wall
   E. None of the above
3. Which of the following are NOT symptoms or clinical presentations of NPC (more than one correct answer possible)?
   A. Acute otitis media
   B. Epistaxis
   C. Anosmia
   D. Cervical lump
   E. Diplopia
4. What are the potential therapies for NPC (more than one correct answer possible)?
   A. Surgery
   B. Radiation
   C. Chemotherapy
   D. Immunotherapy
   E. All of the above
5. Plasma EBV DNA assessment (more than one correct answer possible):
   A. It is a prognostic pretreatment marker.
   B. It is a recurrence marker.
   C. It is used for screening asymptomatic individuals for NPC.
   D. It has a sensitivity and specificity for NPC >95%.
   E. All of the above.

Answers

1. **A, C, E**

The global distribution of NPC is highly imbalanced, with most cases concentrated in East and Southeast Asia. Incidence rates range from 3.0 per 100,000 in China to 0.4 per 100,000 in predominantly white populations [1]. Indigenous populations in Southeast Asia, the Arctic region, North Africa, and the Middle East also show intermediate NPC rates. Males consistently have a two- to threefold higher incidence of NPC compared to females [2]. In China, males experience an incidence rate approximately 2.5 times higher than females [1]. High-risk populations typically peak in NPC incidence between ages 50 and 60, while low-risk populations have a smaller peak during young adulthood (ages 15–24) and a larger peak around ages 65–79 [2, 3]. The International Agency for Research on Cancer (IARC) identifies EBV infection, preserved food consumption, and tobacco smoking as established environmental factors contributing to NPC [2]. EBV infection is considered the primary causal factor [1]. Although HPV and hepatitis B and C viruses have been studied, no definitive causal links with NPC have been established [2]. HPV, more commonly associated with non-endemic NPC, may contribute to both keratinizing and non-keratinizing nasopharyngeal carcinoma, especially among white individuals [3]. Processed food consumption, particularly Chinese-style salted fish, is classified as a known cause [2, 4]. The carcinogenic mechanism of Chinese-style salt-preserved fish is believed to involve dietary exposure to substances like N-nitrosamines, bacterial mutagens, direct genotoxins, and agents that reactivate EBV [2].

2. **B**

   The most common site from which NPC arises is the pharyngeal recess known as the fossa of Rosenmüller. This specific location is situated superior and posterior to the torus tubarius, which is the cartilage covering the Eustachian tubes in the upper and posterior regions [1, 5].

3. **C**

   The clinical presentation and symptoms of NPC can vary depending on the specific anatomical structures affected by the tumor. The presence of a tumor mass in the nasopharynx can lead to symptoms such as epistaxis, nasal obstruction, and nasal discharge. Dysfunction of the Eustachian tube, due to the tumor's extension into the paranasopharyngeal space, may cause symptoms such as ear pain, tinnitus, and hearing loss. If the tumor extends superiorly, it can erode the skull base and result in cranial nerve involvement, leading to symptoms like headache, diplopia, facial pain, and numbness. The most commonly affected cranial nerves are the third, fifth, sixth, and twelfth nerves. Commonly, the presence of neck masses, particularly in the upper neck and involving the retropharyngeal and level II neck nodes, is frequently observed. Nodal metastasis in the neck occurs in approximately three-quarters of patients [3, 6]. Uncommonly, patients with nasopharyngeal carcinoma experience symptoms like anorexia and weight loss, which may indicate distant spread of the disease. A study examining symptoms at presentation identified neck mass as the most prevalent symptom (76%), followed by nasal dysfunction (73%), aural dysfunction (62%), headache (35%), diplopia (11%), facial numbness (8%), weight loss (7%), and trismus (3%). Enlarged neck nodes (75%) and cranial nerve palsy (20%) were the primary physical signs noted during diagnosis [6, 7].

4. **B, C, D**

   The extensive implementation of intensity-modulated radiotherapy, along with the optimization of chemotherapy strategies (including induction, concurrent, and adjuvant approaches), has significantly contributed to improved survival rates while minimizing the negative effects of treatment in NPC [1]. Radiotherapy remains the cornerstone in the management of nonmetastatic NPC. Over time, photon-based radiotherapy techniques have progressed from conventional two-dimensional (2D) methods to 3D conformal radiotherapy, with intensity-modulated radiotherapy (IMRT) currently being the most widely utilized technique [1, 8, 9]. In the case of early-stage nasopharyngeal carcinoma, radiotherapy alone serves as the primary curative treatment. The integration of chemotherapy with radiotherapy has emerged as a vital development in the treatment of locally advanced disease [1]. According to guidelines, there is evidence supporting both concurrent chemoradiotherapy with adjuvant chemotherapy or induction chemotherapy followed by concurrent chemoradiation for stage II–IVA nasopharyngeal carcinoma [10]. Immune checkpoint therapies have made significant advancements in treating recurrent or metastatic NPC, offering a promising future for the management of this condition. Tumor immunotherapy, including strategies such as EBV-directed vaccination, adoptive T-cell therapy, and immune checkpoint blockade, holds great promise as a therapeutic approach for NPC [1].

5. **E**

Plasma EBV DNA has demonstrated utility in various aspects of NPC management. It has been utilized for screening asymptomatic individuals in endemic areas for NPC. Additionally, it is employed in the pretreatment evaluation of patients to determine prognosis. Moreover, it plays a role in post-treatment management by assessing the likelihood of disease progression or recurrence. This aids in identifying patients who may benefit from adjuvant treatment or require closer monitoring. Plasma EBV DNA is also valuable for early detection of disease recurrence during follow-up in successfully treated patients. In cases of recurrent/metastatic NPC, it serves as a tool to monitor disease progression, evaluate response to palliative therapy, and potentially assess life expectancy [1, 11]. Real-time polymerase chain reaction (PCR) is the preferred method for measuring EBV DNA levels [11]. Lastly, a recent study demonstrated the usefulness of plasma EBV DNA detection, yielding a sensitivity of 97.1% and specificity of 98.6% [12].

References

1. Chen YP, Chan ATC, Le QT, Blanchard P, Sun Y, Ma J. Nasopharyngeal carcinoma. Lancet. 2019;394(10192):64–80.
2. Chang ET, Ye W, Zeng YX, Adami HO. The evolving epidemiology of nasopharyngeal carcinoma. Cancer Epidemiol Biomarkers Prev. 2021;30(6):1035–47.
3. Chua MLK, Wee JTS, Hui EP, Chan ATC. Nasopharyngeal carcinoma. Lancet. 2016;387(10022):1012–24.
4. Feng H, Zhou Y, Wang L, Wang Y, Zhou S, Tian F. Consumption of processed food and risk of nasopharyngeal carcinoma: a systematic review and meta-analysis. Transl Cancer Res. 2022;11(4):872–9.
5. Jeyakumar A, Brickman TM, Jeyakumar A, Doerr T. Review of nasopharyngeal carcinoma. Ear Nose Throat J. 2006;85(3):168–70, 172–3, 184.
6. Wei WI, Sham JS. Nasopharyngeal carcinoma. Lancet. 2005;365(9476):2041–54.
7. Lee AWM, Foo W, Law SCK, et al. Nasopharyngeal carcinoma-presenting symptoms and duration before diagnosis. HK Med J. 1997;3:355–61.
8. Zhang B, Mo Z, Du W, Wang Y, Liu L, Wei Y. Intensity-modulated radiation therapy versus 2D-RT or 3D-CRT for the treatment of nasopharyngeal carcinoma: a systematic review and meta-analysis. Oral Oncol. 2015;51:1041–6.
9. Co J, Mejia MB, Dizon JM. Evidence on effectiveness of intensity-modulated radiotherapy versus 2-dimensional radiotherapy in the treatment of nasopharyngeal carcinoma: meta-analysis and a systematic review of the literature. Head Neck. 2016;38(suppl 1):E2130–42.
10. Colevas AD, Yom SS, Pfister DG, et al. NCCN guidelines insights: head and neck cancers, version 1.2018. J Natl Compr Cancer Netw. 2018;16:479–90.
11. Chan KCA, Woo JKS, King A, et al. Analysis of plasma Epstein-Barr virus DNA to screen for nasopharyngeal cancer. New Engl J Med. 2017;377:513–22.
12. Trevisiol C, Gion M, Vaona A, Fabricio ASC, Roca E, Licitra L, Alfieri S, Bossi P. The appropriate use of circulating EBV-DNA in nasopharyngeal carcinoma: comprehensive clinical practice guidelines evaluation. Oral Oncol. 2021;114:105128.

Sinonasal Malignancy

38

Konstantinos Geronatsios

Abstract

Sinonasal malignant tumors are rare, accounting for less than 1% of all malignancies and approximately 3–5% of head and neck malignancies. The most common type is squamous cell carcinoma, followed by adenocarcinoma. Other less common types are adenoid cystic carcinoma, esthesioneuroblastoma, mucosal malignant melanoma, and undifferentiated carcinoma. Common symptoms of sinonasal malignancy include nasal obstruction, episodes of epistaxis, recurrent sinusitis, sinus pain, otalgia, rhinorrhea, tearing from one nostril, loss of smell, and facial swelling. Other symptoms such as an asymptomatic neck mass, facial paresthesia, cranial nerve palsy (paralysis), proptosis, diplopia - visual disturbances, loosening of teeth, and trismus may indicate advanced disease. The clinical diagnostic process includes anterior rhinoscopy, nasendoscopy, examination of the oral cavity, neck palpation, cranial nerve examination, and ophthalmologic examination. MRI scan and CT scan are the preferred imaging tools for assessing and planning surgical treatment for malignant sinonasal tumors. Intestinal type adenocarcinoma of the paranasal sinuses is considered an occupational disease, particularly affecting workers exposed to wood or leather dust. Smoking is also associated with sinonasal malignancies. Adenocarcinoma typically arises from the ethmoid sinuses, in contrast to SCC, which usually arises from the maxillary sinuses. Most sinonasal malignant tumors are treated surgically. For patients with advanced disease, a multimodality treatment approach including surgery and chemoradiotherapy should be considered.

Case Presentation

A 75-year-old male was referred to the ENT clinic with complaints of right nasal obstruction, nasal discharge, recurrent unilateral epistaxis, numbness, and a feeling of pressure on the right side of his face. He also reports recent-onset diplopia. In terms of his medical history, he is a former smoker and has a history of dyslipidemia and hypertension. He worked as a woodworker in a furniture industry for 35 years. During the examination, a large irregular soft tissue mass is observed, occupying the right nasal cavity. The patient also exhibits hypoesthesia on the right side of his face. Medial rectus muscle palsy and mild proptosis are noted on the right side. A CT sinus scan was requested for further evaluation (Fig. 38.1).

K. Geronatsios (✉)
ENT Head and Neck Surgery Department,
424 General Military Hospital, Thessaloniki, Greece

N. Tsetsos et al. (eds.), *Otolaryngology Study Guide*, https://doi.org/10.1007/978-3-031-77374-7_38

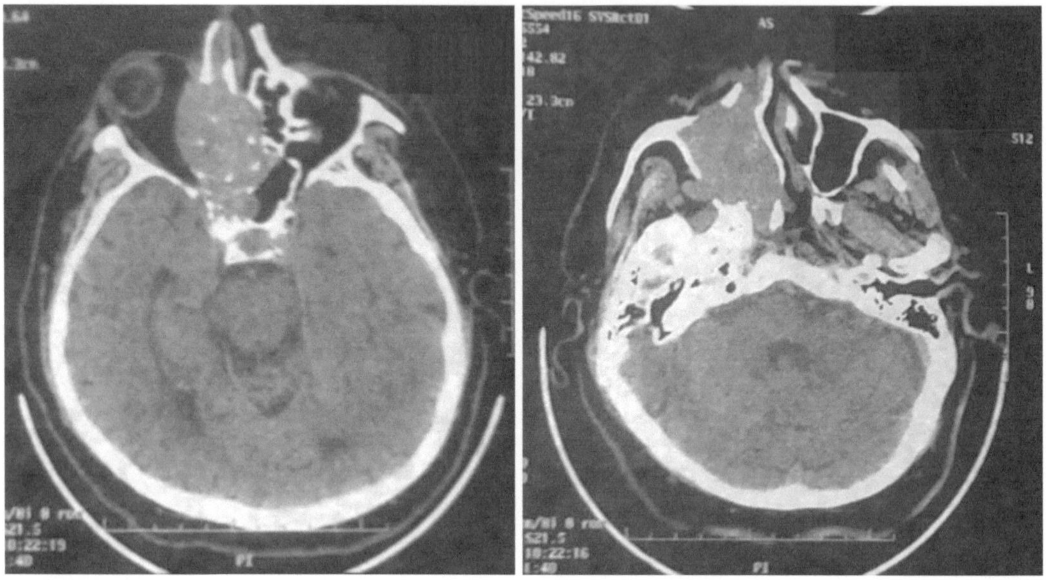

Fig. 38.1 Large soft tissue density mass occupying the maxillary and ethmoid sinuses on the right nasal cavity. You can also notice the invasion of lamina papyracea and right medial rectus muscle

Questions

1. Which of the following statements are true about malignant sinonasal tumors (more than one correct answer possible)?
   A. Squamous cell carcinoma is the commonest malignant sinonasal tumor.
   B. Proptosis and diplopia are not considered signs of advanced disease.
   C. Unilateral epistaxis and obstruction are "red flag symptoms" of sinonasal tumors.
   D. Cranial nerve examination should be performed in all cases of suspected sinonasal malignancy.
   E. In cases of sinonasal malignancy, c-ANCA test may be positive.
2. Which imaging study would you prefer preoperatively to exclude perineural invasion and to distinguish the tumor from the surrounding secretions?
   A. Plain X-ray of the sinuses
   B. Sinus CT scan
   C. Whole-body PET/CT scan
   D. Sinus MRI scan
   E. Gallium-67 scintigraphy
3. Which is the most possible diagnosis, based on the medical history and the clinical and radiological findings, for the above patient?
   A. Squamous cell carcinoma
   B. Adenocarcinoma
   C. Malignant sinonasal melanoma
   D. Undifferentiated carcinoma
   E. Nasal lymphoma
4. How would you stage the above sinonasal tumor, based on the TNM system?
   A. T2
   B. T1
   C. T3
   D. Tis (in situ)
   E. T4
5. Which of the following statements are correct for the treatment of malignant sinonasal tumors (more than one correct answer possible)?
   A. Surgical treatment is indicated in most cases of sinonasal carcinomas.
   B. Adenocarcinomas are usually radiosensitive, and radiotherapy is one of the best treatment options.

C. Chemoradiotherapy can be offered as adjuvant treatment in patients with advanced disease.
D. Topical application of 5-FU is an effective topical treatment option in patients with sinonasal adenocarcinoma.
E. Chemotherapy and radiotherapy are not indicated in cases of sinonasal lymphoma.

Answers

1. **A, C, D**

   Sinonasal malignant tumors are rare, accounting for less than 1% of all malignancies and about 3–5% of head and neck malignancies [1, 2]. The commonest type is squamous cell carcinoma (50–55%), followed by adenocarcinoma (10–15%). Adenoid cystic carcinoma, esthesioneuroblastoma, mucosal malignant melanoma, undifferentiated carcinoma and other histological types are less common [1–3]. Common symptoms of sinonasal malignancy are nasal obstruction, episodes of epistaxis, recurrent sinusitis, sinus pain, headaches, otalgia, rhinorrhea, tearing from one side, loss of smell, and facial swelling. These are considered as "red flag symptoms," especially if they are unilateral and of recent onset. Other symptoms, such as asymptomatic neck mass, facial paresthesia, cranial nerve palsy—paralysis, proptosis, and diplopia—change in vision, loosening of teeth, and trismus, are signs of advanced disease [1, 4–6]. The clinical diagnostic process includes anterior rhinoscopy, nasendoscopy, examination of the oral cavity, neck palpation, cranial nerve examination, and ophthalmology examination if indicated. In many cases, biopsy under local anesthesia can be done in clinic, if there are no contraindications and there are no signs of vascular lesions, such as a juvenile angiofibroma [1, 4, 5]. C-ANCA screening is not recommended in cases of suspected malignancy. C-ANCA can be positive in cases of suspected vasculitis [7].

2. **D**

   MRI scan and CT scan are the preferable imaging tools for the assessment and surgical treatment planning in cases of sinonasal malignant tumors. CT scan is more efficient in evaluating possible bone invasion and destruction. On the other hand, MRI scan is useful in evaluating the size and the type of the malignant tumor, distinguishing the tumor form the surrounding secretions, and detecting perineural spread or dura invasion. Plain X-rays are not recommended. PET/CT scan is indicated only in cases of suspected distal metastasis. Scintigraphy is not indicated in these cases [8, 9]. For staging purposes, after histopathology is confirmed, we recommend MRI scan of the neck and CT scan of the thorax and the upper abdomen [1].

3. **B**

   The possible diagnosis in this case, based on the medical history, clinical and radiological findings, is adenocarcinoma of the right ethmoid sinuses, invading the right maxillary sinus, the orbit, the right sphenoid sinus, the right medial rectus muscle, and the subcutaneous tissues at the level of the right eyebrow. Intestinal type adenocarcinoma of the paranasal sinuses is considered as an occupational disease, affecting especially workers who are exposed to wood or leather dust. Smoking is also associated with sinonasal malignancies [4, 10–12]. Adenocarcinoma usually arises from the ethmoid sinuses, in contrast to SCC, which usually arises from the maxillary sinuses. Nickel dust, formaldehyde and chromium exposure are considered as potential risk factors for sinonasal malignancy [11, 12]. HPV infection is also a possible pathogenic factor for sinonasal SCC [13].

4. **E**

   The T (primary tumor) staging for the malignant tumors of the ethmoid sinuses and nasal cavity is the following:

- Tx—Primary tumor cannot be assessed.
- Tis—Carcinoma in situ.
- T1—Tumor restricted to any one subsite, with or without bony invasion.
- T2—Tumor invading two subsites in a single region or extending to involve an adjacent region within the nasoethmoidal complex, with or without bony invasion.
- T3—Tumor extends to invade the medial wall or floor of the orbit, maxillary sinus, palate, or cribriform plate.
- T4a—Moderately advanced local disease. Tumor invades any of the following: anterior orbital contents, skin of nose or cheek, minimal extension to anterior cranial fossa, pterygoid plates, and sphenoid or frontal sinuses.
- T4b—Very advanced local disease. Tumor invades any of the following: orbital apex, dura, brain, middle cranial fossa, cranial nerves other than V2, nasopharynx, or clivus [14].

5. **A, C, D**

   Most sinonasal malignant tumors are treated surgically. Complete surgical excision can be achieved endoscopically or sometimes by external approaches. For patients with advanced disease, multimodality treatment including surgery and chemoradiotherapy should be offered [1]. Unfortunately, adenocarcinomas may be radioresistant, which means that the role of radiotherapy is usually limited to palliative treatment of patients with unresectable tumors. Topical application of 5-FU is an effective topical treatment option in patients with sinonasal adenocarcinoma [4]. Sinonasal lymphomas are usually type B-cell non-Hodgkin lymphomas. Chemotherapy and radiotherapy are the mainstay of treatment [15].

References

1. Khalil HS. Sino-nasal squamous cell carcinoma. In: Stavrakas M, Khalil HS, editors. Rhinology and anterior skull base surgery. Cham: Springer; 2021.
2. Turner JH, Reh DD. Incidence and survival in patients with sinonasal cancer: a historical analysis of population-based data. Head Neck. 2012;34(6):877–85.
3. Dutta R, Dubal PM, Svider PF, Liu JK, Baredes S, Eloy JA. Sinonasal malignancies: a population-based analysis of site-specific incidence and survival. Laryngoscope. 2015;125(11):2491–7.
4. Khalil HS, Mackie S, Malik T. Sino-nasal intestinal type adenocarcinoma. In: Stavrakas M, Khalil HS, editors. Rhinology and anterior skull base surgery. Cham: Springer; 2021.
5. Khan T, El-Sockary Y, Hamilton WT, Shephard EA. Recognizing sinonasal cancer in primary care: a matched case-control study using electronic records. Fam Pract. 2022;39(3):354–9.
6. Harvey RJ, Dalgorf DM. Chapter 10: Sinonasal malignancies. Am J Rhinol Allergy. 2013;27(Suppl 1):S35–8.
7. Guchelaar NAD, Waling MM, Adhin AA, van Daele PLA, Schreurs MWJ, Rombach SM. The value of anti-neutrophil cytoplasmic antibodies (ANCA) testing for the diagnosis of ANCA-associated vasculitis, a systematic review and meta-analysis. Autoimmun Rev. 2021;20(1):102716.
8. Kawaguchi M, Kato H, Tomita H, Mizuta K, Aoki M, Hara A, Matsuo M. Imaging characteristics of malignant Sinonasal tumors. J Clin Med. 2017;6(12):116.
9. Eggesbø HB. Imaging of sinonasal tumours. Cancer Imaging. 2012;12:136–52.
10. Bimbi G, Saraceno MS, Riccio S, Gatta G, Licitra L, Cantù G. Adenocarcinoma of ethmoid sinus: an occupational disease. Acta Otorhinolaryngol Ital. 2004;24(4):199–203.
11. Cantu G, Solero CL, Mariani L, Lo Vullo S, Riccio S, Colombo S, Pompilio M, Perrone F, Formillo P, Quattrone P. Intestinal type adenocarcinoma of the ethmoid sinus in wood and leather workers: a retrospective study of 153 cases. Head Neck. 2011;33(4):535–42.
12. Binazzi A, Ferrante P, Marinaccio A. Occupational exposure and sinonasal cancer: a systematic review and meta-analysis. BMC Cancer. 2015;15:49.
13. Chang Sing Pang KJW, Mur T, Collins L, Rao SR, Faden DL. Human papillomavirus in Sinonasal squamous cell carcinoma: a systematic review and meta-analysis. Cancers (Basel). 2020;13(1):45.
14. Amin MB, Edge S, Greene F, Byrd DR, Brookland RK, Washington MK, Gershenwald JE, Compton CC, Hess KR, et al., editors. AJCC cancer staging manual. 8th ed. Springer International Publishing: American Joint Commission on Cancer; 2017.
15. Peng KA, Kita AE, Suh JD, Bhuta SM, Wang MB. Sinonasal lymphoma: case series and review of the literature. Int Forum Allergy Rhinol. 2014;4(8):670–4.

Part IV

Skin/Facial Plastics

Basal Cell Carcinoma

39

Aikaterini Tsentemeidou and Elena Sotiriou

Abstract

Basal cell carcinoma (BCC) is the most common cancer of the Caucasian race and arises in the skin. The primary risk factor for BCC is ultraviolet radiation, which explains why most tumours are located to sun-exposed areas, such as the face. BCC typically grows slowly over years, and 10-year survival of patients is actually higher than that of the general population. However, BCC can rarely be locally advanced with local, occasionally extensive, tissue destruction or even metastasis. It typically first appears as a small, inconspicuous, skin-coloured, pearly papule that slowly progresses into an ulcerated nodule (nodular subtype, "rodent ulcer"). Localized BCCs are categorized into low and high risk based on a set of clinical and histopathological criteria, and this guides therapeutic decisions (the TNM system is not used). The treatment recommended for low-risk primary tumours is standard surgical excision. Mohs micrographic surgery is superior to standard excision for tumours of the face (primary or recurrent) in terms of recurrences. It should be considered for primary high-risk BCCs and is recommended as first-line treatment for recurrent BCCs with at least one more high-risk feature, especially high-risk location. Radiotherapy should be considered for (preferably) adults ≥60 years of age with low- or high-risk BCCs, in case MMS and standard excision are unsuitable. Vismodegib per os, a Hedgehog-signalling pathway inhibitor, is the first-line treatment for metastatic BCC, and cemiplimab, a monoclonal antibody, is recommended for locally advanced or metastatic BCCs, in case vismodegib has failed.

Case Presentation

A 72-year-old, Fitzpatrick skin type 2 male presents to the clinic with a lesion to the right side of his nose (Fig. 39.1). He says that he has had it for about 2 years, during which the lesion has been slowly growing. It has recently started to bleed, when scratched. The patient has spent a lot of time outdoors due to his profession (fisherman) and is not in the habit of applying sunscreen or using a wide-brimmed hat. He has a history of hypertension and benign prostate hyperplasia, but is otherwise very fit. On clinical examination, an 8 mm skin-coloured, pearly, ulcerated nodule is seen. No enlarged lymph nodes are found on neck examination.

A. Tsentemeidou (✉) · E. Sotiriou
1st Department of Dermatology and Venereology, School of Medicine, Aristotle University, Thessaloniki, Greece

N. Tsetsos et al. (eds.), *Otolaryngology Study Guide*, https://doi.org/10.1007/978-3-031-77374-7_39

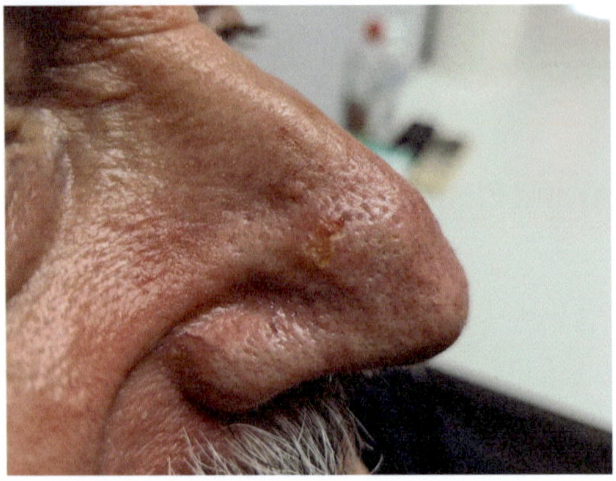

Fig. 39.1 A 72-year-old male with slow-growing, ulcerated nodule to the right side of his nose

Questions

1. Which of the following statements regarding basal cell carcinoma (BCC) are correct (one or more answers may be correct)?
   A. BCC is the most common type of oropharyngeal cancer
   B. Exposure to ultraviolet radiation is the main risk factor for BCC development
   C. BCC is a fast-growing aggressive cancer
   D. 10-year survival is not lower than that of the general population
   E. BCC is never metastatic
2. Which of the following statements regarding basal cell carcinoma (BCC) are correct (one or more answers may be correct)?
   A. Morphoeic BCC is the most common subtype
   B. Nodular subtype is more common in the head and neck area
   C. Diagnosis is seldom made clinically
   D. Biopsy is warranted in tumours that have high-risk features or have recurred
   E. Excisional biopsy is the standard biopsy method
3. Which of the following statements regarding basal cell carcinoma (BCC) are correct (one or more answers may be correct)?
   A. The TNM system is traditionally used for the staging of BCCs
   B. An 8 mm (greatest diameter) tumour on the nose is low risk
   C. A local recurrence of a previously treated tumour is always considered high risk
   D. Immunosuppression status must be considered when determining a tumour's risk
   E. Nodular histopathologic subtype is high risk
4. Which of the following statements regarding basal cell carcinoma (BCC) are correct (one or more answers may be correct)?
   A. Topical treatment is recommended as the treatment of choice for high-risk BCCs
   B. A 5 mm margin of clinically uninvolved skin around the lesion is recommended for low-risk tumours
   C. Mohs micrographic surgery is superior to standard excision for high-risk BCCs
   D. Standard excision of high-risk BCCs should not be performed without complete margin assessment
   E. Flaps should not be performed after standard excision of high-risk BCCs, unless histological margins are confirmed negative prior to repair
5. Which of the following statements regarding basal cell carcinoma (BCC) are correct (one or more answers may be correct)?
   A. Radiotherapy should be considered in young patients
   B. Radiotherapy should be considered if Mohs micrographic surgery or standard excision is unsuitable
   C. Radiotherapy can be repeated after tumour recurrence
   D. Vismodegib is a drug administered orally for locally advanced or metastatic BCC
   E. Cemiplimab is a monoclonal antibody administered for locally advanced or metastatic BCC, in case vismodegib has failed or is unsuitable

Answers

1. **B, D**

Basal cell carcinoma (BCC) is the most common cancer of the Caucasian race and arises in the epidermis, which is the outermost layer of the skin [1]. Its incidence has been found to be 76.21/100,000 person-years in England, while the highest incidence has been documented in Australia, followed by Europe and the USA [1]. Worldwide incidence is rising rapidly [2, 3]. Men are affected twice as frequently as women [1]. The primary risk factor for BCC is mutation-inducing ultraviolet (UV) radiation, which explains why most tumours are located to sun-exposed areas, such as the face [1]. Other risk factors are light skin phototype, older age, genetic skin diseases, BCC in the family and immunosuppression (especially solid organ transplantation) [1]. BCC typically grows slowly over years, and there is enough time to diagnose and treat it [1]. According to a German study, the 5- and 10-year survival rate of BCC patients was 3–6% higher than that of the general population [1]. However, BCC can rarely be locally advanced (laBCC, 0.8% of all BCC cases) with local, occasionally extensive, tissue destruction or even metastasis (mBCC) [1].

2. **B, D**

   BCC clinical presentation may vary, but it typically first appears as a small, inconspicuous, skin-coloured, pearly papule, most often located at the head and neck area; this grows slowly and steadily, usually over the course of years, into a nodule (nodular subtype) [1]. At this stage, ulceration is common (BCC is also called "rodent ulcer") [1]. The superficial subtype presents as a well-demarcated patch or plaque, typically located at the trunk, which is scaly and erythematous and has a characteristic rolled border and numerous small erosions [1]. Morphoeic BCC, a rarer subtype, is typically flat, yellow-whitish, with ill-defined borders, firm to the touch (scar-like), depressed or elevated, and frequently ulcerates [4]. Dermatologists are usually able to make a clinical diagnosis (good lighting and stretching of skin are helpful) [5]. Dermoscopy significantly improves sensitivity and specificity of clinical diagnosis (91.2% and 95%, respectively) [1]. In case clinical diagnosis is doubtful, the tumour has high-risk features and histological subtype is likely to influence treatment or to confirm there is recurrence after previous treatment, biopsy is warranted [5]. No single biopsy method is considered optimal; punch, shave or curette biopsy with sufficient size and depth is performed in most cases [2, 5].

3. **C, D**

   The TNM system is not used for the staging of BCCs, as regional and distant metastases are very uncommon [2, 6]. Localized BCCs are categorized into low and high risk based on a set of criteria (Table 39.1), and this guides therapeutic decisions [2]. According to the European Guidelines, BCCs could alternatively be classified into "easy to treat" (>95% of cases) and "difficult to treat" (Table 39.2) [1].

4. **C, D, E**

   A wide array of treatment modalities are available for BCCs and can have good results, if properly selected [7]. Decisions regarding treatment should be made by a skin cancer multidisciplinary team [5]. Surgical excision is associated with lower risk of recurrence compared to topical treatment, radiotherapy or other destructive treatments, such as cryosurgery and curettage and electrocautery [7]. According to the American Guidelines for BCC management, the treatment recommended for low-risk primary tumours is standard surgical excision with a 4 mm margin of clinically uninvolved skin around the lesion and as deep as the mid-subcutaneous layer [7]. Standard excision may be considered for high-risk tumours too (there is no recommendation for excision margins), provided that complete margin assessment is performed. Linear repair, skin graft and secondary healing are preferred over flaps, unless negative histological margins are confirmed prior to repair [7]. Mohs micrographic surgery (MMS) was superior to standard excision for tumours of the face (primary or recurrent) at the 5- and 10-year follow-up mark [7]. MMS should be considered for primary high-risk BCCs and is recommended as first-line treatment for recurrent BCCs with at least one more high-risk feature, especially high-risk location [5].

Table 39.1 Criteria for categorization of localized basal cell carcinomas (BCCs) into low and high risk

BCC features	Low risk	High risk
Clinical		
Site and size[a]	Trunk and extremities (area L), <2 cm	Trunk and extremities (area L), ≥2 cm
	Cheeks, forehead, scalp, neck and pretibia (area M[b]), <10 mm	Cheeks, forehead, scalp, neck and pretibia (area M), ≥10 mm
		Central face, eyelids, eyebrows, periorbital skin, mandible, periauricular skin, ear, temple, genitalia, hands, feet (area H[c])
Borders	Well defined	Poorly defined
Recurrence	No	Yes
Immunosuppression	No	Yes
Prior radiotherapy	No	Yes
Histopathology		
Type	Nodular, superficial, keratotic, infundibulocystic, fibroepithelioma of Pinkus	Morpheaform, basosquamous (metatypical), sclerosing, mixed infiltrative, micronodular features in any portion of the tumour
Perineural involvement	No	Yes

[a] Size: greatest tumour diameter
[b] Area M: may constitute high risk regardless of size
[c] Area H: regardless of size

Table 39.2 Staging of basal cell carcinomas (BCCs) by the European Association of Dermato-Oncology

EADO[a] stage	Description
I	Easy to treat and low risk for recurrence
IIA	Somewhat difficult to treat because of the location, borders, recurrence or patient status/wishes
IIB	Difficult to treat because of multiple tumours
IIIA	Large and/or destructive tumours in non-critical areas
IIIB	Large and/or destructive tumours in critical areas
IIIC	Giant and/or deeply invasive tumours with extracutaneous involvement
IV	Distant metastases

[a] *EADO* European Association of Dermato-Oncology

Imaging may be performed to rule out deep structural involvement in case of large tumours [7].

5. **B, D, E**

Radiotherapy should be considered for (preferably) adults ≥60 years of age with low- or high-risk BCCs, in case MMS and standard excision are unsuitable and the patient feels positive about RT [5]. RT should not be considered, in case the tumour is a recurrence after previous RT, is associated with a genetic syndrome such as Gorlin syndrome, is located at an area of poor blood supply and has invaded bone or cartilage [5]. Vismodegib per os, a Hedgehog-signalling pathway inhibitor, has been approved by the US Food and Drug Administration (FDA) as the first-line treatment for metastatic BCC [7]. It should be considered for locally advanced BCCs, in case MMS, standard excision or radiotherapy (RT) are unsuitable [5]. Cemiplimab, a monoclonal antibody blocking the PD-1/PD-L1 pathway, is recommended for locally advanced BCCs, in case curative surgery or radiotherapy is not feasible and vismodegib has failed/is not appropriate, and for metastatic BCCs, in case vismodegib has failed/is not appropriate [2].

References

1. Peris K, Fargnoli MC, Garbe C, Kaufmann R, Bastholt L, Seguin NB, et al. Diagnosis and treatment of basal cell carcinoma: European consensus-based interdisciplinary guidelines. Eur J Cancer. 2019;118:10–34. https://pubmed.ncbi.nlm.nih.gov/31288208/

2. Mai Nguyen N, Lynn B, Chrysalyne-Schmults BD II, Blitzblau R, Chair V, et al. NCCN guidelines version 1.2022 basal cell skin cancer continue NCCN guidelines. 2021. https://www.nccn.org/home/member-.
3. Fernández-Figueras MT, Malvehi J, Tschandl P, Rutten A, Rongioletti F, Requena L, et al. Position paper on a simplified histopathological classification of basal cell carcinoma: results of the European consensus project. J Eur Acad Dermatol Venereol. 2022;36(3):351–9.
4. Inamura Y, Imafuku K, Kitamura S, Hata H, Shimizu H. Morphoeic basal cell carcinoma with ring-form ulceration. Int J Dermatol. 2016;55(7):e415–6. https://pubmed.ncbi.nlm.nih.gov/26967584/.
5. Nasr I, McGrath EJ, Harwood CA, Botting J, Buckley P, Budny PG, et al. British Association of Dermatologists guidelines for the management of adults with basal cell carcinoma 2021. Br J Dermatol. 2021;185(5):899–920. https://doi.org/10.1111/bjd.20524.
6. Grob JJ, Gaudy-Marqueste C, Guminski A, Malvehy J, Basset-seguin N, Bertrand B, et al. Position statement on classification of basal cell carcinomas. Part 2: EADO proposal for new operational staging system adapted to basal cell carcinomas. J Eur Acad Dermatology Venereol. 2021;35(11):2149–53. https://doi.org/10.1111/jdv.17467.
7. Bichakjian C, Armstrong A, Baum C, Bordeaux JS, Brown M, Busam KJ, et al. Guidelines of care for the management of basal cell carcinoma. J Am Acad Dermatol. 2018;78(3):540–59. https://doi.org/10.1016/j.jaad.2017.10.006.

Cutaneous Squamous Cell Carcinoma

40

Aikaterini Tsentemeidou and Elena Sotiriou

Abstract

Cutaneous squamous cell carcinoma (cSCC) is the second most frequent cancer of the skin and most often arises in sun-exposed anatomic sites of individuals with fair skin, like the head and neck; ear and lip tumours can be particularly aggressive. The most important risk factors are cumulative sun exposure and organ transplantation-induced immunosuppression. Invasive cSCC can be flat, nodular or a plaque with flesh-like or red colour, hyperkeratosis and ulceration with oozing/bleeding/crusting. Clinical diagnosis can be supported through dermoscopy (white circles) and confirmed through incisional biopsy. Classification of cSCCs into low risk, high risk and very high risk based on clinical and histopathological criteria helps guide treatment and follow-up. First-line gold standard treatment for primary resectable cutaneous SCC is surgical excision. If there is clinical suspicion of lymph node involvement, ultrasonography-guided aspiration should be offered. In case of confirmed metastasis, therapeutic regional lymphadenectomy should be performed after TNM staging via imaging. Levels of neck dissection depend on the location of the primary tumour. In case of nodal metastasis of the parotid gland, therapeutic parotidectomy (usually superficial) along with neck dissection should be performed. Radiotherapy can be used as primary or adjuvant treatment. Immune checkpoint inhibitors are first-line treatment for patients with locally advanced or metastatic cSCC, excluding patients with organ transplantation.

Case Presentation

A 90-year-old, Fitzpatrick skin type 2 male presents to the clinic with a progressively growing tumour to the scalp. He believes the tumour first appeared approximately 1 year ago. It is now itchy, oozing and bleeding (Fig. 40.1). He says that he has been bald for the past 40 years and has had multiple lumps and bumps on his head for the past couple of decades, but none like the one for which he is having this consultation. He seldom wears a hat. He has high blood pressure and walks with a stick due to osteoarthritis. On clinical examination, there is a firm, flesh-coloured, ulcerated, non-tethered tumour to the scalp, measuring 4.2 mm in its greatest diameter. No palpable lymph nodes are found on clinical examination.

A. Tsentemeidou (✉) · E. Sotiriou
1st Department of Dermatology and Venereology, School of Medicine, Aristotle University, Thessaloniki, Greece

N. Tsetsos et al. (eds.), *Otolaryngology Study Guide*, https://doi.org/10.1007/978-3-031-77374-7_40

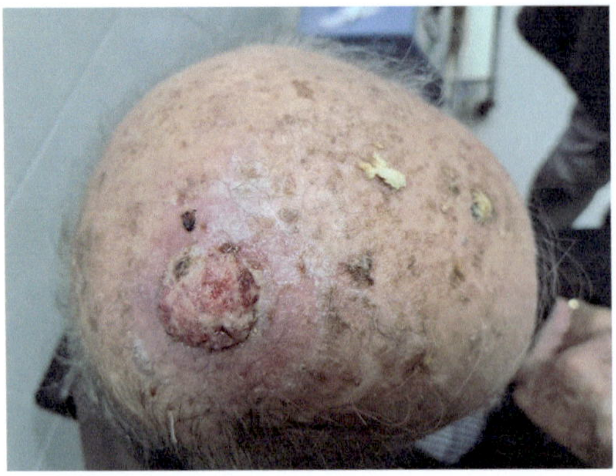

Fig. 40.1 A 90-year-old man with a bleeding, progressively growing lesion to the scalp. History of decade-long sun exposure

Questions

1. Which of the following statements regarding cutaneous squamous cell carcinoma (cSCC) are correct (one or more answers may be correct)?
   A. The most important risk factor for cSCC development is chronic inflammation
   B. Ear and lip cSCCs can be particularly aggressive
   C. cSCC practically always has excellent prognosis
   D. cSCC first metastasizes to regional lymph nodes
   E. Biopsy must include peripheral and deep margins
2. Which of the following statements regarding cutaneous squamous cell carcinoma (cSCC) are correct (one or more answers may be correct)?
   A. At least three low-risk criteria need to be met, for a tumour to be low risk
   B. Any single high-risk factor denotes a high-risk tumour
   C. Located at ear or lip is a high-risk factor
   D. Thickness >7 mm is a "very-high-risk" factor
   E. Close but not involved margins are always low risk
3. Which of the following statements regarding cutaneous squamous cell carcinoma (cSCC) are correct (one or more answers may be correct)?
   A. First-line gold standard treatment is surgical excision with 2 mm radial margin and deep margin down to the subcutaneous tissue
   B. Cryotherapy can be considered for the treatment of small, low-risk, well-defined tumours
   C. In case of involved or close (<1) margins, decisions regarding further treatment should be made following multidisciplinary team (MDT) discussion
   D. In case of clinically suspicious regional lymph nodes, ultrasonography-guided aspiration should be offered
   E. Adjuvant radiotherapy can be considered for completely excised pT3 tumours with multiple high-risk factors and incompletely excised or recurrent tumours
4. Which of the following statements regarding cutaneous squamous cell carcinoma (cSCC) are correct (one or more answers may be correct)?
   A. In case of symptomatic perineural invasion, aggressive surgical excision by head and neck specialists should be performed
   B. Superficial parotidectomy should be performed, in case of nodal metastasis of the parotid gland along with neck dissection
   C. Superficial nodes should always be preserved
   D. Regional lymphadenectomy is useless in case of metastatic cSCCs
   E. Patients with organ transplantation cannot receive immune checkpoint inhibitors
5. Which of the following statements regarding cutaneous squamous cell carcinoma (cSCC) are correct (one or more answers may be correct)?
   A. Patients with low-risk cSCCs do not need long-term follow-up
   B. Patients with high-risk cSCCs should be followed up for a total of 2 years
   C. Very-high-risk cSCCs should be followed up for a total of 5 years
   D. Organ transplant recipients should be followed up for a total of 5 years
   E. Patients with metastatic cSCCs should be followed up every 3 months for 5 years

Answers

1. **B, D, E**

   Squamous cell carcinoma (SCC) is the second most frequent cancer of the skin and arises in epidermal keratinocytes [1, 2]. The lifetime incidence of cutaneous SCC (cSCC) is 9–14% and 4–9% for men and women in the USA, respectively, and it has been steadily increasing throughout the world [3]. The most important risk factor for developing cSCC is cumulative sun exposure, which accounts for its higher incidence in sun-exposed anatomic sites of individuals with fair skin, like the head and neck, while ear and lip tumours can be particularly aggressive [3–5]. cSCC, however, can also develop in darker-skinned individuals (even in sun-protected sites) [3, 4]. Other risk factors are immunosuppression, especially as a result of solid-organ transplantation, male sex and older age [3, 6]. cSCC can be associated with pre-existing actinic keratosis or arise de novo or on skin with chronic inflammation or ulceration [4, 7]. In most cases, surgical removal leads to an excellent prognosis; however, cSCC can be a significant cause of morbidity, especially in the elderly [4, 6]. Some tumours carry increased risk of local recurrence, while, unlike basal cell carcinoma (BCC), cSCC can metastasize to regional lymph nodes and then haematogenically to distant sites, with poor prognosis [4, 7]. In situ cSCC (Bowen's disease) presents as one or more erythematous, scaly lesions that grow slowly and mimic inflammatory skin diseases [5]. Invasive cSCC can be flat, nodular or a plaque with flesh-like or red colour, hyperkeratosis and ulceration with oozing/bleeding/crusting [8]. There can be induration on palpation, while the tumour may be painful and tender, which could be the result of perineural invasion [8]. Clinical diagnosis can be supported through dermoscopy (white circles) and confirmed through incisional biopsy, which should be full thickness and include the peripheral as well as the deep margins [9, 10].

2. **B, C**

   As with basal cell carcinoma (BCC), classification of cSCCs into low risk and high risk, rather than the TNM (tumour–nodes–metastasis) grading system, is used to guide treatment (Table 40.1). However, as cSCCs have greater potential for lymphogenic and haematogenic metastasis than BCCs, the TNM grading system can be used for the staging of patients with SCC (Table 40.2) [10].

3. **C, D, E**

   First-line gold standard treatment for primary resectable cutaneous SCC is surgical excision; clinical radial margins depend on risk factors (at least 4, 6 and 10 mm for low-risk, high-risk and very-high-risk SCCs, respectively), and deep margin should always be down to the next clean surgical plane (the galea in case of scalp tumours, perhaps muscle, bone, etc. in case of fixed tumours) [1, 10]. All histological margins should be at least 1 mm clear, and they should be checked prior to reconstruction, e.g. with flaps, after resection of central face tumours. Completely resected low-risk T1 SCCs without additional clinical risk factors are considered cured (no MDT discussion needed). If margins are close (<1 mm) but clear in the absence of clinical risk factors, observation could be considered. In high-risk patients, however, or in case of involved margins, MDT discussion should decide on further wide local excision, Mohs micrographic surgery or adjuvant radiotherapy. Curettage and cautery, but not cryotherapy, can be considered for primary tumours, which are low risk, well defined and small (<1 cm), with further MDT discussion in case high-risk factors are subsequently identified. Mohs can be considered in selected patients with indistinct tumour margins or where tissue preservation is key [10].

   Ultrasonography imaging of regional lymph nodes can be offered to patients with very-high-risk tumours (such as greater lip ones) [10].

Table 40.1 Criteria for low-risk, high-risk and very-high-risk cutaneous squamous cell carcinoma

Low risk[a]	High risk[b]	Very high risk[c]
Patient factors		
Immunocompetent	Immunosuppression due to medical therapy including biologic agents; frailty and/or comorbidities causing some degree of immunosuppression, stabilized HIV infection under HAART	As for high risk, but especially solid-organ transplantation, haematological malignancy or other significant immunosuppression
Tumour factors		
Diameter ≤20 mm (pT1)	Diameter >20–40 mm (pT2)	Diameter >40 mm (pT3)
Thickness ≤4 mm	Thickness >4 to 6 mm	Thickness >6 mm
Invasion into dermis	Invasion into subcutaneous fat	Invasion beyond subcutaneous fat
No perineural invasion	Dermal perineural invasion (nerve diameter <0.1 mm)	Any bone invasion
No lymphovascular invasion	Lymphovascular invasion	Invasion of named nerve, nerve ≥1 mm, nerve beyond dermis
Well or moderately differentiated	Poorly differentiated	High-grade histological subtype: adenosquamous, desmoplastic, spindle/sarcomatoid/metaplastic
	Located at ear or lip	In-transit metastasis
	Located at the area of scarring or chronic inflammation	
Histopathologic margins		
All clear (≥1 mm)	For pT1: one or more involved or close margins (<1 mm)	One or more involved or close margins (<1 mm) in a high-risk tumour
	For pT2: one or more close margins (<1 mm)	

[a]All mentioned criteria need to be met for a tumour to be low risk
[b]Any single factor denotes high-risk tumour
[c]Any single factor denotes very-high-risk tumour

Table 40.2 TNM (tumour–nodes–metastasis) classification for cutaneous squamous cell carcinoma

T categories	
T1	≤2 cm in greatest dimension
T2	>2 to 4 cm in greatest dimension
T3	>4 cm in greatest dimension or minor bone erosion or specified perineural invasion (≥0.1 mm diameter and/or deeper than the dermis and/or a named nerve) or deep invasion (thickness >6 mm and/or beyond the subcutaneous fat)
T4a	Tumour with gross cortical bone/marrow invasion
T4b	Tumour with skull base or axial skeleton invasion including foraminal involvement and/or vertebral foramen involvement to the epidural space
N categories for head and neck region	
N1	Metastasis in a single ipsilateral lymph node ≤3 cm in greatest dimension without ENEa
N2a	Metastasis in a single ipsilateral lymph node >3 cm but <6 cm in greatest dimension without ENE
N2b	Metastasis in multiple ipsilateral lymph nodes, where none are >6 cm in greatest dimension without ENE
N2c	Metastasis in bilateral or contralateral lymph nodes, where none are >6 cm in greatest dimension without ENE
N3a	Metastasis in a single or multiple lymph nodes >6 cm in greatest dimension without ENE
N3b	Metastasis in a single or multiple lymph nodes with ENE
M categories	
M0	No distant metastasis
M1	Distant metastasis

ENE extranodal extension, clinical or pathological

If there is clinical suspicion of lymph node involvement, ultrasonography-guided aspiration should be offered; if aspiration is negative, core or open biopsy should be offered. In case of confirmed metastasis, therapeutic regional lymphadenectomy should be performed after TNM staging via computed tomography (CT) or magnetic resonance (MRI) of the tumour area and (at least) the chest [10].

Radiotherapy can be offered as primary treatment, if the patient prefers it or the tumour cannot be surgically removed on aesthetic or functional grounds. Cases where adjuvant radiotherapy can be considered are close but clear margins (<1 mm), completely excised pT3 tumours with more than one high-risk factor (e.g. thickness >6 mm and invasion beyond the subcutaneous fat), incompletely excised tumours (patient preference, impossible further surgery, high risk of recurrence as in perineural invasion >0.1 mm or of known nerve), high-risk nodal metastasis (e.g. two or more nodes), recurrent tumours and immunocompromised patients. Radiotherapy should not be offered for completely excised pT1 or T2 tumours, or in case of perineural invasion <0.1 mm.

4. **A, B, E**

Imaging of the cSCC area should be performed, in case of in-transit metastasis (lymphatic spread between primary tumour and regional lymph nodes), perineural invasion of named nerves, locally advanced and/or metastatic cSCC or relapse of such tumour after lymphadenectomy [10].

In case of nodal metastasis of the parotid gland, in the absence of neck involvement, therapeutic parotidectomy (usually of only the superficial lobe) along with selective neck dissection (I–III) should be performed [10]. Superficial parotidectomy can be considered for temporal or anterior scalp primary tumours with neck nodal metastasis [10]. Levels of neck dissection depend on the location of the primary tumour: posterior tumour → preservation of level I, central lower face tumour → preservation of level V [10]. Superficial nodes such as occipital and external jugular should also be dissected based on primary tumour location [10].

Locally recurrent cSCC can be treated with surgical resection with or without adjuvant radiotherapy or primary radiotherapy [10]. In case of metastatic disease, regional disease control could be attempted through regional lymphadenectomy or irradiation of nodal basin [10]. Treatment of locally advanced (where resection or irradiation is not reasonable) or metastatic cSCC should commence with immune checkpoint inhibitors, excluding patients with organ transplantation or significant autoimmune conditions [10]. In these cases, systemic chemotherapy or epidermal growth factor receptor inhibitors can be considered, with poor responses [10]. Electrochemotherapy is an option for locally advanced disease as palliative care or if other treatments are not appropriate [10].

5. **A, B**

Patients with cSCC should be followed up based on their risk factors [10]. Every follow-up visit should include full skin examination and lymph node check (or any other clinical examination deemed appropriate) [10]. In case of low-risk cSCCs, one post-treatment appointment suffices for patient education on self-examination of skin and nodes, including taking digital photographs of treatment area [10]. In case of high-risk factors (especially multiple), patients should be followed up every 4 months for a year and then every 6 months for another year [10]. In case of very-high-risk tumours, follow-up visits should be scheduled 4-monthly for 2 years and then 6-monthly for another year [10]. Patients with high risk of developing new high-risk, primary cSCCs, like organ transplant recipients, should be under surveillance throughout the course of their lives [10]. In case of metastatic cSCCs, follow-up appointments should be scheduled 3-monthly for 2 years and then 6-monthly for another 3 years (with potential longer term surveillance) [10].

References

1. Woo WA, Suarez M, Falero B, Keohane SG. Summary of the updated 2020 guidelines for cutaneous squamous cell carcinoma. Clin Exp Dermatol. 2021;46(6):1174–7. https://pubmed.ncbi.nlm.nih.gov/33729596/.
2. Skulsky SL, O'Sullivan B, McArdle O, Leader M, Roche M, Conlon PJ, et al. Review of high-risk features of cutaneous squamous cell carcinoma and discrepancies between the American joint committee on cancer and NCCN clinical practice guidelines in oncology. Head Neck. 2017;39(3):578–94. https://doi.org/10.1002/hed.24580.
3. Alam M, Armstrong A, Baum C, Bordeaux JS, Brown M, Busam KJ, et al. Guidelines of care for the management of cutaneous squamous cell carcinoma. J Am Acad Dermatol. 2018;78(3):560–78. https://pubmed.ncbi.nlm.nih.gov/29331386/.
4. Motaparthi K, Kapil JP, Velazquez EF. Cutaneous squamous cell carcinoma: review of the eighth edition of the American joint committee on cancer staging guidelines, prognostic factors, and histopathologic variants. Adv Anat Pathol. 2017;24(4):171–94. https://pubmed.ncbi.nlm.nih.gov/28590951/.
5. Prieto-Granada C, Rodriguez-Waitkus P. Cutaneous squamous cell carcinoma and related entities: epidemiology, clinical and histological features, and basic science overview. Curr Probl Cancer. 2015;39(4):206–15.
6. Leiter U. What is new in the 2020 British guidelines for cutaneous squamous cell carcinoma? Br J Dermatol. 2021;184(3):384–5. https://doi.org/10.1111/bjd.19861.
7. Peris K, Alaibac M, Argenziano G, Di Stefani A, Fargnoli MC, Frascione P, et al. Cutaneous squamous cell carcinoma. Italian guidelines by SIDeMaST adapted to and updating EADO/EDF/EORTC guidelines. G Ital Dermatol Venereol. 2018;153(6):747–62. https://pubmed.ncbi.nlm.nih.gov/29898593/.
8. Howell JY, Ramsey ML. Squamous cell skin cancer. StatPearls; 2022. https://www.ncbi.nlm.nih.gov/books/NBK441939/.
9. Sgouros D, Theofili M, Damaskou V, Theotokoglou S, Theodoropoulos K, Stratigos A, et al. Dermoscopy as a tool in differentiating cutaneous squamous cell carcinoma from its variants. Dermatol Pract Concept. 2021;11(2):e2021050. https://pubmed.ncbi.nlm.nih.gov/33954021/.
10. Keohane SG, Botting J, Budny PG, Dolan OM, Fife K, Harwood CA, et al. British Association of Dermatologists guidelines for the management of people with cutaneous squamous cell carcinoma 2020*. Br J Dermatol. 2021;184(3):401–14.

Melanoma

41

Aikaterini Tsentemeidou
and Polychronia Eftychidou

Abstract

Cutaneous melanoma arises in skin melanocytes. Albeit largely resistant to available therapeutic options when advanced, it is curable at an early stage. Most melanoma cases are associated with previous exposure to ultraviolet radiation, especially in fair-skinned individuals. Clinical subtypes of melanoma are superficial spreading, nodular, lentigo maligna, acral lentiginous and desmoplastic neurotropic. Lentigo maligna develops on the head and neck of elderly individuals and follows a lengthy pre-invasive course. Diagnosis must always be confirmed through full-thickness excisional biopsy with minimal clinical margins. Breslow (tumour) thickness in millimetres and presence of ulceration determine the T (tumour) part of the TNM staging system (tumour, node, metastasis). BRAF gene mutations are present in a significant number of patients and are actionable. Following histologic confirmation of diagnosis, wide local excision (WLE) is performed with clinical margins dependent on thickness. Systemic treatment can be administered on an adjuvant basis in cases of resectable primary tumours with clinically occult nodal metastasis or on a first-line basis in case of metastatic disease. PD-1 inhibitors (nivolumab, pembrolizumab) and BRAF inhibitors (vemurafenib, dabrafenib, encorafenib) are the main systemic drugs for melanoma, but a number of other agents are used or being studied in clinical trials.

A. Tsentemeidou (✉) · P. Eftychidou
1st Department of Dermatology and Venereology, School of Medicine, Aristotle University, Thessaloniki, Greece

Case Presentation

Case A: A 69-year-old, Fitzpatrick skin type 2 woman presents with a raised, 2.9 cm, pigmented lesion to the top of her scalp (Fig. 41.1). She has had it for many years (almost a decade), during which time the lesion has been slowly growing and changing in appearance. It has also recently started bleeding. The patient has spent a lot of time in the sun and has not been in the habit of wearing a hat. Regional lymph nodes are normal on palpation. Full-thickness excision with minimal clinical margin is scheduled immediately. Histopathology report shows a superficial spreading melanoma with 4.2 mm Breslow thickness and ulceration. The patient is then scheduled for wide local excision with 2 cm clinical margin, sentinel lymph node biopsy, whole-body PET/CT and brain MRI for complete staging, which is eventually determined as IIIC. She is then started on nivolumab and enters remission.

Case B: An 82-year-old, Fitzpatrick skin type 2 man presents with a flat, 1.9 cm, pigmented

N. Tsetsos et al. (eds.), *Otolaryngology Study Guide*, https://doi.org/10.1007/978-3-031-77374-7_41

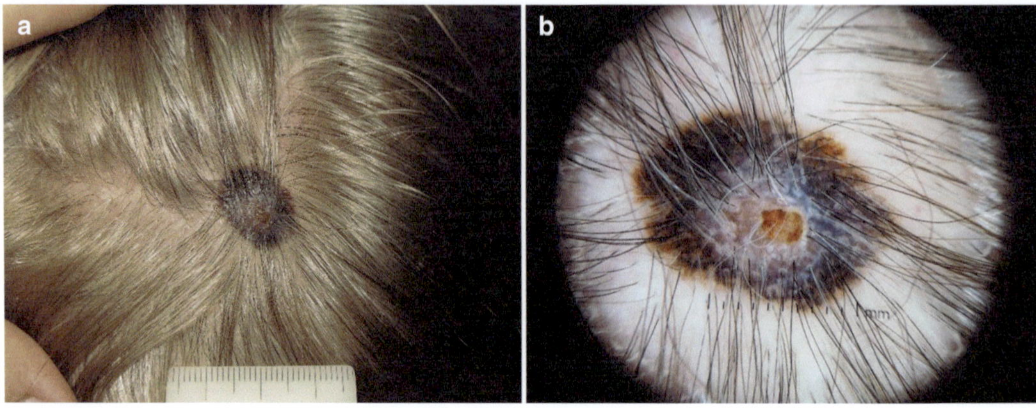

Fig. 41.1 (**a**) Superficial spreading melanoma to the top of the scalp of a 69-year-old woman. (**b**) Dermoscopic image with visible melanoma criteria: blue-white veil, irregular pigmentation, atypical pigment network

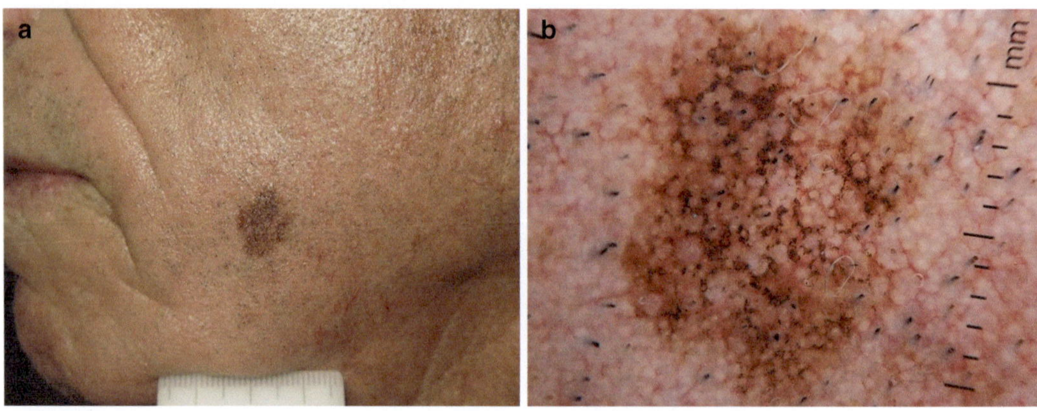

Fig. 41.2 (**a**) Lentigo maligna melanoma to the left cheek of an 82-year-old man. (**b**) Dermoscopic image with "inverse approach" criteria: absence of scales, rosettes, brown parallel lines, moth-eaten borders, seborrheic keratosis features, obliteration of follicular openings by pigment

lesion to his left cheek (Fig. 41.2). He has had it for more than a decade, during which time the lesion has been very slowly becoming larger and somewhat darker, but is otherwise asymptomatic. The patient has spent a lot of time outdoors since a young age and has not been using sunscreen. Regional lymph nodes are normal on palpation. Full-thickness excision with minimal clinical margin is scheduled immediately. Histopathology report shows a lentigo maligna with 0.7 mm Breslow thickness without ulceration. Wide local excision with 1 cm clinical margin is performed, and imiquimod is then prescribed for topical application 7 days a week for 6 weeks.

Questions

1. Which of the following statements regarding cutaneous melanoma are correct (one or more answers may be correct)?
   A. Melanoma is mostly a non-life-threatening cancer of the skin
   B. Individuals with darker skin are most susceptible to melanoma development
   C. Lentigo maligna is a type of slow-growing melanoma that typically develops on the head and neck of elderly individuals
   D. ABCDE is a list of features of early melanoma

   E. Dermoscopy has enabled early melanoma detection and prevention of unnecessary excisions of benign lesions
2. Which of the following statements regarding cutaneous melanoma are correct (one or more answers may be correct)?
   A. If a lesion is suspicious for melanoma, a punch or shave biopsy can quickly confirm diagnosis
   B. Histologic information used to stage melanoma is Breslow thickness and ulceration
   C. In-transit metastasis is located within 2 cm of the primary tumour
   D. Ultrasound of regional lymph nodes is not required for pT1a tumours
   E. BRAF gene mutation testing is mandatory for high-risk stage IIC, III and IV disease
3. Which of the following statements regarding cutaneous melanoma are correct (one or more answers may be correct)?
   A. Following resection of primary melanoma, wide local excision (WLE) must be performed
   B. Lentigo maligna can alternatively be treated with radiotherapy or adjuvant topical imiquimod, as it can be rather large in diameter
   C. Sentinel lymph node biopsy (SNB) must be performed in cases of stage III disease or higher
   D. Complete lymph node dissection must be performed in case of positive SNB
   E. In case of non-resectable satellite or in-transit metastasis, systemic treatment is warranted
4. Which of the following statements regarding cutaneous melanoma are correct (one or more answers may be correct)?
   A. Stage IIIA disease can be treated with adjuvant nivolumab
   B. According to current guidelines, SNB-negative pT4 melanoma should be treated with adjuvant nivolumab
   C. Oligometastatic disease can be treated with resection of primary tumour and distant metastasis along with systemic treatment
   D. Non-resectable stage III/IV BRAF-mutated melanoma should be treated with BRAF and MEK inhibitors
   E. Neurosurgery is a potential option for brain metastases depending on the individual
5. Which of the following statements regarding cutaneous melanoma are correct (one or more answers may be correct)?
   A. There is no evidence suggesting that melanoma patients should take precautions against further ultraviolet radiation exposure, as they have already developed skin cancer
   B. Skin self-examination is essential as melanoma patients have a high risk of developing further skin cancer
   C. Follow-up should be performed 4-monthly for 5 years
   D. Lymph node ultrasound should be performed once yearly for the rest of a patient's life
   E. Whole-body PET scan is recommended for stage IIA disease

Answers

1. **C, E**

Cutaneous melanoma arises in skin melanocytes [1]. Its incidence has been rising over recent decades, but prognosis has been improving due to earlier diagnosis and treatment [1]. Melanoma is the major cause of skin cancer-induced mortality [1]. Albeit largely resistant to available therapeutic options when advanced, it is curable at an early stage [1]. Most melanoma cases are associated with previous exposure to ultraviolet radiation, especially at a young age, in susceptible individuals [1]. Very fair skin with red (or fair) hair and freckles are associated with a three times greater risk of developing melanoma [1]. Clinical subtypes of melanoma with distinct morphologic and prognostic characteristics are the following: superficial spreading, nodular, lentigo maligna, acral lentiginous and desmoplastic neurotropic [1]. With the exception of acral lentiginous melanoma, all other types can occur in the head and neck area; lentigo maligna develops on the head and neck of elderly individuals and follows a lengthy pre-invasive course, while desmoplastic neurotropic melanoma, a type linked with peri-neural invasion and higher propensity for local recurrence, predominantly develops in the head and neck area [1]. The staple of melanoma clinical diagnosis (ABCDE checklist—large, elevated, asymmetric, pigmented (or not) lesion with irregular borders and at least two different colours) may not apply to early lesions—at least when examined with the naked eye—as those often look no different than melanocytic nevi (moles) [2]. Dermoscopy performed by trained individuals has significantly increased cases of early melanoma detection while reducing unnecessary excisions [2, 3].

2. **B, D, E**

Diagnosis must always be confirmed through full-thickness excisional biopsy with minimal clinical margins [2]. Information regarding clinical subtype, anatomical site and presence of sun damage to surrounding skin must be provided to the histopathologist [2]. Histology report must include Breslow thickness in millimetres, presence of ulceration, surgical margin clearance, mitotic rate and regression (the last two no longer determine stage but have prognostic value) [2]. Regarding disease staging, thorough physical examination should be performed to identify other suspicious pigmented lesions, satellite (within 2 cm of primary site) and in-transit (further along the lymphatic course towards the lymph nodes) metastases, involved regional lymph nodes or distant metastases [2]. The eighth edition of the American Joint Committee on Cancer (AJCC) Tumor, Node, Metastasis (TNM) staging is currently used to stage melanoma (Tables 41.1 and 41.2) [2]. Imaging tests are performed in pT1b-pT4b tumours and include ultrasound (US) of the regional lymph node basin, computed tomography (CT), positron emission tomography (PET) and brain magnetic resonance imaging (MRI)—the latter only for pT3b-pT4b tumours [2]. Testing for BRAF gene mutations, and other actionable mutations, must be performed in patients with high-risk stage IIC, stage II and IV disease [2].

Table 41.1 Melanoma TNM staging according to the eighth edition of the American Joint Committee on Cancer (AJCC) staging

T—primary tumour	Thickness	Ulceration[a]
Tx	Unknown, e.g. curettage	–
T0	No tumour found	–
Tis	Melanoma in situ	–
T1a	<0.8 mm	
	<0.8 mm	With
T1b	0.8–1 mm	With or without
T2a	>1 to 2 mm	Without
T2b	>1 to 2 mm	With
T3a	>2 to 4 mm	Without
T3b	>2 to 4 mm	With
T4a	>4 mm	Without
T4b	>4 mm	With
N—lymph nodes	**Node metastasis**	**In-transit and/or satellite metastasis**
NX	Not assessed	–
N0	Not detected	No
N1a	Clinically occult	No
N1b	1 node clinically detected	No
N1c	Not detected	Yes

(continued)

Table 41.1 (continued)

T—primary tumour	Thickness	Ulceration[a]
N2a	2–3 clinically occult	No
N2b	2–3, at least 1 clinically detected	No
N2c	1 clinically occult/detected	Yes
N3a	≥4 clinically occult	No
N3b	≥4, at least 1 clinically detected or any matted ones	No
N3c	≥2 clinically occult/detected and/or any matted ones	Yes
M—metastasis	**Anatomic site**	**LDH[b] levels[a]**
M0	None detected	–
M1a(0)	Skin, soft tissue including muscle and/or non-regional lymph node	Not elevated
M1a(1)		Elevated
M1b(0)	Distant metastasis to lung with or without M1a sites of disease	Not elevated
M1b(1)		Elevated
M1c(0)	Distant metastasis to non-CNS[c] visceral sites with or without M1a or M1b sites of disease	Not elevated
M1c(1)		Elevated
M1d(0)	Distant metastasis to CNS with or without M1a, M1b or M1c sites of disease	Not elevated
M1d(1)		Elevated

[a] If unknown, stage is not characterised with a lower case letter, e.g. M1
[b] *LDH* lactate dehydrogenase
[c] *CNS* central nervous system

Table 41.2 Final melanoma staging according to the eighth edition of the American Joint Committee on Cancer (AJCC) staging

T	N	M	Stage
Tis[a]	N0	M0	0
T1a[a]	N0	M0	IA
T1b[a]	N0	M0	IA
T2a	N0	M0	IB
T2b	N0	M0	IIA
T3a	N0	M0	IIA
T3b	N0	M0	IIB
T4a	N0	M0	IIB
T4b	N0	M0	IIC
T0	N1b, N1c	M0	IIIB
T0	N2b, N2c, N3b or N3c	M0	IIIC
T1a/b–T2a	N1a or N2a	M0	IIIA
T1a/b–T2a	N1b/c or N2b	M0	IIIB
T2b/T3a	N1a–N2b	M0	IIIB
T1a–T3a	N2c or N3a/b/c	M0	IIIC
T3b/T4a	Any N ≥ N1	M0	IIIC
T4b	N1a–N2c	M0	IIIC
T4b	N3a/b/c	M0	IIID
Any T, Tis	Any N	M1	IV

[a] Tis and T1 only require clinical (not pathological) evaluation of lymph nodes to determine the final AJCC stage

3. **A, B**

   Following histologic confirmation of diagnosis, wide local excision (WLE) is performed with the following clinical margins: in situ melanoma → 0.5 cm, Breslow thickness ≤2 mm → 1 cm, Breslow thickness >2 mm → 2 cm (slow Mohs micrographic surgery for facial melanomas can result in smaller margins) [2]. Lentigo maligna can be quite large, and radiotherapy (RT) is a potential curative option in cases where surgery would be unacceptable [2]. An alternative approach, currently not officially recommended in guidelines, is application of imiquimod prior to or following simple excision, instead of performing WLE [4]. Sentinel lymph node biopsy (SNB) is recommended for pT1b tumour stage or higher; this should only be performed in specialised centres that fulfil certain quality criteria [2]. Complete lymph node dissection (CLND) after positive SNB is no longer recommended, as it has no impact on survival [2]. In case of clinically (macroscopically) detected nodal metastasis and absence of distant metastasis as determined through appropriate imaging, CLND is recommended, as sole removal of involved lymph node(s) is not sufficient [2]. Patients with non-resectable satellite or in-transit metastasis or primary tumour of the limbs without other metastases are candidates for topical treatment, such as melphalan and talimogene laherparepvec [2]. Adjuvant RT for local control of disease (primary tumour site and nodal basin) is not routinely recommended but can be considered in certain cases of head and neck melanoma, where local disease control is critical [2].

4. **A, C, D, E**

   The impact of adjuvant systemic treatment for stages IIB/C and III has been investigated in many well-designed clinical trials [2]. Stage IIIA (SNB >1 mm) BRAF-mutated melanoma can be treated with adjuvant anti-PD-1 treatment (nivolumab, pembrolizumab) or dabrafenib/trametinib [2]. Decisions on an individual basis should be made for SNB <1 mm [2]. PD-1 blockade is the only recommended adjuvant systemic treatment for BRAF wild-type (negative) melanoma [2]. It seems that SN-negative pT3b and pT4 melanoma carries a high risk of relapse with 20% mortality at 10 years; consequently, PD-1 blockade or dabrafenib/trametinib could benefit such patients, although clinical trial evidence is currently lacking [2]. Some stage IV patients have resectable, oligometastatic disease, and surgical removal of primary tumour and single distant metastasis, along with systemic treatment, is a viable option [2]. Resection and stereotactic irradiation in fit patients are also options for locoregional recurrence and can offer long-term disease control [2]. First-line treatments for non-resectable stage III/IV disease is PD-1 blockade (nivolumab, pembrolizumab), nivolumab combined with ipilimumab (CTLA-4 blockade) and BRAF inhibitors (vemurafenib, dabrafenib, encorafenib) combined with MEK inhibitors (cobimetinib, trametinib, binimetinib) for BRAF-mutated melanoma [2]. Talimogene laherparepvec (T-VEC) is also an option [2]. Brain metastasis is associated with very poor prognosis and can be treated with the following options depending on the case: neurosurgery, stereotactic radiosurgery, a combination of BRAF and MEK inhibitors, and immunotherapy [2].

5. **B**

   Melanoma patients need to be educated on how to protect their skin from ultraviolet radiation (avoid prolonged exposure, wear protective clothing, use high-SPF sunscreen, check and maintain healthy vitamin D levels) and regularly self-examine their skin and lymph nodes [2]. They have increased risk of a second melanoma or other skin tumour; their family members have an increased risk for melanoma too [2]. Follow-up appointments should be scheduled for whole-body skin check, lymph node check, imaging and blood tests, but there is currently no consensus regarding the frequency of such appointments (a common plan is 3 monthly for the first 3 years and then 6 monthly or yearly) [2]. Imaging tests (US of lymph nodes, CT, whole-body PET or PET/CT) should be reserved for high-risk patients, such as those with thick primary tumours or metastases [2]. Patients with positive SNB should definitely be followed up frequently with US [2]. The only blood test of possible value in melanoma follow-up is serum S100 protein (rather than LDH, due to higher specificity for disease progression) [2].

References

1. Ahmed OA, Kelly C. Head and neck melanoma (excluding ocular melanoma): United Kingdom National Multidisciplinary Guidelines. J Laryngol Otol. 2016;130:S133–41. https://doi.org/10.1017/S0022215116000852.
2. Michielin O, Van Akkooi ACJ, Ascierto PA, Dummer R, Keilholz U. Cutaneous melanoma: ESMO clinical practice guidelines for diagnosis, treatment and follow-up. Ann Oncol Off J Eur Soc Med Oncol. 2019;30:1884–901. https://doi.org/10.1093/ANNONC/MDZ411.
3. Lallas A, Apalla Z, Chaidemenos G. New trends in dermoscopy to minimize the risk of missing melanoma. J Skin Cancer. 2012;2012:1–5. https://doi.org/10.1155/2012/820474.
4. Fosko SW, Navarrete-Dechent CP, Nehal KS. Lentigo Maligna-challenges, observations, imiquimod, confocal microscopy, and personalized treatment. JAMA Dermatol. 2018;154:879–81. https://doi.org/10.1001/JAMADERMATOL.2018.0531.

42 Rhinoplasty

John Goudakos

Abstract

The removal of a dorsal nasal hump is a commonly performed procedure in rhinoplasty. It is crucial and essential to reconstruct the middle vault in order to stabilize the function of the nasal valve and achieve the desired aesthetic lines of the dorsal area. The nasal midvault consists of the upper lateral cartilages and their attachment to the nasal septum and bones. The keystone area, which is the junction of the quadrangular cartilage to the nasal bones and the attachment of the upper lateral cartilages (ULCs), is a critical structure in the middle vault. Failure to restore the middle vault after hump removal can lead to functional complications such as internal nasal valve collapse, saddle deformity, and inverted-V deformity, as well as aesthetic issues. Patients with a tension nose (high nasal dorsum combined with a long caudal edge and stretching of the skin and soft tissue), dorsal hump (short nasal bones and long ULCs), and midvault asymmetry and deviation are suitable candidates for middle vault restoration. Spreader grafts, which are two strips of cartilage placed between the dorsal septum and ULCs, are currently considered the gold standard for middle vault restoration. Another technique, known as spreader flaps, involves inward folding of the ULCs and can also be effective in reconstructing the nasal middle vault.

J. Goudakos (✉)
ENT Head and Neck Surgery Department,
424 General Military Hospital, Thessaloniki, Greece

Case Presentation

A 32-year-old male presents to your practice with the main concern of improving the aesthetic shape of their nose, specifically addressing the dorsal hump. They do not report any functional issues related to nasal breathing. Upon physical examination, it is observed that the patient has a straight nasal septum and normal volume of the inferior turbinates. On the lateral view, there is a prominent dorsal hump and a "tension" nose deformity characterized by an overprojected nasal tip, an obtuse nasolabial angle, and a short upper lip (Fig. 42.1).

Questions

1. Which of the following is not a potential complication of a nonrestoration of middle vault after rhinoplasty?
   A. Inverted-V deformity
   B. Internal nasal valve collapse
   C. Saddle nose
   D. Narrowed nasal dorsum
   E. External nasal valve collapse

N. Tsetsos et al. (eds.), *Otolaryngology Study Guide*, https://doi.org/10.1007/978-3-031-77374-7_42

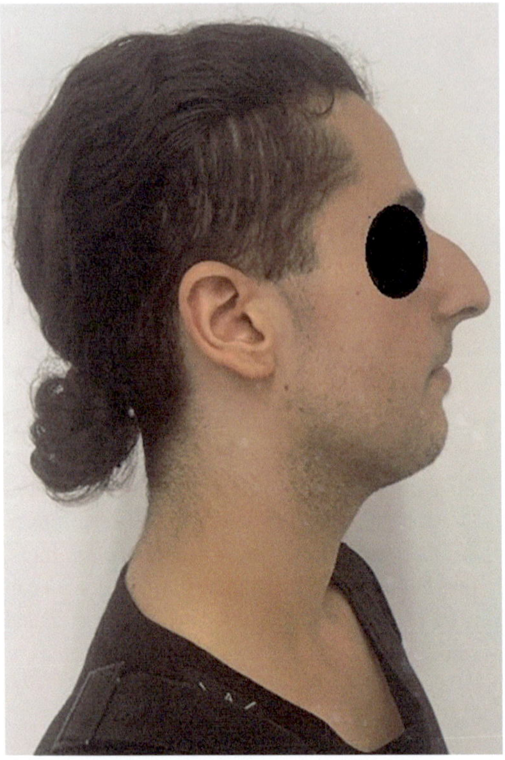

Fig. 42.1 The male patient with a prominent dorsal hump and a "tension" nose deformity characterized by an over-projected nasal tip, an obtuse nasolabial angle, and a short upper lip

2. Which of the following is not part of the keystone area?
   A. Quadrangular cartilage
   B. Low lateral cartilages
   C. Nasal bones
   D. Nasal septum
   E. Upper lateral cartilages

3. Which statement describes better the inverted-V deformity after rhinoplasty?
   A. Disassociation between the ULCs and the nasal bones
   B. Widening of the middle third of nose
   C. Loss of nasal dorsal height
   D. Nasal dorsum convexity
   E. Internal nasal valve collapse
4. Which two are the main advantages of spreader grafts in reconstruction of middle vault?
   A. Increase in middle vault width
   B. Stabilization of middle vault
   C. Increase of internal nasal valve angle
   D. Need to harvest cartilage
   E. Stiffness of the nose
5. Which of the following is not an indication for middle vault restoration after rhinoplasty?
   A. Tension nose deformity
   B. Dorsal hump reduction
   C. Crooked nose
   D. Middle vault asymmetry
   E. Ptotic nasal tip

Answers

1. **E**

   In fact, hump removal involves the removal of the upper lateral cartilages, septum, and nasal bones. Over-resection without preserving the underlying mucosa can lead to complications such as saddle nose, inverted-V deformity, internal nasal valve collapse, and an overly narrowed middle vault [1–3].
2. **B**

   The keystone area, as its name suggests, is crucial for maintaining the structural integrity of the nasal middle vault and plays a role in the dorsal aesthetic lines. It consists of the junction of the nasal bones with the quadrangular cartilage, along with contributions from the perpendicular ethmoid plate and upper lateral cartilages (ULCs) [4].
3. **A**

   Failure to reconstruct the nasal middle vault after hump removal can potentially result in the collapse of the upper lateral cartilages, leading to a saddle deformity of the middle vault known as inverted-V deformity. This occurs because the spreader effect of the Y-shaped dorsal septum is not addressed. The underlying pathophysiology of this deformity involves the dislocation of the ULCs from the nasal bones [5, 6].
4. **B, C**

   The spreader grafts, popularized by Sheen in the 1980s, are now considered the gold standard for middle vault reconstruction. These grafts are strips of cartilage that are placed and sutured along the anterior septal border [7]. They are typically placed bilaterally and serve to stabilize and widen the internal nasal valve. In cases of a crooked nose or asymmetries, they can also be performed unilaterally. An alternative technique known as the autospreader graft or spreader flaps, introduced by Oneal and Bergowitz in the 1990s, involves folding the excess upper lateral cartilages inward and suturing them to the upper septum [8]. Similar to spreader grafts, these flaps enhance the strength of the middle vault and prevent internal valve collapse. Their main advantages are that they mimic the natural anatomy and do not require harvesting additional cartilage.

5. **E**

Dorsal hump removal is one of the most commonly performed maneuvers in rhinoplasty, involving the removal of the bony cap, part of the nasal bones, upper lateral cartilages, and septum. These structures contribute to the formation of the internal nasal valve, and any reduction in size without proper restoration can potentially affect valve patency. Patients with a dorsal hump and short nasal bones, as well as those with a tension nose deformity (overprojected nasal tip, obtuse nasolabial angle, and short upper lip), are at a higher risk. Middle vault restoration using unilateral or bilateral spreader grafts can also be utilized in cases of a crooked nose when the deviation involves the upper lateral cartilages. Asymmetric middle vault is another indication for reconstruction using spreader grafts or flaps [1–8].

References

1. Lee MR, Unger JG, Rohrich RJ. Management of the nasal dorsum in rhinoplasty: a systematic review of the literature regarding technique, outcomes, and complications. Plast Reconstr Surg. 2011;128:538e–50e.
2. Rohrich RJ, Muzaffar AR, Janis JE. Component dorsal hump reduction: the importance of maintaining dorsal aesthetic lines in rhinoplasty. Plast Reconstr Surg. 2004;114:1298–308; discussion 1309–1312.
3. Fischer H, Gubisch W. Nasal valves—importance and surgical procedures. Facial Plast Surg. 2006;22(4):266–80.
4. Palhazi P, Daniel RK, Kosins AM. The osseocartilaginous vault of the nose: anatomy and surgical observations. Aesthet Surg J. 2015;35(3):242–51.
5. Sykes JM, Tapias V, Kim J-E. Management of the nasal dorsum. Facial Plast Surg. 2011;27(2):192–202.
6. Most SP. Trends in functional rhinoplasty. Arch Facial Plast Surg. 2008;10(6):410–3.
7. Sheen JH. Spreader graft: a method of reconstructing the roof of the middle nasal vault following rhinoplasty. Plast Reconstr Surg. 1984;73(2):230–9.
8. Oneal RM, Berkowitz RL. Upper lateral cartilage spreader flaps in rhinoplasty. Aesthet Surg J. 1998;18(5):370–1.

Part V

Paediatric ENT

Microtia/Anotia

43

Nikolaos I. Sakellaris, Eleni I. Sakellari, and Marios Stavrakas

Abstract

Microtia, a malformation disorder resulting from incomplete embryonic development of external ear structures, is relatively rare, is more prevalent in males, and often affects the right side in unilateral cases. It ranges in severity from minor abnormalities to complete absence of the auricle (anotia). Microtia can occur as an isolated condition or as part of syndromes like the oculo-auriculo-vertebral spectrum (OAVS) and has strong genetic associations, with common syndromes including Treacher Collins, Townes-Brock-Goldenhar, and Nager syndrome. Initial treatment typically involves non-interventional techniques and prosthetics, with surgical repair performed at older ages, using techniques such as autologous rib cartilage-based reconstruction. Conductive hearing loss is common in microtia cases, necessitating early auditory evaluation with auditory brainstem response (ABR) testing and consideration of hearing devices before the age of 4 months and surgical intervention after the age of 5. While CT scans are not recommended in early infancy, they are valuable for assessing temporal bone structure and detecting associated anomalies like congenital cholesteatoma. Renal abnormalities are frequently observed in microtia patients, suggesting the importance of routine early ultrasound examinations in these cases.

N. I. Sakellaris
Department of Otolaryngology, "G. Gennimatas" General Hospital of Athens, Athens, Greece

E. I. Sakellari
Faculty of Health Sciences, Aristotle University of Thessaloniki, AHEPA University Hospital, Thessaloniki, Greece

M. Stavrakas (✉)
ENT Head and Neck Surgery Department, University Hospitals Plymouth NHS Trust, Plymouth, UK

Case Presentation

A 1-year-old boy, diagnosed with Treacher Collins syndrome and microtia, was referred to the MDT pediatric ENT clinic. The child had been diagnosed with Treacher Collins syndrome (TCS) shortly after birth based on characteristic craniofacial features, including microtia. Family history revealed no known genetic disorders or hearing impairments. Physical examination confirmed the presence of bilateral microtia and identified conductive hearing loss on the right side. Otoscopy revealed a small, malformed right external auditory canal, suggestive of atresia. Audiological evaluation using brainstem auditory evoked response (BAER) testing indicated bilateral conductive hearing loss, with more

N. Tsetsos et al. (eds.), *Otolaryngology Study Guide*, https://doi.org/10.1007/978-3-031-77374-7_43

severe impairment on the right side. Computed tomography (CT) imaging of the temporal bones confirmed the presence of bilateral microtia and revealed associated middle ear anomalies, including ossicular malformations and a hypoplastic mastoid cavity on the right side.

Questions

1. Which of the following statements are true about microtia (more than one correct answer possible)?
   A. The incidence of this malformation is estimated to be 1:6000 to 12,000 live births.
   B. Bilateral microtia is more common than unilateral.
   C. Bilateral microtia indicates higher risk for other anomalies.
   D. It is more common in males.
   E. The unilateral form is frequently on the left side.
2. In which of the following Marx classifications is the “peanut ear” observed?
   A. Grade I
   B. Grade II
   C. Grade III
   D. Grade IV
   E. None of the above
3. Which syndrome may be associated with this pathology?
   A. Treacher Collins syndrome
   B. Trichorhinophalangeal syndrome
   C. Fragile X syndrome
   D. Börjeson–Forssman–Lehmann syndrome
   E. None of the above
4. Which is currently the most frequently used approach?
   A. Observational (non-interventional) approach
   B. Alloplastic reconstruction
   C. Autologous rib cartilage-based reconstruction
   D. Porous polyethylene frameworks such as Medpor
   E. None of the above
5. Which of the following statements are true about microtia?
   A. Diagnostic audiological assessment should be completed by the age of 6 months.
   B. Conductive hearing loss should be treated immediately surgically.
   C. At birth, in children with any grade of microtia, kidney ultrasound should be performed.
   D. Early at age, a CT scan should be performed.
   E. None of the above.

Answers

1. **A, C, D**

   Microtia is a malformation disorder caused by incomplete embryonic development of external ear structures [1]. It is an uncommon disease, and its incidence is estimated to be 1:6000–12,000 live births [1]. It occurs more frequently in male gender with an estimation of 20–40% and on the right side in approximately 60% of unilateral cases [1, 2]. Bilateral microtia appears approximately only in 10% of the cases [1]; however, it is associated with a higher risk of other congenital anomalies or underlying syndromes [1, 2].
2. **C**

   Microtia as a complex malformation ranged in severity. Several grading systems exist for microtia, but the Marx classification is widely used (Table 43.1) [2, 3].

   There is a strong correlation between the degree of microtia and the severity of the mid-

Table 43.1 Marx classification for microtia

Grade	Definition
Grade I	Slightly smaller auricle (at least two standard deviations below normal), but all subunits are present
Grade II	The auricle is smaller. Subunits are severely underdeveloped or absent. The upper half of the ear is often less developed than the lower half
Grade III	Only a small piece of cartilage is present in the superior remnant of the ear, and the lobule is rotated anterosuperiorly; this configuration is the most common and is often colloquially referred to as a “peanut ear”
Grade IV	Complete absence of the auricle and lobule (anotia)

Grade of microtia and their definition according to Marx classification [2, 3]

dle ear dysplasia, as during the first and second branchial arches of embryogenesis, there is an interconnected development [3, 4]. In 55–93% of cases, it can be associated with atresia or stenosis of the ear canal resulting in the loss of conductive hearing [4]. However, in more than 90% of cases, the bone conduction remains intact [4].

3. **A**

   Microtia can appear as an isolated condition or as part of a spectrum of clinical manifestations, such as anomalies seen in the oculo-auriculo-vertebral spectrum (OAVS). OAVS is characterized by microtia, microphthalmia, macrostomia, ear tags, and epibulbar dermoids, or it can be associated with other syndromes [2–4]. Microtia has strong genetic association and is related to many genetic syndromes, which may have autosomal dominant or recessive inheritance, or caused by chromosomal abnormalities such as trisomies 13 and 18 [3, 4]. The most common hereditary causes of microtia are Treacher Collins, Townes-Brock-Goldenhar, and Nager syndrome [1, 4, 5].

   Genetic syndromes as fragile X, Börjeson–Forssman–Lehmann, and trichorhinophalangeal are associated with larger ear [6, 7].

4. **D**

   Non-interventional techniques and prosthetics are used as initial treatment. Surgical repair is usually performed at older ages [1]. The indications for surgical correction of microtia concern not only functionality but also cosmetics, as they often impact the social environment [1]. The autologous rib cartilage-based method is the most widespread surgical technique [1]. It is mainly performed after the age of 6 years and includes several stages. Another technique used after the age of 3, carried out as a single-stage surgery, involves alloplastic reconstruction [1, 5]. However, it is associated with a reduction in popularity due to its many long-term complications, including a higher overall risk of extrusion, fractures, and infections [1, 5]. Finally, porous polyethylene frameworks, such as Medpor, have been used, providing satisfactory aesthetic results [8].

5. **C**

   Conductive hearing loss is the most common finding in pediatric cases of microtia [5]. Therefore, hearing evaluation with auditory brainstem response (ABR) testing is important to be completed by the age of 2–3 months, as the period between 3 and 6 months is critical for the development of speech and language skills [5]. Worn hearing devices are recommended to be used before the age of 4 months, especially in cases of bilateral microtia [5]. Surgical intervention is recommended later as some implanted devices are approved and used after the age of 5 [5].

   CT scan for the evaluation of the temporal bone is not recommended during early stages, such as infancy. It is best performed before surgical procedures or in cases with an increased risk of cholesteatoma [5]. Conducting CT scans at earlier stages may yield inaccurate results due to the incomplete maturation of the external ear and the pneumatization of the mastoid bone [8]. Furthermore, CT scans are essential for assessing atresia, ruling out the presence of a canal, and detecting congenital cholesteatoma in the middle ear [5, 8].

   Further image investigation is also important as microtia is correlated with other congenital anomalies [5]. The most common are renal abnormalities, macrostomia, oral clefts, facial asymmetry, cardiac defects, microphthalmia, holoprosencephaly, polydactyly, and vertebral anomalies [2]. Renal abnormalities are frequently observed in patients with isolated microtia, as well as in many syndromes genetically correlated with microtia [5]. Therefore, a routine early ultrasound examination in these children could be beneficial [5, 9].

References

1. Hartzell LD, Chinnadurai S. Microtia and related facial anomalies. Clin Perinatol. 2018;45(4):679–97. https://doi.org/10.1016/j.clp.2018.07.007.
2. Luquetti DV, Heike CL, Hing AV, Cunningham ML, Cox TC. Microtia: epidemiology and genetics. Am J Med Genet A. 2012;158A(1):124–39. https://doi.org/10.1002/ajmg.a.34352.
3. Alnujaim NH, Alnujaim MH. Review of microtia: a focus on current surgical approaches. Egypt J Hosp Med. 2017;69(1):1698–705. https://doi.org/10.12816/0040136.
4. Alasti F, Van Camp G. Genetics of microtia and associated syndromes. J Med Genet. 2009;46(6):361–9. https://doi.org/10.1136/jmg.2008.062158.
5. Truong MT, Liu YC, Kohn J, et al. Integrated microtia and aural atresia management. Front Surg. 2022;9:944223. https://doi.org/10.3389/fsurg.2022.944223.
6. Gécz J, Turner G, Nelson J, et al. The Börjeson–Forssman–Lehman syndrome (BFLS, MIM #301900). Eur J Hum Genet. 2006;14:1233–7. https://doi.org/10.1038/sj.ejhg.5201639.
7. Maas S, Shaw A, Bikker H, et al. Trichorhinophalangeal syndrome. In: Adam MP, Mirzaa GM, Pagon RA, et al., editors. GeneReviews®. Seattle, WA: University of Washington, Seattle; 2017; 1993–2023. https://www.ncbi.nlm.nih.gov/books/NBK425926/.
8. Ali K, Mohan K, Liu YC. Otologic and audiology concerns of microtia repair. Semin Plast Surg. 2017;31(3):127–33. https://doi.org/10.1055/s-0037-1603957.
9. Kini S, Barton GW, Carol Liu Y-C. Renal anomalies and microtia: determining the clinical utility of screening affected children. Int J Pediatr Otorhinolaryngol. 2020c;133:109957. https://doi.org/10.1016/j.ijporl.2020.109957.

Congenital Hearing Loss

44

Konstantinos Garefis and Konstantinos Markou

Abstract

Congenital hearing loss (CHL) refers to hearing loss present at birth and has significant implications for a child's development and quality of life. In the United States, CHL affects approximately 2–3 out of every 1000 children. The majority of cases involve sensorineural hearing loss, with causes categorized as genetic, nongenetic/acquired factors, or idiopathic in nature. Genetic causes account for around half of congenital or childhood hearing loss cases and can be further classified as syndromic or non-syndromic. Nongenetic CHL is commonly associated with infectious diseases such as cytomegalovirus (CMV), toxoplasmosis, rubella, herpes, syphilis, as well as factors like ototoxicity, prematurity, and asphyxiation. Early diagnosis is crucial for minimizing the impact of CHL. Full-term newborns typically undergo hearing screening using methods such as otoacoustic emissions (OAEs). If an infant does not pass the initial screening, a follow-up screening is recommended. If the second screening results in a referral, diagnostic auditory brainstem response (ABR) testing is advised. If the ABR results indicate hearing loss, comprehensive audiological and etiological assessments are necessary. These assessments should include a review of the family history, imaging studies such as magnetic resonance imaging (MRI) or computed tomography (CT) scans, virological examinations, and genetic tests based on the suspected cause. Management and treatment of CHL depend on the severity and underlying cause. Options for hearing restoration include implantable or non-implantable devices such as conventional hearing aids, cochlear implants, and bone-anchored hearing aids.

K. Garefis (✉) · K. Markou
2nd Academic ORL, Head and Neck Surgery Department, Aristotle University of Thessaloniki, Papageorgiou Hospital, Thessaloniki, Greece

Case Presentation

A 1-month-old male infant was brought to the Ear, Nose, Neck (ENT) Department by his parents due to a previous referral for OAE testing. The infant had undergone OAE testing on the third day after birth, which resulted in a referral for both ears. The infant was born full-term without any complications, and the mother had a healthy pregnancy with no reported infections or exposure to ototoxic substances. There was a family history of hearing loss on the mother's side and possibly on the father's side as well. The physical examination of the infant revealed no visible abnormalities in the external ear, ear canal, or tympanic membrane. Tympanometry

N. Tsetsos et al. (eds.), *Otolaryngology Study Guide*, https://doi.org/10.1007/978-3-031-77374-7_44

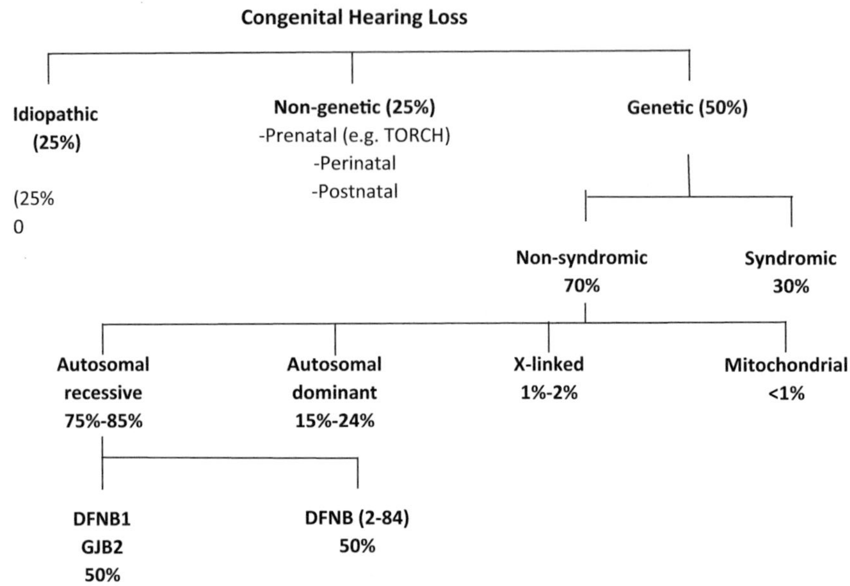

Fig. 44.1 Etiology of congenital hearing loss

results were normal. However, upon further evaluation with OAE testing, the results again showed a referral for both ears (Fig. 44.1).

Questions

1. Which of the following statements are true about CHL (more than one correct answer possible)?
   A. Genetic causes account for about 30% of CHL
   B. The majority of genetic CHL cases are autosomal recessive
   C. Mutations in GJB2 are strongly associated with CHL
   D. Prematurity is responsible for the majority of CHL
   E. Syndromes are related to CHL
2. Which is the most common cause of infection-related CHL?
   A. Herpes zoster
   B. Rubella
   C. Moraxella
   D. CMV
   E. None of the above
3. Which of the following syndromes can cause CHL (more than one correct answer possible)?
   A. Pendred
   B. Usher
   C. Waardenburg
   D. Treacher Collins
   E. All of the above
4. Which is the next diagnostic step in the infant described above?
   A. Pure-tone audiometry
   B. Magnetic resonance imaging
   C. ABR testing
   D. Tympanometry
   E. CMV saliva detection
5. The infant described was diagnosed with profound hearing loss in both ears. Genetic testing revealed mutations in GJB2. What is the appropriate treatment for this condition?
   A. Hearing aids
   B. Bilateral cochlear implantation
   C. Bone-anchored hearing aids
   D. Antivirals and corticosteroids
   E. Speech therapy

Answers

1. **B, C, E**

   A significant proportion of congenital or childhood hearing loss, estimated to be at least 50%, is attributed to genetic causes. Another 25% is considered idiopathic, meaning the exact cause is unknown. The remaining cases are caused by environmental factors such as infections, prematurity, and exposure to ototoxic substances. Among cases of genetic hearing loss, approximately 70% are classified as non-syndromic. Within this category, around 80% are autosomal recessive, 15% are autosomal dominant, and 1–2% are either mitochondrial or X-linked. It is worth noting that syndromic genetic hearing loss accounts for about 30% of all genetic cases [1]. One specific gene associated with congenital hearing loss is GJB2, which encodes the connexin-26 protein [2]. Mutations in GJB2 are responsible for around 50% of severe-to-profound autosomal recessive non-syndromic hearing impairment in European countries [3, 4].

2. **D**

   TORCHES infections, which include toxoplasmosis, rubella, CMV, herpes, and syphilis, are recognized as risk factors for sensorineural hearing loss. Among these infectious causes, congenital CMV infection is the most prevalent non-hereditary cause of sensorineural hearing loss. In industrialized countries, the prevalence of congenital CMV infection is approximately 0.58%, while in developing countries with higher rates of maternal seroprevalence, this figure can range from 1 to 6% [4, 5].

3. **E**

   Pendred syndrome is an inherited disorder with an autosomal recessive pattern, featuring a spectrum of sensorineural hearing loss ranging from mild to profound, vestibular dysfunction, and presence of euthyroid goiter. Additional indicators may involve both sides of the vestibular aqueduct, cochlear hypoplasia, and manifestation of an abnormal perchlorate discharge test [6–8]. Usher syndrome is identified as one of the prevalent causes of autosomal recessive syndromic hearing loss and retinitis pigmentosa [7, 8]. Waardenburg syndrome is recognized as a common contributor to syndromic sensorineural hearing loss, with this primary feature observed in up to 71% of affected individuals [7]. Other distinctive features may include heterochromia iridium (pale blue eyes), a white forelock, synophrys, a broad nasal root, hypoplasia of the alae nasi, a patent metopic suture line, and a square jaw [8]. Treacher Collins syndrome is characterized by distinct craniofacial abnormalities and typically presents with moderate-to-severe conductive hearing loss [7, 8]. Anomalies affecting the external and middle ear encompass microtia, stenosis, or atresia of the external auditory canal, hypoplastic middle ear cavity, and presence of dysmorphic or aberrant ossicular chains [8].

4. **C**

   As per the guidelines provided by the American Academy of Pediatrics' Joint Committee on Infant Hearing, it is recommended that all newborns undergo screening test (OAE, automated ABR) within the first month of their birth to screen for hearing loss. If a newborn does not pass this initial screening, it is further recommended that they undergo a comprehensive audiological evaluation, which includes ABR testing, by the time they reach 3 months of age [9]. Additionally, infants who have spent more than 5 days in the neonatal intensive care unit should have ABR testing included as part of their screening process [5]. Nonetheless, it is important to note that passing the initial neonatal hearing screening does not guarantee the absence of progressive, late-onset, or mild CHL (30–40 dB hearing loss) that may go undetected. In cases where children have risk factors for hearing loss or if their parents express concerns about their child's hearing abilities, it is crucial to provide regular follow-up evaluations. This is necessary as hearing loss can develop later in life depending on the underlying cause [4].

5. **B**

Determining the underlying cause can aid in selecting the appropriate therapeutic or management approach. In cases of conductive hearing loss in children with congenital anomalies like external auditory canal atresia, bone-anchored hearing aids have been utilized to improve or restore hearing [4]. For individuals with mild-to-severe sensorineural hearing loss, conventional hearing aids have proven effective in facilitating hearing rehabilitation. However, when hearing loss reaches severe-to-profound levels, these devices no longer offer sufficient clarity for meaningful speech comprehension. In such cases, cochlear implantation has become the standard treatment for children with profound congenital hearing loss. Unilateral cochlear implants have demonstrated improved hearing abilities and quality-of-life scores, while bilateral cochlear implants have shown substantial enhancements in sound localization and speech perception in noisy environments. Due to superior vocabulary outcomes, speech perception, and sound localization, an increasing number of countries now provide reimbursement for a second implant in children [4, 10]. Notably, the age for initial implantation has progressively decreased, and many children now receive implants before their first birthday [11].

References

1. Yang T, Guo L, Wang L, Yu X. Diagnosis, intervention, and prevention of genetic hearing loss. Adv Exp Med Biol. 2019;1130:73–92.
2. Kiang DT, Jin N, Tu ZJ, Lin HH. Upstream genomic sequence of the human connexin26 gene. Gene. 1997;199(1–2):165–71.
3. Kenneson A, Van Naarden BK, Boyle C. GJB2 (connexin 26) variants and non-syndromic sensorineural hearing loss: a HuGE review. Genet Med. 2002;4(4):2.
4. Korver AM, Smith RJ, Van Camp G, Schleiss MR, Bitner-Glindzicz MA, Lustig LR, Usami SI, Boudewyns AN. Congenital hearing loss. Nat Rev Dis Primers. 2017;3:16094.
5. Belcher R, Virgin F, Duis J, Wootten C. Genetic and non-genetic workup for pediatric congenital hearing loss. Front Pediatr. 2021;9:536730.
6. Smith RJ, Bale JF Jr, White KR. Sensorineural hearing loss in children. Lancet. 2005;365(9462):879–90.
7. Casazza G, Meier JD. Evaluation and management of syndromic congenital hearing loss. Curr Opin Otolaryngol Head Neck Surg. 2017;25(5):378–84.
8. Gettelfinger JD, Dahl JP. Syndromic hearing loss: a brief review of common presentations and genetics. J Pediatr Genet. 2018;7(1):1–8.
9. American Academy of Pediatrics, Joint Committee on Infant Hearing. Year 2007 position statement: principles and guidelines for early hearing detection and intervention programs. Pediatrics. 2007;120(4):898–921.
10. Gaylor JM, et al. Cochlear implantation in adults: a systematic review and meta-analysis. JAMA Otolaryngol Head Neck Surg. 2013;139:265–72.
11. Fitzpatrick EM, Ham J, Whittingham J. Pediatric cochlear implantation: why do children receive implants late? Ear Hear. 2015;36:688–94.

Glue Ear

45

Nikolaos I. Sakellaris, Eleni I. Sakellari, and Marios Stavrakas

Abstract

Glue ear or otitis media with effusion (OME) is a common pathology in children, impacting approximately 90% of them before they reach school age, with a higher frequency observed between the ages of 6 months and 4 years. The etiology of OME differs between children and adults. In children, OME is mainly linked to conditions such as poor Eustachian tube function, resulting from an upper respiratory infection or an inflammatory response following a prior episode of acute otitis media. In contrast, in adults, it can be linked to conditions such as a nasopharyngeal tumor; therefore, careful assessment is essential. The main presenting symptoms of OME in children consist of hearing impairment and a feeling of fullness in the ear. Many episodes are asymptomatic and therefore are not always detected. Once diagnosed, clinically and audiologically, the treatment options vary and include a period of watchful waiting, hearing aid provision, and insertion of ventilation tubes, sometimes in combination with adenoidectomy.

N. I. Sakellaris
Department of Otolaryngology, "G. Gennimatas" General Hospital of Athens, Athens, Greece

E. I. Sakellari
Faculty of Health Sciences, Aristotle University of Thessaloniki, AHEPA University Hospital, Thessaloniki, Greece

M. Stavrakas (✉)
ENT Head and Neck Surgery Department, University Hospitals Plymouth NHS Trust, Plymouth, UK

Case Presentation

A 4-year-old boy has been referred to the ENT clinic with concerns over speech and hearing. He had speech and language therapy, and his speech is improving. There are still concerns about his hearing, but he does not have any history of recurrent ear infections or discharge. He has no other ENT problems. He was a full-term baby that passed his newborn hearing screening assessment, and he is up to date with his vaccines. On examination, he had grade 3 tonsils, and ears bilaterally showed an intact tympanic membrane with no obvious retraction. His hearing assessment shows bilateral mild conductive hearing loss with type B tympanograms bilaterally and normal ear canal volumes. We have discussed management options including watchful waiting, hearing aids, and grommet insertion. We agreed to repeat the hearing test in 3 months and reassess the child clinically (Fig. 45.1).

N. Tsetsos et al. (eds.), *Otolaryngology Study Guide*, https://doi.org/10.1007/978-3-031-77374-7_45

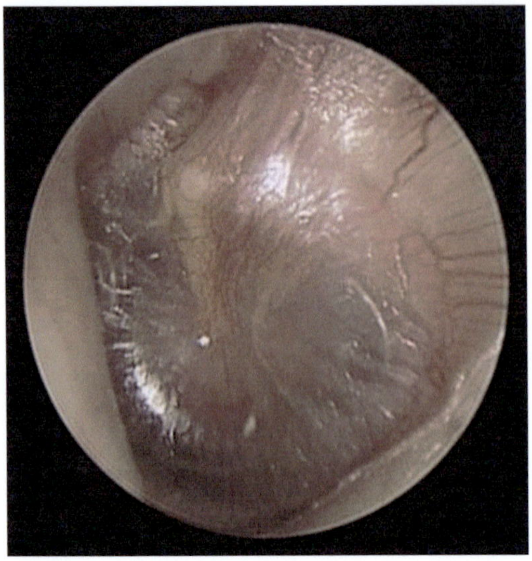

Fig. 45.1 Endoscopic photograph demonstrating middle ear effusion

Questions

1. Which of the following statements are true about otitis media with effusion (OME) (more than one correct answer possible)?
   A. An otitis media with effusion is always an acute inflammatory situation.
   B. The majority of children are affected by OME at least once before the age of 12.
   C. Most frequently, OME occurs between the ages of 6 months and 4 years.
   D. Fever is a common symptom.
   E. Can occur due to poor Eustachian tube function.
2. What is the first-line treatment for mild cases of OME?
   A. Steroids
   B. Antibiotics
   C. Antihistamines
   D. Decongestants
   E. Watchful waiting
3. Which of the following statements are true for hearing assessment in OME (more than one correct answer possible)?
   A. Hearing test should be performed in all patients with the initial diagnosis.
   B. Down syndrome requires more frequent hearing assessment.
   C. Conventional audiometry is recommended for children up to 6 months of age.
   D. If hearing loss is ≤20 dB, hearing test is repeated in 3–6 months.
   E. All of the above.
4. Which of the following surgical options is most suitable for children under 4 years old?
   A. Adenoidectomy.
   B. Tympanostomy tubes.
   C. Adenoidectomy plus tympanoscopy tubes.
   D. Adenotonsillectomy.
   E. None of the above.
5. Which of the following is a correct indication for tympanostomy tube insertion?
   A. Children with bilateral chronic OME regardless of hearing impairment.
   B. Children with unilateral chronic OME and documented hearing difficulties.
   C. Children with recurrent acute otitis media regardless of OEM signs.
   D. Children with recurrent acute otitis media and bilateral OEM.
   E. None of the above.

Answers

1. **B, C, E**

   Otitis media with effusion (OME), also referred to as glue ear, is lacking of inflammatory signs or symptoms [1, 2]. It is crucial to differentiate OME from acute otitis media, which presents with signs and symptoms of middle ear inflammation [1]. OME is a common condition among children, impacting approximately 90% of them before they reach school age, with a higher frequency observed between the ages of 6 months and 4 years [1]. Many episodes are asymptomatic and therefore are not always detected [1].

   The etiology of OME differs between children and adults [3]. In children, OME is mainly linked to conditions such as poor Eustachian tube function, resulting from an upper respiratory infection or an inflammatory response following a prior episode of acute otitis media. In contrast, in adults, it can be linked to conditions such as a nasopharyngeal tumor; therefore, adults who present with unilateral glue ear require thorough clinical examination including endoscopic evaluation of the nasopharynx [1, 3]. The main presenting symptoms of OME in children consist of hearing impairment and a feeling of fullness in the ear [3].

2. **E**

   To confirm the presence of OME, pneumatic otoscopy or tympanometry should be performed, especially when the diagnosis is uncertain with otoscopy alone [1, 2, 4]. Children with mild case of OME who are not identified as being at higher risk for speech, language, and learning problems should undergo a watchful waiting process for 3 months after the date of diagnosis [1, 2, 4]. Since OME often resolves spontaneously, interventions such as antibiotics, intranasal or systemic steroids, decongestants, and antihistamines are usually unnecessary [1, 4]. Throughout the active observation period, individuals should be offered guidance on educational and behavioral approaches to mitigate the impacts of their hearing loss [1, 2]. It is crucial to note that the decision for watchful waiting should be made based on a careful assessment by a qualified medical professional, considering the individual patient's age, overall health, potential risk factors, and coexisting causes contributing to hearing impairment [1, 2]. Regular follow-up visits during the observation period are essential to track any changes in the condition and determine the need for further intervention, if required [1, 2].

3. **B, D**

   OME is characterized by the accumulation of fluid in the middle ear, which hinders the conduction of sound through the middle ear and its transmission to the inner ear, leading to conductive hearing loss [1]. Hearing test should be conducted in patients who are at non-risk for developmental problems, if OME persists for more than 3 months [1, 2, 4]. Children diagnosed with developmental disabilities, such as Down syndrome and cleft palate, should undergo regular and more frequent hearing assessments to mitigate potential impacts on their developmental outcomes [1, 2, 4]. Age-appropriate hearing tests should be performed [1, 2]. A comprehensive audiological evaluation is suitable for children aged 6 months to 4 years. Additionally, visual response audiometry is recommended for children aged 6 months to 2.5 years, play audiometry for children aged 2.5–4 years old, and conventional audiometry for children aged up to 4 years old [1, 2]. In cases that hearing levels fall within the normal ranges (≤20 dB), a follow-up hearing test should be scheduled in 3–6 months [1]. Mild-to-moderate hearing loss, whether unilateral or bilateral, may have an impact on everyday life and development [1]. Timely detection and appropriate interventions are essential during this timeframe [1].

4. **B**

   In children under 4 years old, when it is determined that surgical management is necessary for OME, tympanostomy tube insertion is considered the primary procedure of choice [1, 2, 4]. Adenoidectomy is generally not recommended for patients within this specific age group. In certain cases, when specific signs are present, chronic adenoid hypertrophy or chronic adenoiditis leading to nasal obstruction, a concurrent adenoidectomy may be indicated [1, 4].

5. **B, C**

   In cases of bilateral OME, the indication for surgically inserting tympanostomy tubes is the duration of more than 3 months (chronic OME) and documented hearing difficulties [1]. This treatment could also be an option for children with chronic OME and symptoms that reduce their quality of life and development [1]. Furthermore, the only evidence for tube insertion in patients with recurrent acute otitis media is the presence of unilateral or bilateral OME at the time of assessment [1]. After the ventilation tube insertion, hearing ability should be reevaluated [2].

References

1. Rosenfeld RM, Shin JJ, Schwartz SR, et al. Clinical practice guideline: otitis media with effusion (update). Otolaryngol Head Neck Surg. 2016;154(1 Suppl):S1–S41. https://doi.org/10.1177/0194599815623467.
2. National Collaborating Centre for Women's and Children's Health (UK). Surgical Management of Otitis Media with effusion in children. London: RCOG Press; 2008.
3. Hidaka H, Ito M, Ikeda R, et al. Clinical practice guidelines for the diagnosis and management of otitis media with effusion (OME) in children in Japan—2022 update. Auris Nasus Larynx. 2023;50(5):655–99. https://doi.org/10.1016/j.anl.2022.12.004.
4. Lambert M. AAO-HNS releases updated guideline on management of otitis media with effusion. Am Fam Physician. 2016;94(9):747–9.

46 Obstructive Sleep Apnoea

Kidus Eshete and Marios Stavrakas

Abstract

Obstructive sleep apnoea is a sleep disorder that involves cessation or significant decrease in airflow in the presence of breathing effort. It is the most common type of sleep-disordered breathing and is characterised by recurrent episodes of upper airway collapse during sleep. Common risk factors include male sex, age, obesity, cranial facial anatomy resulting in narrow airways and obesity. General symptoms of OSA could be nocturnal, such as snoring, witnessed apnoea, gasping, choking sensations, nocturia and insomnia. Daytime symptoms include non-refreshing sleep, morning headache, excessive daytime sleepiness and fatigue. Diagnosing OSA is dependent on overnight sleep studies or polysomnography. Treatment of OSA partly depends on the patient's severity of sleep-disordered breathing. Those with mild apnoea have more options, whereas people with moderate-to-severe apnoea should be treated with nasal continuous positive airway pressure (CPAP).

K. Eshete
University Hospitals Plymouth NHS Trust, Plymouth, UK

M. Stavrakas (✉)
ENT Head and Neck Surgery Department, University Hospitals Plymouth NHS Trust, Plymouth, UK

Case Presentation

A 42-year-old man, who works as a truck driver for a delivery company, presented to the clinic complaining of excessive daytime sleepiness and having to pull to the side of the road to take frequent multiple breaks. He has gained about 10 kg of weight over the past 6 months, and he barely engages in physical exercises. He smokes about 15 cigarettes/day and consumes alcohol occasionally. He has a family history of type 2 diabetes. His Epworth sleepiness score was 13, and there is a marked increase on the apnoea-hypopnea index on the polysomnography study (Fig. 46.1).

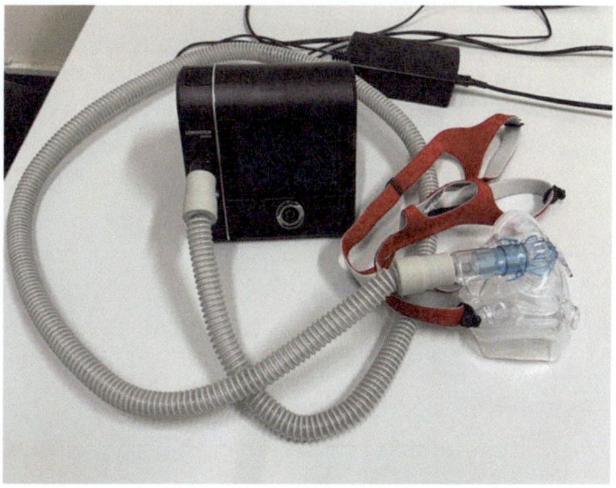

Fig. 46.1 CPAP machine

N. Tsetsos et al. (eds.), *Otolaryngology Study Guide*, https://doi.org/10.1007/978-3-031-77374-7_46

Questions

1. Which of the following statements about obstructive sleep apnoea is true?
   A. OSA occurs secondary to respiratory secretions accumulating in the respiratory tract
   B. Presence of severity of OSA is quantified by the apnoea-hypopnea index
   C. OSA is more prevalent among women than men
   D. Symptoms of OSA are limited to night-time symptoms
   E. The gold standard diagnostic method is pulse oximetry
2. Which of the following is the most common presenting complaint of OSA?
   A. Unrefreshing sleep, with excessive fatigue
   B. Awakenings accompanied by gasping or choking at night
   C. Morning headache
   D. Snoring
   E. Difficulty falling asleep
3. Which of the following is true about the pathophysiology and associations of OSA?
   A. OSA is linked with increased insulin sensitivity
   B. Low blood pressure is linked with OSA
   C. OSA is associated with arrest in respiratory effort
   D. Patients with cardiovascular disease have a higher risk of OSA
   E. Exercise worsens OSA
4. What is the standard diagnostic screening test for OSA?
   A. Polysomnography
   B. The Epworth Sleepiness Scale
   C. Home sleep apnoea test
   D. Oximetry
   E. STOP-Bang Questionnaire
5. Which of the following is shown to help in improving OSA?
   A. Avoid sleeping in supine position
   B. Regular aerobic exercise
   C. Bariatric surgery
   D. Continuous positive airway pressure (CPAP)
   E. All of the above

Answers

1. **B**

   Obstructive sleep apnoea (OSA) occurs when there are recurrent episodes of upper airway collapse and obstruction during sleep associated with arousals with or without oxygen desaturations. The oropharynx in the back of the throat collapses during OSA events to cause arousal or oxygen desaturation or both, resulting in fragmented sleep [1]. Common risk factors include obesity, male gender, old age and smoking [2]. There are several common sleep and daytime symptoms associated with OSA though patients vary in the number and combination of symptoms reported [3]. During sleep, snoring is one of the most common symptoms [1]. According to the apnoea-hypopnea index (AHI), OSA could be divided into mild (AHI 5–15), moderate (AHI 15–30) or severe (AHI >30). This may determine if a patient with OSA needs to be treated or not [1].

2. **A**

   The most common symptom of OSA is unrefreshing sleep, with excessive sleepiness reported by up to 90% of patients with OSA referred to sleep clinics [4, 5]. Patients may also report fatigue, tiredness or lack of energy [6]. Excessive daytime sleepiness is feeling very drowsy or very sleepy at times, whereas fatigue is feeling tired, low on energy and unmotivated. During sleep, snoring is one of the most common symptoms [1]. Other important elements in the history are nasal symptoms, associated medical conditions such as atrial fibrillation, congestive heart failure, hypertension, chronic lung disease, pregnancy, acromegaly, hypothyroidism and Parkinson's. Especially in the paediatric population, the clinician should enquire about comorbidities associated with OSA, which include Down syndrome, neuromuscular disease, craniofacial abnormalities, achondroplasia, mucopolysaccharidosis and Prader-Willi syndrome [7].

3. **D**

   Intermittent hypoxemia, particularly with concomitant hypercapnia, activates the sympathetic nervous system and is the major contributor to both acute and chronic elevation of blood pressure [8, 9]. Increased catecholamine levels decrease insulin sensitivity and, in animal models, promote pancreatic beta-cell apoptosis, suggesting a possible mechanism underlying the association of OSA with type 2 diabetes mellitus [10]. Repetitive episodes of hypoxemia increase reactive oxygen species, which may further contribute to vascular disease, metabolic abnormalities, and inflammation [8]. Unlike OSA, where there is a physical obstruction of the airway, in central apnoea, there is no respiratory effort [1].

4. **A**

   Screening patients for OSA starts with a good sleep history to identify symptoms, risk factors and comorbid conditions, as well as a physical examination for OSA-related features. The Epworth Sleepiness Scale and STOP-Bang Questionnaire are brief, effective screening tools that can inform the need for further testing [1]. However, the standard diagnostic test is laboratory-based polysomnography, during which both sleep and respiratory parameters are monitored [11].

5. **E**

   Effective treatments for OSA include behavioural measures, medical devices, and surgery. For mild OSA with no symptoms or symptoms that do not affect usual daytime activities, behavioural measures include abstinence from alcohol, regular aerobic exercise, weight loss and sleep advice, which are usually enough [2, 12]. For mild OSA with symptoms that affect quality of life and usual daytime activities or moderate/severe OSA, consideration of CPAP in addition to lifestyle changes is recommended. Other treatment options include a customised or semi-customised mandibular advancement splint in people aged 18 and over with optimal dental and periodontal health, a positional modifier for mild or moderate positional OSA or referral for assessment for oropharyngeal surgery for moderate or severe OSA. The clinician may consider tonsillectomy if the person has large obstructive tonsils and BMI <35 kg/m^2. If the patient suffers from rhinitis, appropriate medical treatment with an intranasal corticosteroid spray should be initiated. In case of significant nasal obstruction, nasal surgery can be considered aiming to improve the anatomical obstruction [12].

References

1. Rundo JV. Obstructive sleep apnea basics. Cleveland Clinic J Med. 2019;86(9 Suppl 1):2–9.
2. Gottlieb DJ, Punjabi NM. Diagnosis and management of obstructive sleep apnea: a review. JAMA. 2020;323(14):1389–400.
3. Adult Obstructive Sleep Apnea Task Force of the American Academy of Sleep Medicine. Clinical guideline for the evaluation, management and long-term care of obstructive sleep apnea in adults. J Clin Sleep Med. 2009;5(3):263–76.
4. Davies RJ, Ali NJ, Stradling JR. Neck circumference and other clinical features in the diagnosis of the obstructive sleep apnoea syndrome. Thorax. 1992;47(2):101–5.
5. Guilleminault C, et al. A clinical investigation of obstructive sleep apnea syndrome (OSAS) and upper airway resistance syndrome (UARS) patients. Sleep Med. 2000;1(1):51–6.
6. Chervin RD. Sleepiness, fatigue, tiredness, and lack of energy in obstructive sleep apnea. Chest. 2000;118(2):372–9.
7. Manjaly J, Kullar PJ, editors. Advanced ENT training: a guide to passing the FRCS (ORL-HNS) examination. CRC Press; 2019.
8. Dempsey JA, et al. Pathophysiology of sleep apnea. Physiol Rev. 2010;90(1):47–112.
9. Somers VK, et al. Sleep apnea and cardiovascular disease: an American heart association/American College of cardiology foundation scientific statement from the American heart association council for high blood pressure research professional education committee, council on clinical cardiology, stroke council, and council on cardiovascular nursing in collaboration with the national heart, lung, and blood institute national center on sleep disorders research (national institutes of health). Circulation. 2008;118(10):1080–111.
10. Briançon-Marjollet A, et al. The impact of sleep disorders on glucose metabolism: endocrine and molecular mechanisms. Diabetol Metab Syndrome. 2015;7(1):1–16.
11. Kapur VK, et al. Clinical practice guideline for diagnostic testing for adult obstructive sleep apnea: an American Academy of Sleep Medicine clinical practice guideline. J Clin Sleep Med. 2017;13(3):479–504.
12. Guideline NG202 NI. Obstructive sleep apnoea/hypopnoea syndrome and obesity hypoventilation syndrome in over 16s. Methods. 2021.

Tonsillectomy

47

Kidus Eshete and Marios Stavrakas

Abstract

Tonsillectomy is a common procedure performed to alleviate various throat-related conditions. Palatine tonsils are located on each side of the throat and can become enlarged or infected, leading to recurrent tonsillitis, obstructive sleep apnoea, and other respiratory issues. The surgery is typically recommended for patients experiencing frequent or severe throat infections or OSA or in case malignancy is suspected. Tonsillectomy is often considered a safe and effective intervention with a relatively straightforward recovery process. However, potential risks and complications, such as post-operative bleeding and infection, warrant careful post-operative monitoring and adherence to appropriate aftercare instructions. As with any surgical procedure, patients and healthcare providers must weigh the benefits and risks to determine the most suitable course of action for individual cases.

K. Eshete
University Hospitals Plymouth NHS Trust, Plymouth, UK

M. Stavrakas (✉)
ENT Head and Neck Surgery Department, University Hospitals Plymouth NHS Trust, Plymouth, UK

Case Presentation

A 5-year-old male patient was referred to the ENT service by his GP due to disordered sleep and witnessed apnoeic episodes, lasting for about 10 s. The child is otherwise fit and well, with clear perinatal history. Clinical examination revealed grade III tonsils, and it was decided to proceed with tonsillectomy. He underwent a bilateral tonsillectomy (Fig. 47.1) with uneventful recovery, and the patient demonstrated complete resolution of symptoms.

Questions

1. Which of the following arteries supply the palatine tonsil?
   A. Internal carotid artery
   B. Ophthalmic artery
   C. Ascending pharyngeal artery
   D. Sphenopalatine artery
   E. None of the above
2. Which of the following are indications for tonsillectomy?
   A. 6 episodes of tonsillitis in the past 12 months
   B. 4 episodes of tonsillitis in each of the preceding 2 years
   C. 3 episodes of tonsillitis in each of the preceding 3 years
   D. History of one peri-tonsillar abscess
   E. Halitosis

N. Tsetsos et al. (eds.), *Otolaryngology Study Guide*, https://doi.org/10.1007/978-3-031-77374-7_47

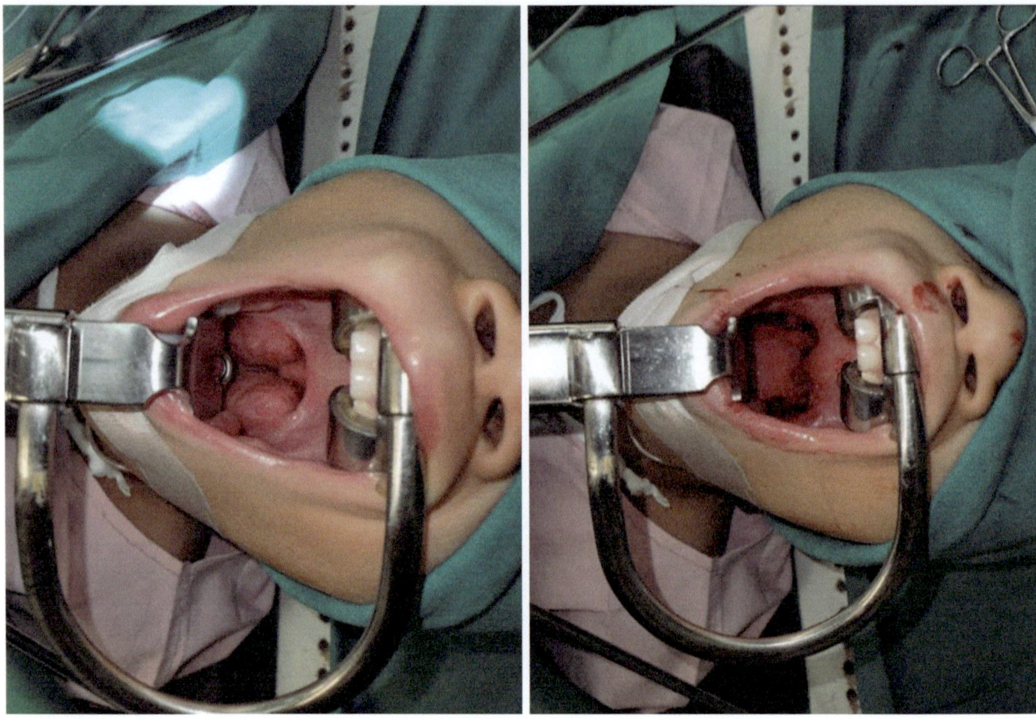

Fig. 47.1 Pre- (left) and post-tonsillectomy (right) photographs

3. Which of the following is true about post-tonsillectomy haemorrhage (more than one correct answer possible)?
   A. Primary haemorrhage is bleeding in the first week post-tonsillectomy
   B. Secondary haemorrhage occurs following the separation of the eschar from the tonsillar bed
   C. Older age is a risk factor for post-tonsillectomy bleeding
   D. Risk of haemorrhage on patients with infectious mononucleosis is significantly high
   E. All of the above
4. Which of the following statement is NOT TRUE?
   A. Palatopharyngeal insufficiency is a possible post-tonsillectomy complication
   B. The risk of post-tonsillectomy haemorrhage is lower if tonsillectomy is done in less than 3 weeks from an episode of acute tonsillitis
   C. The incidence of post-tonsillectomy haemorrhage is about 2–3%
   D. There is no evidence that antibiotics have a role in preventing recurrent tonsillitis
   E. Coblation intracapsular tonsillectomy is an acceptable method for recurrent tonsillitis and OSA in children
5. Which of the following are surgical instruments used in tonsillectomy?
   A. Boyle Davis mouth gag
   B. Draffin rods
   C. Mollison pillar retractor
   D. Negus knot pusher
   E. All of the above

Answers

1. **C**

The tonsils consist of lymphoid tissue covered by respiratory epithelium. The term "tonsil" refers specifically to the palatine tonsils, and the term "adenoids" refers to the pharyngeal tonsils. Waldeyer's ring is the ring of lymphoid tissues in the pharynx formed by the palatine tonsils, pharyngeal tonsils, and lingual tonsils [1]. The blood supply comes from the external carotid artery, with numerous branches that penetrate the superior pharyngeal constrictor muscle. More specifically, the inferior pole is supplied primarily by the tonsillar artery, branch of the facial artery, and also branches of the lingual artery. The ascending palatine artery, another branch of the facial artery, divides distally into two branches, one of which also supplies the palatine tonsil. The superior pole is supplied primarily by tonsillar branches of the ascending pharyngeal artery and by the descending palatine artery, a branch of the internal maxillary artery [2].

2. **C**

   The following are recommended as indications for consideration of tonsillectomy in both children and adults: suspected malignancy, OSA, seven or more well documented, clinically significant, adequately treated sore throats in the preceding year, five or more such episodes in each of the preceding 2 years or three or more such episodes in each of the preceding 3 years, and two or more episodes of peritonsillar abscess [3]. A recent large-scale trial demonstrated that compared with conservative management, immediate tonsillectomy is clinically effective and cost effective in adults with recurrent acute tonsillitis [4].

3. **B, C, D**

   Post-tonsillectomy haemorrhage in most studies is defined as primary when occurring less than 24 h post-operatively and secondary when occurring after 24 h post-operatively. Primary haemorrhage occurs most commonly within 6 h of surgery. It is often severe and is more likely to require returning to the operating room than secondary haemorrhage. Secondary haemorrhage is most likely to occur between the fifth and 14th post-operative days. This is the time when the tonsillar bed eschar separates, exposing small surface vessels to local trauma [1].

   Risk factors for bleeding include the tonsillectomy technique, older age (adult vs. child) [5, 6], and presence of inflammation (chronic tonsillitis, peritonsillar abscess at the time of tonsillectomy) [7]. The risk of haemorrhage in patients with infectious mononucleosis was 20% in one study, illustrating why tonsillectomy is generally avoided in this population [8].

4. **B**

   Delaying tonsillectomy surgeries for at least 3 weeks following an episode of tonsillitis permits recuperation and also reduces the risk of post-operative haemorrhage.

   Apart from haemorrhage, other complications of tonsillectomy include infection, injury to teeth/lips/gums/TMJ, persistent pharyngitis, palatopharyngeal insufficiency, and glossopharyngeal neuralgia. Coblation intracapsular tonsillectomy, according to a recent study, carries an additional risk of symptomatic regrowth, requiring revision tonsillectomy (approximately 1.1% at 2 years and 2.2% at 5 years). The same study compares the outcomes of the National Prospective Tonsillectomy Audit (2015), where overall haemorrhage rates were 4.6% for coblation (extracapsular), 4.6% for bipolar dissection, 2.7% for cold steel and bipolar haemostasis, and 1.7% for cold steel and packs or ties. The overall bleeding rate in this study (intracapsular coblation tonsillectomy) was 1.3% [9].

5. **E**

   Cold steel tonsillectomy has been the standard practice for several years and remains an option for dissection tonsillectomy. Other variations include bipolar cautery and more recently coblation. The surgical steps are the following:

   - The patient is under general anaesthesia, with the neck extended using a shoulder bag.
   - A Boyle Davis gag is used to hold the mouth open and allow access to the tonsils.
   - Draffin rods are used to secure the Boyle Davis gag in position.
   - The surgeon starts by incision of the anterior pillar, to dissect the upper pole and ligate the vessels.

- The tonsil is freed by using a Gwynne-Evans tonsil dissector or bipolar diathermy to allow simultaneous haemostasis too.
- The lower pole can be then either clamped or ligated with an appropriate tie and the tonsil removed.
- Haemostasis is achieved using ties ± bipolar diathermy.
- The gag is then released to check for tension-related haemostasis, and any bleeding points are controlled.
- The postnasal space and pyriform fossae are suctioned with a flexible nasal catheter to remove any clots.
- The teeth and TMJ should be checked for any damage and documented in the operation notes [10].

References

1. Jose W Ruiz. Tonsillectomy in adults: surgery. UpToDate; 2012.
2. Arambula A, Brown JR, Neff L. Anatomy and physiology of the palatine tonsils, adenoids, and lingual tonsils. World J Otorhinolaryngol. 2021;7(03):155–60.
3. SIGN. Management of sore throat and indications for tonsillectomy. April 2010.
4. Wilson JA, O'Hara J, Fouweather T, Homer T, Stocken DD, Vale L, Haighton C, Rousseau N, Wilson R, McSweeney L, Wilkes S. Conservative management versus tonsillectomy in adults with recurrent acute tonsillitis in the UK (NATTINA): a multicentre, open-label, randomised controlled trial. Lancet. 2023;401(10393):2051–9.
5. Lowe D. National prospective tonsillectomy audit tonsillectomy technique as a risk for postoperative haemorrhage. Lancet. 2004;364:697–702.
6. Lowe D, et al. Key messages from the national prospective tonsillectomy audit. Laryngoscope. 2007;117(4):717–24.
7. Paradise JL. Tonsillectomy and adenoidectomy. Pediatric Otolaryngol. 1996;2:1054–65.
8. Windfuhr JP, Chen YS, Remmert S. Hemorrhage following tonsillectomy and adenoidectomy in 15,218 patients. Otolaryngol Head Neck Surg. 2005;132(2):281–6.
9. Powell S, Tweedie DJ, Jonas NE, Bateman ND, Keltie K, Sims AJ. Coblation intracapsular tonsillectomy: a cohort study of NHS practice in England using Hospital Episode Statistics. Clin Otolaryngol. 2022;47(3):471–7. https://doi.org/10.1111/coa.13929. Epub 2022 Mar 22. Erratum in: Clin Otolaryngol. 2022;47(6):707. PMID: 35289094; PMCID: PMC9310914
10. Yao A, Cameron M, McIntyre C, Allen J, Khalid-Raja M, Doshi J, Robson A, Karamchandani D, Hettige R, Shamil E, Syed I. Ear nose and throat: the official handbook for medical students and junior doctors. London: ENT UK; 2018.

48 Down Syndrome

Eleni I. Sakellari, Nikolaos I. Sakellaris, and Fotini Ieridou

Abstract

Down syndrome, or trisomy 21, is the most common chromosomal anomaly in children born alive. It presents with distinct clinical and facial features and is related to various medical challenges, including otolaryngological issues and obstructive sleep apnea. Otolaryngological problems such as stenotic ear canals, chronic ear disease, internal auditory canal and cochlear nerve hypoplasia, laryngomalacia, and subglottic stenosis predispose to a high incidence of cerumen impaction, middle ear effusion, acute otitis media with effusion, and conductive, sensorineural, or mixed hearing loss in Down syndrome patients. Due to the multiple problems related to otolaryngology, it is crucial to perform frequent evaluations, even at birth, including otoscopy, brainstem auditory testing, and tympanometry. Furthermore, obstructive sleep apnea can be diagnosed with polysomnography, and adenotonsillectomy can be considered as an optimal treatment.

Case Presentation

A 6-year-old girl with Down syndrome referred to our clinic complaining of hearing difficulties. Otoscopic examination revealed bilateral middle ear effusions consistent with glue ear, and audiometric testing confirmed bilateral conductive hearing loss. There was a consideration of installing a pressure equalization (PE) tube in the tympanic membrane, but ultimately hearing aids were offered as the primary management option. She was additionally referred to a speech and language therapist for communication support. With comprehensive care and regular follow-up, her condition improved significantly.

Questions

1. Which of the following are common facial clinical characteristics of Down syndrome (more than one correct answer possible)?
   A. Flat nasal bridge
   B. Broad forehead
   C. Cleft palate
   D. Micrognathia
   E. None of the above

E. I. Sakellari (✉)
Faculty of Health Sciences, Aristotle University of Thessaloniki, AHEPA University Hospital, Thessaloniki, Greece

N. I. Sakellaris
Department of Otolaryngology, "G. Gennimatas" General Hospital of Athens, Athens, Greece

F. Ieridou
University Hospitals Plymouth NSH Trust, Plymouth, UK

N. Tsetsos et al. (eds.), *Otolaryngology Study Guide*, https://doi.org/10.1007/978-3-031-77374-7_48

2. Which of the following is a common ENT problem in patients with Down syndrome?
   A. Chronic ear disease
   B. Hearing loss
   C. Obstructive sleep apnea
   D. Laryngomalacia
   E. All of the above
3. Which of the following statements are true regarding the hearing in patients with Down syndrome (more than one correct answer possible)?
   A. The first hearing evaluation should be performed at birth.
   B. If the child passes the first screening test, they are reevaluated yearly.
   C. If the child failed the first screening test, proceed immediately with tympanometry.
   D. Behavioral audiogram may be attempted at first year of age.
   E. The hearing usually fluctuates.
4. Which of the following statements are true for adenotonsillectomy in patients with Down syndrome (more than one correct answer possible)?
   A. The patient needs normal hospitalization as other patients.
   B. Preoperative evaluation includes the atlantoaxial instability.
   C. Before the surgery, polysomnography should be performed.
   D. After the surgery, most of the patients have fully recovered from obstructive sleep apnea.
   E. There is lower risk for complications.
5. Which is the first-line treatment for hearing impairment due to glue ear in patients with Down syndrome?
   A. Tympanostomy tube insertion
   B. Tonsillectomy
   C. Hearing aid
   D. Adenoidectomy
   E. None of the above

Answers

1. **A, D**

   Down syndrome, also known as trisomy 21, is the most common chromosome anomaly in children who are born alive [1]. There are many distinct facial features related to this syndrome. Among the most common features are small brachycephalic head, midface hypoplasia, small mouth with macroglossia which may be relative to micrognathia, shortened palate, smaller pinna approximately 2 standard deviations than general population, flat nasal bridge, and epicanthal folds [1–3]. Other common clinical characteristics include generalized hypotonia, a single transverse palmar crease, and clinodactyly of the fifth finger which appears smaller [2]. There are also a small number of cases with Down syndrome and congenital cleft palate, but it is not a common feature for this syndrome [4].
2. **E**

   There are several morphological abnormalities related to this syndrome that lead to otorhinolaryngological problems. Approximately 50% of newborns with Down syndrome are estimated to have stenotic ear canals, which predispose them to cerumen impaction and increase the incidence of middle ear effusion [1, 3]. Furthermore, these patients have an increased incidence of chronic ear disease which is multifactorial [1]. Factors predisposing to chronic ear disease include impaired immune system function and generalized hypotonia. The latter impacts the function of the tensor veli palatini muscle, leading to tube narrowing and poor aeration of the middle ear space [1]. All the previous factors predispose to increased prevalence for otitis media with effusion [1]. There are also abnormalities of inner ear, such as internal auditory canal and cochlear nerve hypoplasia [1]. For all the previous reasons, up to 75% of Down syndrome patients may have hearing loss conductive, sensorineural, or mixed [1, 3, 5, 6].

   A large number of children with Down syndrome experience severe obstructive sleep apnea, primarily due to their massive hypotonia, macroglossia, tonsillar hypertrophy, narrowing of the oropharynx, and chronic rhinosinusitis resulting from abnormalities in the paranasal sinuses and adenoid hypertrophy [1, 3, 6]. Furthermore, laryngomalacia and subglottic stenosis, which may present as inspiratory stridor, are also common issues in children with Down syndrome [1].

3. **A, D**

Brainstem auditory evoked response [BAER, ABR] or otoacoustic emission testing is recommended for all neonates including children with Down syndrome. In children with Down syndrome, due to their anatomical abnormalities such as the narrowing of the auditory canal as well as their greater possibility for acute otitis media with fluid, chronic ear disease, and hearing loss, the reevaluation despite the first successful screening must be repeated at the age of 6 months [7]. If the first test fails, then it should be tested for stenotic external canals to determine if there is a middle ear abnormality [7]. Frequent examination should be performed, every 3–6 months, either by a pediatrician or by an otolaryngologist in case of a narrowing auditory canal [7]. When the tympanic membrane is completely visible, then the tympanogram is performed [7]. A behavioral audiogram can be attempted at the age of 1 year, and in case of failure to complete, the BAER test is repeated [7]. Hearing test auditory thresholds, tympanometry, and otoscopy should be performed every 6 months until bilaterally normal hearing levels are achieved and then annually [7].

4. **B, C**

The anatomical abnormities such as the adenotonsillar hypertrophy account for Down syndrome patients as increased risk for obstructive sleep disorders [8]. Adenotonsillectomy is an option for the patient's improvement [8]. Preoperatively, it is recommended to perform a polysomnography, but also due to the concomitant anatomical abnormalities, a carefully preoperative evaluation should include also the exclusion of atlantoaxial instability [9]. Furthermore, patients with Down syndrome have a greater risk of postoperative complications, including velopharyngeal insufficiency, nasopharyngeal stenosis, and referred otalgia, often necessitating longer hospitalization [9].

5. **C**

Children with Down syndrome have higher rates of glue ears (otitis media with effusion) [10]. The management is often difficult as it appears at a young age, can lead to chronic problems, and has a greater risk of complications. Hearing loss is a common finding, often attributed to glue ears, requiring immediate treatment due to the risk of speech, language, and learning difficulties [3, 10]. Hearing aids are offered as first-option management [10]. Ventilation tubes are considered an alternative option due to challenges in placement resulting from a narrow ear canal, increased risk of subsequent otorrhea, and higher expulsion rates. Risks also encompass surgical difficulties arising from coexisting anatomical abnormalities and potential comorbidities [10].

References

1. Chin CJ, Khami MM, Husein M. A general review of the otolaryngologic manifestations of down syndrome. Int J Pediatr Otorhinolaryngol. 2014;78(6):899–904. https://doi.org/10.1016/j.ijporl.2014.03.012.
2. Bull MJ, Committee on Genetics. Health supervision for children with down syndrome [published correction appears in Pediatrics. 2011;128(6):1212]. Pediatrics. 2011;128(2):393–406. https://doi.org/10.1542/peds.2011-1605.
3. Rodman R, Pine HS. The otolaryngologist's approach to the patient with down syndrome. Otolaryngol Clin N Am. 2012;45(3):599–629, vii-viii-viii. https://doi.org/10.1016/j.otc.2012.03.010.
4. Cabanas CC, Falconi S, Jones H, Subhani M, Adesanya OA. Cleft palate in a newborn with trisomy 21: a case report. Cureus. 2023;15(5):e39107.
5. Data statistics on Down Syndrome. Centers for Disease Control and Prevention. https://www.cdc.gov/ncbddd/birthdefects/downsyndrome/data.html.
6. Shott SR. Down syndrome: common otolaryngologic manifestations. Am J Med Genet Part C Semin Med Genet. 2006;142C:131–40.
7. Bull MJ, Trotter T, Santoro SL, et al.; AAP Council on GeneticsHealth supervision for children and adolescents with down syndrome. Pediatrics. 2022;149(5):e2022057010.
8. Ali KI. Role of adenotonsillectomy and tonsillectomy in children with down syndrome who develop obstructive sleep apnea by obesity as a risk factor. Int J Pediatr. 2022;2022:8074094. Published 2022 May 6. https://doi.org/10.1155/2022/8074094.
9. Mitchell RB, Archer SM, Ishman SL, et al. Clinical practice guideline: tonsillectomy in children (update)-executive summary. Otolaryngol Head Neck Surg. 2019;160(2):187–205. https://doi.org/10.1177/0194599818807917.
10. National Collaborating Centre for Women's and Children's Health (UK). Surgical management of otitis media with effusion in children. London: RCOG Press; 2008.

49 Choanal Atresia

Nikolaos Tsetsos and Marios Stavrakas

Abstract

Choanal atresia (CA) is an uncommon clinical entity with an estimated incidence of 1:5000–7000 births. Interestingly, the characteristics of CA follow a "2–1" rule, namely the ratio of unilateral to bilateral CA, female to male, and right-sided to left-sided CA. Multiple congenital anomalies are commonly encountered among these patients, with CHARGE syndrome accounting approximately for 25% of the cases. In case of bilateral CA, infants can have acute respiratory distress with intermittent cyanosis characteristically relieved by crying. Feeding difficulty can be the initial alerting event in which the infants can present with progressive airway obstruction and choking during feeding because of their inability to breathe and feed simultaneously. Infants with unilateral CA, rarely present with neonatal respiratory distress, are often diagnosed later on in life. The most common presentation is chronic unilateral nasal obstruction, persistent mucoid rhinorrhea, and/or a history of chronic sinusitis. Occasionally, the correct diagnosis could not be reached until adulthood. Given the relatively low morbidity of unilateral CA, its definitive treatment is usually delayed until later age. Five main CA surgical approaches have been described: trans-palatal, trans-antral, transseptal, sublabial, and trans-nasal. The trans-nasal endoscopic approach is currently the most frequently used.

Case Presentation

You are called to see a neonate in respiratory distress. The obstetric history and birth were uncomplicated. You are told that the neonate became distressed and cyanotic soon after birth. The cyanosis appeared to settle on crying but resumed when crying stopped. Currently, there is an oropharyngeal airway in situ, and the neonate appears well and settled. Nasal mist test is negative, and the neonatal ICU team has obtained a CT scan (Fig. 49.1).

N. Tsetsos
ENT Head and Neck Surgery Department,
424 General Military Hospital, Thessaloniki, Greece

M. Stavrakas (✉)
ENT Head and Neck Surgery Department,
University Hospitals Plymouth NHS Trust,
Plymouth, UK

N. Tsetsos et al. (eds.), *Otolaryngology Study Guide*, https://doi.org/10.1007/978-3-031-77374-7_49

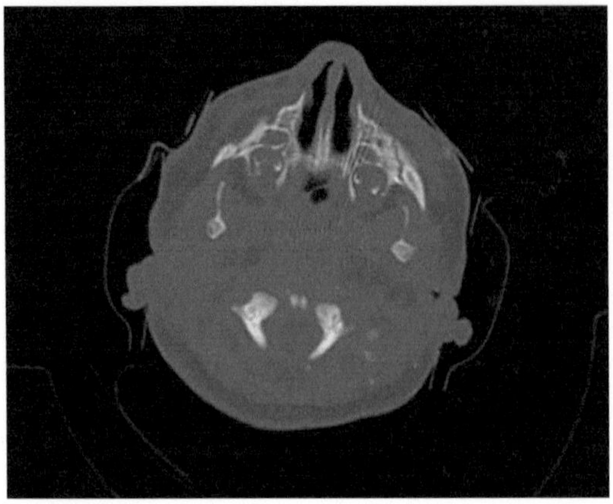

Fig. 49.1 CT scan

Questions

1. Which of the following statements are true about choanal atresia (CA) (more than one correct answer possible)?
   A. The incidence of this malformation is between 1:5000 and 1:7000 live births.
   B. Bilateral atresia is more common than unilateral.
   C. The malformation is made up of 90% bony and 10% membranous tissue.
   D. It is more common in males.
   E. The unilateral form is frequently on the right side.
2. Which of the following anatomic structures can cause the syndrome?
   A. The undersurface of the body of the sphenoid bones
   B. The medial pterygoid lamina
   C. The vomer
   D. The horizontal portion of the palatal bone
   E. All of the above
3. Which syndrome may be associated with this pathology?
   A. Down's syndrome
   B. Turner's syndrome
   C. Marfan's syndrome
   D. Bardet-Biedl syndrome
   E. None of the above
4. Which of the following statements are true (more than one correct answer possible)?
   A. Unilateral atresia can cause mild or no symptoms.
   B. Many times, diagnosis of unilateral CA cannot be reached until adulthood.
   C. Cyclical cyanosis is a characteristic of unilateral choanal atresia.
   D. Intermittent cyanosis characteristically deteriorated by crying.
   E. Feeding difficulty occurs only rarely in bilateral CA.
5. Which is currently the most frequently used surgical approach?
   A. Trans-palatal
   B. Trans-antral
   C. Transseptal
   D. Trans-nasal endoscopic
   E. None of the above

Answers

1. **A, E**

   Choanal atresia, defined as the anatomical closure of the posterior choanae in the nasal cavity, is a relatively uncommon disease entity with an estimated incidence of 1:5000–7000 births. Past reports mention that the malformation was made up of 90% bony and 10% membranous tissue [1]. CT workup and histologic specimens show approximately 30% pure bone atresia and 70% mixed membranous and bone atresia with no purely membranous anomalies present. Interestingly, the characteristics of CA follow a "2–1" rule, namely the ratio of unilateral to bilateral CA, female to male, and right-sided to left-sided CA [2, 3].
2. **E**

   Anatomic boundaries of the posterior choanae include the undersurface of the body of the sphenoid bones superiorly, the medial pterygoid lamina laterally, the vomer medially, and the horizontal portion of the palatal bone inferiorly. The actual narrowing could be caused by one of the abovementioned bony components [4].

3. **E**

Multiple congenital anomalies are commonly encountered among these patients, especially in those with bilateral CA [4]. Airway abnormalities, such as tracheomalacia, laryngomalacia, and subglottic stenosis, may be encountered, and about 20% present with craniofacial abnormalities including Treacher Collins, Pfeiffer, Apert, mandibulofacial dysostosis, and Crouzon syndromes; however, the most common relationship is with CHARGE syndrome accounting approximately for 25% of the cases (coloboma, heart defects, choanal atresia, growth retardation, genitourinary abnormalities, ear abnormalities) [5].

4. **A, B**

Due to the elevated laryngeal position compared to the adult counterpart, newborns are obligate nose breathers until mouth breathing is established with the descent of the larynx approximately 4–6 weeks of life [6, 7]. In case of bilateral CA, infants can have acute respiratory distress with intermittent cyanosis characteristically relieved by crying. Feeding difficulty can be the initial alerting event in which the infants can present with progressive airway obstruction and choking during feeding because of their inability to breathe and feed simultaneously. Neonates with bilateral CA can also present with a history of multiple failed extubation attempts, especially in those with secondary airway issues [8, 9]. Infants with unilateral CA, rarely present with neonatal respiratory distress, are often diagnosed later on in life. The most common presentation is chronic unilateral nasal obstruction, persistent mucoid rhinorrhea, and/or a history of chronic sinusitis. Occasionally, the correct diagnosis could not be reached until adulthood due to the nonspecific symptoms of unilateral nasal obstruction. Given the relatively low morbidity of unilateral CA, its definitive treatment is usually delayed until later age as the chance of successful surgical repair increases with age (i.e., more favorable anatomy later on in life) [9].

5. **D**

Five main CA surgical approaches are described in the medical literature: transpalatal, trans-antral, transseptal, sublabial, and trans-nasal [10]. The trans-nasal endoscopic approach is currently the most frequently used, due to the modern refinements of endoscopic techniques (it does not affect the growth of the mandibular arch; there are no malocclusions or cosmetic alterations to the face), especially in newborns with bilateral CA [3]. The use of postoperative stents is decreasing in light of the evidence on the increased stent-related complications, such as local infection, synechiae, and granulation tissue formation [10, 11]. The effectiveness of mitomycin C has not been adequately proven based on the current literature [12, 13].

References

1. Ramsden JD, Campisi P, Forte V. Choanal atresia and choanal stenosis. Otolaryngol Clin North Am. 2009;42(2):339–52, x
2. Brown OE, Pownell P, Manning SC. Choanal atresia: a new anatomic classification and clinical management applications. Laryngoscope. 1996;106(1 Pt 1):97–101.
3. Hengerer AS, Brickman TM, Jeyakumar A. Choanal atresia: embryologic analysis and evolution of treatment, a 30-year experience. Laryngoscope. 2008;118(5):862–6.
4. Kwong KM. Current updates on choanal atresia. Front Pediatr. 2015;3:52. Published 2015 Jun 9
5. Burrow TA, Saal HM, de Alarcon A, Martin LJ, Cotton RT, Hopkin RJ. Characterization of congenital anomalies in individuals with choanal atresia. Arch Otolaryngol Head Neck Surg. 2009;135(6):543–7.
6. Murray S, Luo L, Quimby A, Barrowman N, Vaccani JP, Caulley L. Immediate versus delayed surgery in congenital choanal atresia: a systematic review. Int J Pediatr Otorhinolaryngol. 2019;119:47–53.
7. Meleca JB, Anne S, Hopkins B. Reducing the need for general anesthesia in the repair of choanal atresia with steroid-eluting stents: a case series. Int J Pediatr Otorhinolaryngol. 2019;118:185–7.
8. Chan J, Ullas G, Narapa Reddy NVS. Completely endoscopic approach using a skeeter drill to treat bilateral congenital choanal atresia in a 33 week born pre-term baby. Indian J Otolaryngol Head Neck Surg. 2018;70(4):608–10.
9. Newman JR, Harmon P, Shirley WP, Hill JS, Woolley AL, Wiatrak BJ. Operative management of choanal

atresia: a 15-year experience. JAMA Otolaryngol Head Neck Surg. 2013;139(1):71–5.
10. Durmaz A, Tosun F, Yldrm N, Sahan M, Kvrakdal C, Gerek M. Transnasal endoscopic repair of choanal atresia: results of 13 cases and meta-analysis. J Craniofac Surg. 2008;19(5):1270–4.
11. Velegrakis S, Mantsopoulos K, Iro H, Zenk J. Long-term outcomes of endonasal surgery for choanal atresia: 28 years experience in an academic medical centre. Eur Arch Otorhinolaryngol. 2013;270(1):113–6.
12. Uzomefuna V, Glynn F, Al-Omari B, Hone S, Russell J. Transnasal endoscopic repair of choanal atresia in a tertiary care centre: a review of outcomes. Int J Pediatr Otorhinolaryngol. 2012;76(5):613–7.
13. Carter JM, Lawlor C, Guarisco JL. The efficacy of mitomycin and stenting in choanal atresia repair: a 20 year experience. Int J Pediatr Otorhinolaryngol. 2014;78(2):307–11.

50 Pyriform Aperture Stenosis

Konstantinos Garefis
and Angelos Chatziavramidis

Abstract

Congenital nasal pyriform aperture stenosis (CNPAS) is the narrowing of the narrowest part of the nasal cavity, which is an uncommon cause of neonatal nasal obstruction. The incidence is estimated to be approximately 1 in 25,000 live births. It arises due to an excessive growth of bone in the medial nasal process of the maxilla around the fourth month of gestation. CNPAS may present on its own or in conjunction with other anomalies. Infants, being obligatory nose breathers, commonly have nasal airway obstruction, marked by cyclic cyanosis that is alleviated when they cry. Both acute and delayed presentations are possible, exhibiting signs such as aspiration, feeding difficulties, and failure to thrive in addition to apneas, cyanosis, and respiratory distress. Symptoms may appear shortly after birth or in the first few hours of life, depending on the severity of obstruction. The diagnosis is determined through clinical assessment and imaging. Differential diagnoses include choanal stenosis and atresia, nasopharyngeal mass, and septal displacement. For mild cases of obstruction, characterized by a stable airway and no feeding difficulties, conservative treatment is generally satisfactory. Surgical intervention, commonly performed with the sublabial technique, is indicated in severe cases with an inadequate airway, unresponsiveness to conservative treatment, or poor weight gain.

Case Presentation

A female infant, born at 36 weeks gestation, required immediate admission to the neonatal intensive care unit owing to respiratory distress, desaturation, and cyanosis. Her desaturation did not improve with continuous positive airway pressure, and at 1 day old, she was intubated. After 2 days, the otorhinolaryngologist was called to examine the newborn using a pediatric flexible endoscope. However, it could not pass through either nostril. Subsequently, a computed tomography (CT) scan was performed, revealing a pyriform aperture width of approximately 4 mm and a single median central incisor in the maxilla (Figs. 50.1, 50.2, and 50.3).

K. Garefis (✉) · A. Chatziavramidis
2nd Academic ORL, Head and Neck Surgery Department, Aristotle University of Thessaloniki, Papageorgiou Hospital, Thessaloniki, Greece

N. Tsetsos et al. (eds.), *Otolaryngology Study Guide*, https://doi.org/10.1007/978-3-031-77374-7_50

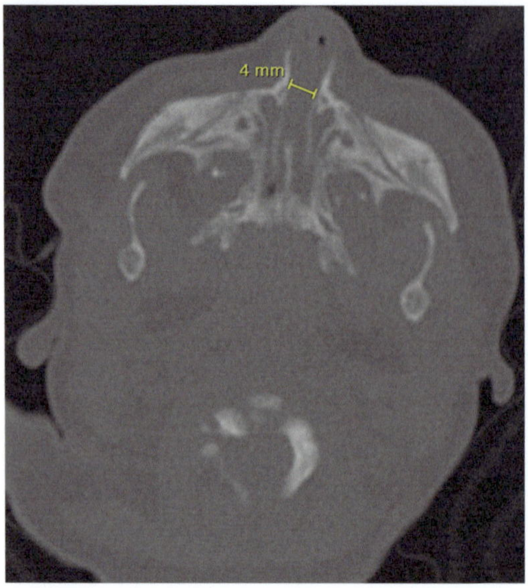

Fig. 50.1 Axial plane of CT showing that the pyriform aperture width is 4 mm

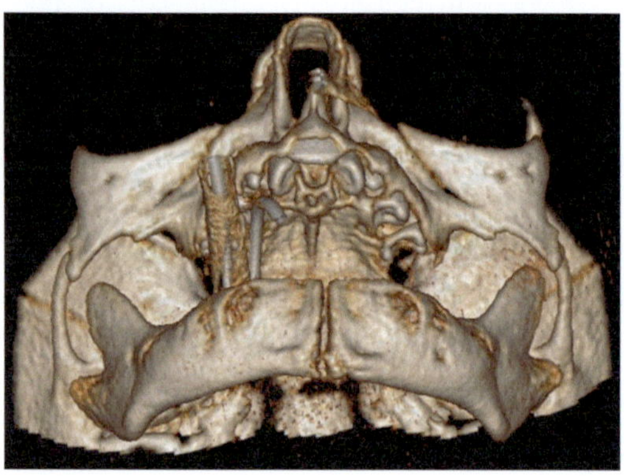

Fig. 50.2 3D CT showing the pyriform aperture stenosis and the single median central incisor in the maxilla

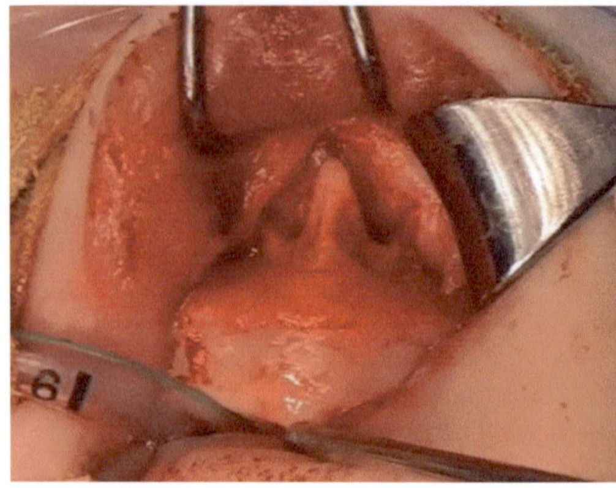

Fig. 50.3 Intraoperative image of the surgery with sublabial technique

Questions

1. Which examination is considered the gold standard for confirming CNPAS diagnosis?
   A. Magnetic resonance imaging (MRI)
   B. Rhinomanometry
   C. CT
   D. X-ray
   E. Flexible endoscopy
2. Which of the following statements are true about CNPAS (more than one correct answer possible)?
   A. It is usually unilateral
   B. It is the result of an excessive growth of the quadrangular cartilage
   C. Choking during feeding is uncommon
   D. A 5–6 Fr nasal catheter fails to pass
   E. Pyriform aperture width is <11 mm in a full-term infant
3. A patient with a single upper incisor and CNPAS most likely associates with:
   A. CHARGE syndrome
   B. Holoprosencephaly
   C. Down syndrome
   D. Hydrocephalus
   E. Goldenhar syndrome
4. Which of the following symptoms and signs should be considered for surgical intervention?
   A. Poor weight gain
   B. Cyanosis
   C. Pyriform aperture <5 mm
   D. Feeding difficulties
   E. All of the above
5. After 10 days, the previously described infant underwent extubation. However, she was reintubated almost immediately due to the recurrence of the same symptoms. What would be the appropriate therapy in this situation?
   A. Decongestants
   B. Extended intubation for another 15 days
   C. Nostril stenting
   D. Surgical intervention using the sublabial technique
   E. Application of topical steroids

Answers

1. **C**

   The preferred imaging modality for verifying CNPAS is a CT scan, covering axial and coronal sections of the nasal and paranasal sinus regions [1, 2]. CT typically reveals a reduced width of the pyriform aperture and may also indicate the existence of a sole central incisor located in the maxilla. Moreover, the use of three-dimensional (3D) CT can offer accurate and useful data for both preoperative and postoperative examination of the nasal pyriform aperture [3]. However, further testing may include electrolyte and endocrine tests in addition to a brain MRI if there are any suspicions of related abnormalities [4, 5].

2. **D, E**

   The pyriform aperture is shaped by the horizontal and nasal processes of the maxilla, the anterior nasal spine, and the nasal bones. CNPAS typically occurs bilateral [6]. It develops around the fourth month of pregnancy due to an overabundance of bone growth in the maxilla's medial nasal process. The first suspicion is raised when a 5–6 Fr nasal catheter is difficult to get into the nose [1, 2]. A full-term infant's pyriform aperture width of less than 11 mm, measured in an axial plane at the level of the inferior turbinate, may be indicative of CNPAS [7]. Additionally, neonates are obligate nasal breathers until around the age of 4 months. Individuals with CNPAS exhibit symptoms of respiratory distress or feeding challenges, including difficulties such as choking during feeding due to their inability to simultaneously breathe and feed [4].

3. **B**

   CNPAS may present either independently or in conjunction with other midline anomalies, including holoprosencephaly. The primary anatomical abnormality associated with CNPAS is the presence of a single median central incisor in the maxilla, observed in up to 60% of cases [8]. These conditions collectively form the holoprosencephaly and solitary median maxillary central incisor syndrome. This syndrome encompasses holoprosencephaly, as well as abnormalities in the pituitary, cardiac, and urogenital systems [4]. The hallmark of holoprosencephaly is the inability of the prosencephalon (forebrain) to split into bilateral cerebral hemispheres, which eventually results in abnormalities in the face's development [6].

4. **E**

   Surgical treatment aims to enlarge the pyriform aperture with careful protection of the nasal mucosa. It becomes necessary in cases where there is an insufficient airway or failure to thrive, an inability to extubate, cyanosis, persistent respiratory distress, sleep apnea, feeding difficulties, inadequate weight gain, a pyriform aperture measuring less than 5.7–6 mm, and failure of conservative treatment. In general, most authors believe that a waiting period of about 2 weeks is adequate [1, 2, 4].

5. **D**

   Saline nasal humidification, topical steroids, and decongestants are the initial treatments for infants experiencing mild nasal obstruction, provided that they have a stable airway and no feeding difficulties. Conservative approach offers short-term relief until the nasal bones enlarge and the stenosis genuinely expands [1, 2]. In serious cases, techniques such as the McGovern nipple, continuous positive airway pressure, or even endotracheal intubation may be employed to stabilize the airway [1, 6]. For definitive therapy, the sublabial technique, either with or without stenting, is the surgical method that is most frequently used. By using this method, the pyriform aperture can be well exposed, allowing for the drilling of the stenosis [1, 2, 4, 6]. Positive surgical outcomes have been shown for both sublabial and endoscopic procedures [2, 6]. An alternative to formal surgery has been suggested: balloon dilatation of the pyriform aperture [4].

References

1. Wormald R, Hinton-Bayre A, Bumbak P, Vijayasekaran S. Congenital nasal pyriform aperture stenosis 5.7 mm or less is associated with surgical intervention: a pooled case series. Int J Pediatr Otorhinolaryngol. 2015;79(11):1802–5.
2. Naina P, Dahiya V, Irodi A, Varghese AM. Congenital nasal pyriform aperture stenosis: same CT dimensions, varied scenarios. Indian J Radiol Imaging. 2022;32(4):591–3.
3. Lee KS, Yang CC, Huang JK, Chen YC, Chang KC. Congenital pyriform aperture stenosis: surgery and evaluation with three-dimensional computed tomography. Laryngoscope. 2002;112(5):918–21.
4. Chakravarty PD, Sim F, Slim MAM, Patel N, Wynne DM, Clement WA. Congenital nasal pyriform aperture stenosis; our experience of 34 cases. Int J Pediatr Otorhinolaryngol. 2023;166:111491.
5. Alvo A, Villarroel G, Sedano C. Neonatal nasal obstruction. Eur Arch Otorrinolaringol. 2021;278(10):3605–11.
6. Tate JR, Sykes J. Congenital nasal pyriform aperture stenosis. Otolaryngol Clin N Am. 2009;42(3):521–5.
7. Belden CJ, Mancuso AA, Schmalfuss IM. CT features of congenital nasal piriform aperture stenosis: initial experience. Radiology. 1999;213(2):495–501.
8. Van Den Abbeele T, Triglia JM, François M, Narcy P. Congenital nasal pyriform aperture stenosis: diagnosis and management of 20 cases. Ann Otol Rhinol Laryngol. 2001;110(1):70–5.

Branchial Cleft Cyst

51

Konstantinos Garefis

Abstract

Branchial cleft cysts (BCCs) occur due to the incomplete disappearance of the pharyngobranchial ducts during the second to seventh weeks of fetal growth. They are the second most prevalent congenital masses in the head and neck region in children, following thyroglossal duct cysts and sinuses. BCCs are categorized into four types based on their embryological roots. The most common type is the second BCC, accounting for up to 90% of all cases. This type is equally common in both genders and typically manifests in the second to fourth decades of life. They often enlarge and become painful due to infection, usually following an upper respiratory tract infection. A second BCC usually presents as a non-painful, round swelling along the anterior edge of the upper third of the sternocleidomastoid muscle. BCCs are filled with a mucoid, yellow-green fluid containing cholesterol crystals and are typically lined by stratified squamous epithelium overlying lymphoid tissue. The preferred treatment is complete surgical removal of the cyst and tract to prevent recurrence and the need for further intervention. However, if a BCC is infected, it should initially be treated with antibiotics, and if the inflammation does not subside, aspiration or another form of drainage should be considered.

Case Presentation

A 23-year-old man was directed to your emergency Ear, Nose, and Throat (ENT) clinic, presenting with a right-sided neck lump that had been growing for 2 weeks. This lump was first noticed during his childhood. Upon examination, a sizable, round mass was found in the right anterior cervical triangle of his neck. The mass was tender to touch and movable. The remainder of the ENT examination showed no abnormalities. A computed tomography (CT) scan was conducted, which identified an infected cystic structure (Fig. 51.1).

Questions

1. Which is the most frequent lateral congenital neck lesion in childhood?
   A. First BCC
   B. Thyroglossal duct cyst
   C. Second BCC

K. Garefis (✉)
2nd Academic ORL, Head and Neck Surgery Department, Aristotle University of Thessaloniki, Papageorgiou Hospital, Thessaloniki, Greece

N. Tsetsos et al. (eds.), *Otolaryngology Study Guide*, https://doi.org/10.1007/978-3-031-77374-7_51

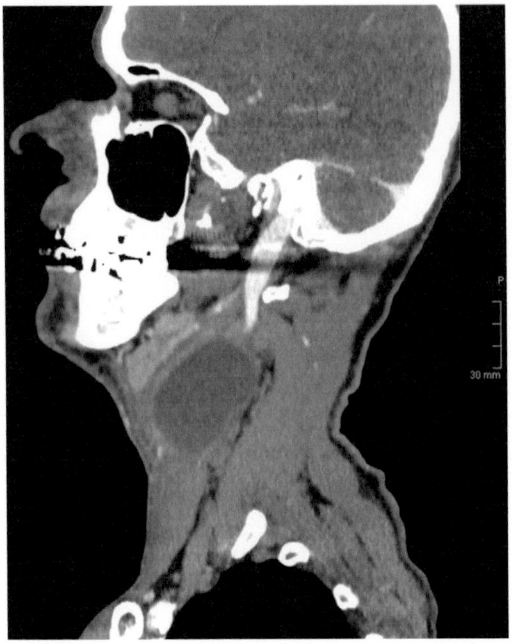

Fig. 51.1 CT scan showing the infected cystic formation

D. Cyst hygroma
E. None of the above

2. Second BCCs are typically found:
   A. Over the angle of the mandible and near parotid gland
   B. In the posterior cervical triangle
   C. High in the neck and deep to the anterior border of the sternocleidomastoid muscle
   D. Near the upper pole of the thyroid gland
   E. In the postauricular region, or near the pinna
3. Which of the following statements are true about second BCCs (more than one correct answer possible)?
   A. They may present with recurrent thyroiditis
   B. They commonly present in the first year of life
   C. It is more common in males
   D. They can be painful and tender
   E. They can by asymptomatic and painless
4. The most appropriate surgical approach for a second BCC is:
   A. Injection of ethanol to sclerose the cyst
   B. Excision of the cyst and tract
   C. Removal of just the cyst itself
   D. Aspiration of the cyst
   E. Excision of the cyst, tract, and tonsillectomy
5. Which nerve can be damaged during excision of a second BCC?
   A. Buccal branch of the facial nerve
   B. Superior laryngeal nerve
   C. Phrenic nerve
   D. Lingual nerve
   E. None of the above

Answers

1. **C**

   BCCs are the most prevalent type of branchial cleft cysts and are the most common congenital lateral neck masses in children [1]. Despite this, thyroglossal duct cysts are the most frequently occurring congenital neck lesions in the pediatric population, with second BCCs ranking second [1–3]. First BCCs represent less than 8% of all branchial anomalies, and the third and fourth types of BCCs are exceedingly rare [4]. The occurrence of cystic hygromas ranges between 1:2000 and 1:4000 live births [5]. Other congenital neck lesions include hemangiomas, teratomas, dermoid cysts, bronchogenic cysts, and thymic cysts [3].
2. **C**

   BCCs are typically found along and deep to the anterior border of the upper third of the sternocleidomastoid muscle. They are classified into four types. Type I BCCs are located anterior to the sternocleidomastoid muscle and do not come into contact with the carotid sheath. Type II BCCs are deep to the sternocleidomastoid muscle and can be either anterior or posterior to the carotid artery (most common). Type III BCCs are situated between the internal and external carotid arteries and are adjacent to the pharynx. Type IV BCCs are medial to the carotid sheath and are in close proximity to the pharynx, adjacent to the tonsillar fossa [2, 6, 7].
3. **D, E**

   These cysts typically appear as painless and asymptomatic lesions on the lateral neck in children and young adults, primarily in the second to fourth decades of life. However, second BCCs can become enlarged, tender, and painful if they become infected [3, 6–8]. Both females and males are equally affected by this condition [6, 9].

4. **B**

 The gold standard of surgical treatment for second BCCs is the complete excision of the cyst along with its tract [6, 10]. However, there is a high incidence of recurrence if the cyst is resected incompletely [3]. Incomplete resection and complications can occur when the surgery takes place during inflammation [11]. Infected cysts should be managed with antibiotics and if the infection persists with aspiration or drainage [1, 11]. Surgical excision should be planned when the acute infection of cyst has resolved, approximately after 6–8 weeks [1]. Care should be taken during ligation and division of the tract, especially near the tonsillar fossa [3, 6]. Other therapies such as repeated incision, drainage, and injection of sclerosing agents to the cyst are considered non-definitive. Moreover, they can increase the recurrence frequency after the surgery [11].

5. **E**

 During the surgical dissection of the second BCC and tract, care must be taken to avoid the injury of nearby structures. These structures include nerves such as hypoglossal, glossopharyngeal, vagus, marginal mandibular branch of the facial nerve, and spinal accessory and vessels such as internal jugular vein and carotid artery [1, 3, 6].

References

1. Christison-Lagay E. Complications in head and neck surgery. Semin Pediatr Surg. 2016;25(6):338–46.
2. Ibrahim M, Hammoud K, Maheshwari M, Pandya A. Congenital cystic lesions of the head and neck. Neuroimaging Clin N Am. 2011;21(3):621–39.
3. Tracy TF Jr, Muratore CS. Management of common head and neck masses. Semin Pediatr Surg. 2007;16(1):3–13.
4. Tarazis K, Garefis K, Garefi M, Nikolaidis V, Chatziavramidis A, Markou K. First branchial cleft anomalies: rare work type I and type II entities. Ear Nose Throat J. 2021;102(8):NP383–5.
5. Perkins JA, Manning SC, Tempero RM, et al. Lymphatic malformations: review of current treatment. Otolaryngol Head Neck Surg. 2010;142(6):795–803.
6. Waldhausen JH. Branchial cleft and arch anomalies in children. Semin Pediatr Surg. 2006;15(2):64–9.
7. Bajaj Y, Ifeacho S, Tweedie D, Jephson CG, Albert DM, Cochrane LA, Wyatt ME, Jonas N, Hartley BE. Branchial anomalies in children. Int J Pediatr Otorhinolaryngol. 2011;75(8):1020–3.
8. Adams A, Mankad K, Offiah C, Childs L. Branchial cleft anomalies: a pictorial review of embryological development and spectrum of imaging findings. Insights Imaging. 2016;7(1):69–76.
9. Chimona TS, Tamiolakis D, Proimos E, Perogamvrakis G, Korres SG, Papadakis CE. Management of second branchial cleft abnormalities in adults. B-ENT. 2007;3(1):39–43.
10. Ho CF, Yang TH, Hsin LJ, Yang SW, Tsai YT, Tsai MS, Yang CT, Lee YC. Postauricular incision versus conventional transcervical incision in second branchial cleft cyst excision: a systematic review and meta-analysis. J Craniofac Surg. 2022;33(8):2365–71.
11. Guldfred LA, Philipsen BB, Siim C. Branchial cleft anomalies: accuracy of pre-operative diagnosis, clinical presentation and management. J Laryngol Otol. 2012;126(6):598–604.

Thyroglossal Duct Cyst

52

Maria Garefi and Konstantinos Garefis

Abstract

Thyroglossal duct cyst (TGDC) is the most commonly encountered mass in the midline anterior neck, often found in the perihyoid area. TGDC represents approximately 75% of all congenital neck masses and typically occurs in children and young adults. TGDCs originate from persistent epithelial remnants of the thyroglossal duct, a structure that guides the descent of the thyroid gland from the foramen caecum to its final position in the anterior neck during embryogenesis. If TGDC remnants persist, they may give rise to cysts or fistula later in life. It is classically described as a painless anterior neck swelling that moves with deglutition and tongue protrusion. Most TGDCs are asymptomatic. Infection and sinus formation are the most common complications of thyroglossal duct cysts. While clinical examination is often sufficient for diagnosing a TGDC, in most cases, imaging such as ultrasound, computed tomography (CT), and magnetic resonance imaging (MRI) is required to identify a normal thyroid gland, appreciate the characteristics of the cyst, and rule out other conditions such as dermoid/epidermoid cysts, ectopic thyroid gland, lymphadenopathy, branchial cleft cysts, ranula, and cystic hygromas. Surgical excision of TGDC with the Sistrunk procedure is the gold standard of treatment.

Case Presentation

A 22-year-old male presented at the otorhinolaryngology clinic with a 3-year history of neck swelling. One month ago, he complained of pain and noted an increase in swelling. His medical history was unremarkable. During the physical examination, a soft, painless, and non-tender mass measuring 3 cm in diameter was observed in the midline of the neck. The remainder of the otorhinolaryngology examination was normal. Neck ultrasonography revealed an echogenic, homogeneous thyroid. Furthermore, it identified a mass above the thyroid gland characterized by a solid connective tissue capsule and an anechoic internal structure (Fig. 52.1).

Questions

1. What is the most common location of a TGDC?
   A. Infrahyoid
   B. Suprasternal
   C. Intralingual

M. Garefi
Department of Paediatrics, Faculty of Medicine, School of Health Sciences, University of Thessaly, Larissa, Greece

K. Garefis (✉)
2nd Academic ORL, Head and Neck Surgery Department, Aristotle University of Thessaloniki, Papageorgiou Hospital, Thessaloniki, Greece

N. Tsetsos et al. (eds.), *Otolaryngology Study Guide*, https://doi.org/10.1007/978-3-031-77374-7_52

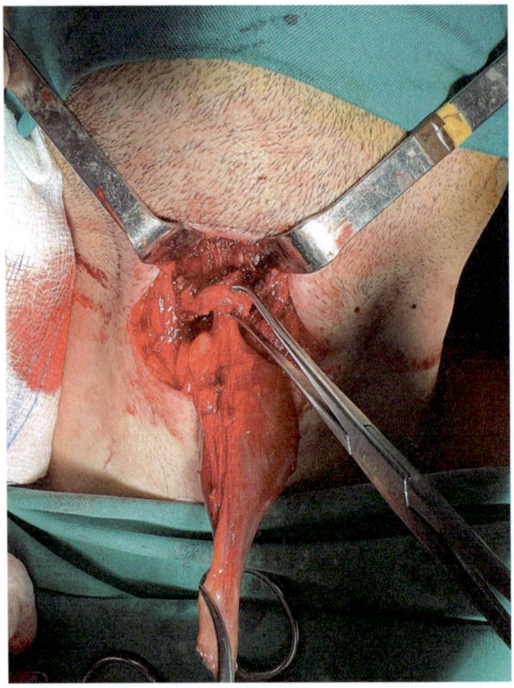

Fig. 52.1 Intraoperative image of the patient showing the cyst and a part of the hyoid bone

D. Suprahyoid
E. In the hyoid

2. Which of the following statements are true about TGDC (more than one correct answer possible)?
   A. It may present with recurrent thyroiditis
   B. They may be present in up to 7% of the adult population
   C. It is more common in males
   D. They may present as lateral neck masses in adults
   E. Development of malignancy can occur in about 9%
3. What imaging modality should be considered for initial diagnosing of TGDC?
   A. MRI
   B. CT scan
   C. X-ray
   D. Ultrasound
   E. PET scan
4. Which of the following treatments could be employed as a definitive treatment for the patient described above (more than one correct answer possible)?
   A. Sistrunk procedure
   B. Ultrasound-guided ethanol ablation
   C. Antibiotics
   D. Cyst marsupialization
   E. Thyroidectomy
5. Which of the following statements about the Sistrunk procedure is true (more than one correct answer possible)?
   A. It includes the resection of the lateral hyoid
   B. It is characterized by a recurrence rate of about 27%
   C. It is recommended for recurrent infections
   D. Hypoglossal nerve can be damaged during operation
   E. It is performed under local anesthesia

Answers

1. **A**

   TGDCs can appear in various anatomical regions along the neck, spanning from the foramen cecum to the base of the tongue and the suprasternal fissure. While the majority of these occurrences are centralized in the midline, less than 1% are located away from this central position [1]. During the developmental and descending phases of the thyroglossal duct, it closely interacts with the hyoid bone. Consequently, most thyroglossal duct cysts are situated either at the level of (15%) or immediately below (65%) the hyoid bone [2]. They are commonly described based on their relationship to the hyoid bone, with approximately 20–25% designated as suprahyoid, 15–50% positioned anteriorly or posteriorly at the hyoid bone level, and 25–65% occurring infrahyoid [1, 3].
2. **B, D**

   TGDCs represent the predominant congenital anomaly in the neck, constituting approximately 70–75% of midline neck swellings in children and appearing in around 7% of adults [1, 3, 4]. While the majority are situated in the midline, 10–24% of these cysts are found laterally in adults, typically on the left side, attributed to the usual presence of the levator glandulae thyroideae muscle on that side [5]. Both male and female patients exhibit a similar prevalence of thyroglossal cysts, suggesting an equal distribution across genders [5]. These cysts can manifest as a midline neck swelling, presenting as either a soft, firm, or hard mass, generally mobile but occasionally exhibiting fluctuations. Due to their anatomical proximity to the oral cavity, TGDCs may be associated with infections, constituting the most prevalent complication [6]. Malignancy within a TGDC is rare, accounting for approximately 1% of cases, with papillary carcinoma being the most common type [3, 5, 7].

3. **D**

   Ultrasound stands as the primary diagnostic tool when a TGDC is clinically suspected, exhibiting a diagnostic sensitivity of 75% in TGDC diagnosis [8]. Particularly in children, it is the investigation of choice, as it is radiation free. Moreover, it can be used preoperatively to identify whether the mass represents the only functional thyroid tissue. An uncomplicated TGDC may manifest as an anechoic, well-defined cyst heightened through transmission or with a pseudosolid appearance [2]. Complementary imaging through CT and MRI serves to more precisely delineate the lesion's anatomy, especially in the case of larger cysts. These modalities are invaluable for characterizing cysts and determining their relationships with surrounding tissues [9]. Radioisotope scanning is infrequently employed, primarily addressing the potential of ectopic thyroid manifestation as a midline neck mass in the absence of a functioning thyroid gland lower in the neck before surgical removal [2]. Conversely, X-rays are insufficient for diagnosing TGDC [9].

4. **A**

   The primary approach for treating TGDC is surgical, with alternative treatment options being seldom recommended. Numerous techniques have been outlined, yet the method introduced by Sistrunk in 1920 remains the established gold standard [1]. Ultrasound-guided ethanol ablation, a minimally invasive office-based procedure widely employed for nonsurgical treatment of various benign cystic lesions, especially benign thyroid cysts, is not a well-established method for TGDC [10]. In cases where a patient with a thyroglossal duct cyst presents with infection or an abscess, the initial treatment involves antibiotics and/or drainage [1]. In instances of severe superinfection, needle aspiration can be undertaken to reduce cyst size, alleviate upper airway pressure, and aid in microbial identification [11]. Sole cyst aspiration or incomplete dissection is linked to a relatively rapid recurrence of TGDC, with rates exceeding 50% [1, 12].

5. **C, D**

   The Sistrunk procedure involves the thorough removal of the thyroglossal duct cyst (TGDC) and a central portion of the hyoid bone, with careful excision of the persistent duct up to the foramen cecum [11]. This treatment is recommended due to the potential for recurrent infections, the rare chance of malignancy, and occasionally for cosmetic considerations [3, 11]. Notably, the Sistrunk procedure has significantly improved the effective management of TGDC, reducing recurrence rates from 45–55% after simple excision to 1–10% [11]. However, it necessitates general anesthesia [13]. The lingual nerve, the stylohyoid muscle, and the hyoglossus muscle are all reached by the hypoglossal nerve as it passes close to the lateral aspect of the hyoid bone. When dissecting the hyoid bone during the Sistrunk surgery, it is important to avoid excessive lateral dissection as this is unnecessary and might cause injuries to the lingual artery and the hypoglossal nerve (cranial nerve XII) [11].

References

1. Oomen KP, Modi VK, Maddalozzo J. Thyroglossal duct cyst and ectopic thyroid: surgical management. Otolaryngol Clin N Am. 2015;48(1):15–27.
2. Ahuja AT, Wong KT, King AD, Yuen EH. Imaging for thyroglossal duct cyst: the bare essentials. Clin Radiol. 2005;60(2):141–8.

3. Chou J, Walters A, Hage R, Zurada A, Michalak M, Tubbs RS, Loukas M. Thyroglossal duct cysts: anatomy, embryology and treatment. Surg Radiol Anat. 2013;35(10):875–81.
4. Yang YJ, Haghir S, Wanamaker JR, Powers CN. Diagnosis of papillary carcinoma in a thyroglossal duct cyst by fine-needle aspiration biopsy. Arch Pathol Lab Med. 2000;124(1):139–42.
5. Allard RH. The thyroglossal cyst. Head Neck Surg. 1982;5(2):134–46.
6. Gioacchini FM, Alicandri-Ciufelli M, Kaleci S, Magliulo G, Presutti L, Re M. Clinical presentation and treatment outcomes of thyroglossal duct cysts: a systematic review. Int J Oral Maxillofac Surg. 2015;44(1):119–26.
7. Rayess HM, Monk I, Svider PF, Gupta A, Raza SN, Lin HS. Thyroglossal duct cyst carcinoma: a systematic review of clinical features and outcomes. Otolaryngol Head Neck Surg. 2017;156(5):794–802.
8. Li W, Ren YP, Shi YY, Zhang L, Bu RF. Presentation, management, and outcome of lingual thyroglossal duct cyst in pediatric and adult populations. J Craniofac Surg. 2019;30(5):e442–6.
9. Gallagher TQ, Hartnick CJ. Thyroglossal duct cyst excision. Adv Otorhinolaryngol. 2012;73:66–9.
10. Ahn D. Ultrasound-guided ethanol ablation for thyroglossal duct cyst: a review of technical issues and potential as a new standard treatment. J Clin Med. 2023;12(17):5445.
11. Righini CA, Hitter A, Reyt E, Atallah I. Thyroglossal duct surgery. Sistrunk procedure. Eur Ann Otorhinolaryngol Head Neck Dis. 2016;133(2):133–6.
12. Urao M, Teitelbaum DH, Miyano T. Lingual thyroglossal duct cyst: a unique surgical approach. J Pediatr Surg. 1996;31(11):1574–6.
13. Goldsztein H, Khan A, Pereira KD. Thyroglossal duct cyst excision—the sistrunk procedure. Oper Tech Otolaryngol. 2009;20:256–9.

53 Subglottic Stenosis

Maria Garefi, Konstantinos Garefis, and Iordanis Konstantinidis

Abstract

Subglottic stenosis (SGS) is a congenital or acquired condition defined by a constriction of the upper airway that spans from slightly underneath the vocal folds to the lower edge of the cricoid cartilage. Congenital SGS is linked to a developmental anomaly during the tenth week of gestation and is commonly associated with other congenital head and neck abnormalities and syndromes. SGS is usually associated with iatrogenic injury or other causes of blunt or penetrating trauma, with 90% of cases attributable to prior or prolonged duration of intubation in both children and adults. Subglottic stenosis typically presents with biphasic stridor as the most common manifestation. In addition, patients may exhibit respiratory distress or recurrent upper respiratory infections, which cause inflammation that further narrows the subglottis. Evaluation in a patient with potential subglottic stenosis starts with a comprehensive medical history and physical assessment, including flexible fiber-optic laryngoscopy, focusing on ruling out airway blockages originating outside the larynx. When SGS is suspected, rigid direct laryngoscopy and bronchoscopy are required. The differential diagnosis typically involves croup, bacterial tracheitis, subglottic hemangioma, subglottic cysts, vocal cord paralysis, and complete tracheal rings. The treatment of SGS depends on the severity of the stenosis. Mild subglottic narrowing is often treated conservatively, while moderate-to-severe cases frequently necessitate surgery. Current treatment approaches include balloon dilation, endoscopic CO_2 laser use, partial cricotracheal resection, laryngotracheal reconstruction, cricoid split, and tracheostomy.

Case Presentation

The ENT clinic has been requested to evaluate a 4-month-old girl who presented at the pediatric clinic with a history of cough and biphasic stridor in the last 3 days. The girl was born through an emergent cesarean section under general anesthesia due to severe fetal respiratory distress. The newborn was intubated for 4 weeks during the neonatal period due to respiratory distress syndrome. After extubation, the infant, while at home, experienced two previous respiratory infections characterized by cough, stridor, and

M. Garefi
Department of Paediatrics, Faculty of Medicine, School of Health Sciences, University of Thessaly, Larissa, Greece

K. Garefis (✉) · I. Konstantinidis
2nd Academic ORL, Head and Neck Surgery Department, Aristotle University of Thessaloniki, Papageorgiou Hospital, Thessaloniki, Greece

N. Tsetsos et al. (eds.), *Otolaryngology Study Guide*, https://doi.org/10.1007/978-3-031-77374-7_53

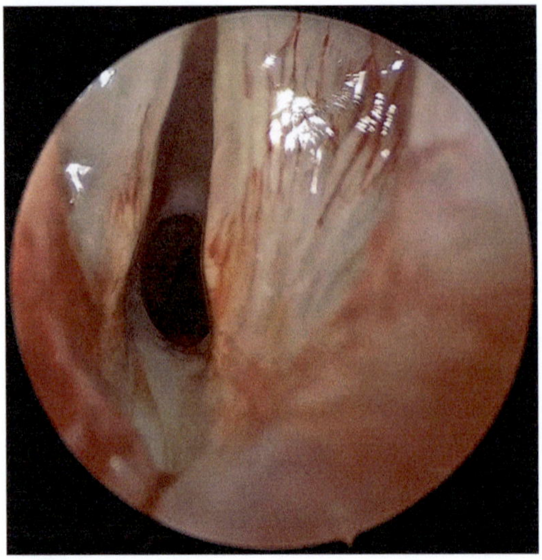

Fig. 53.1 Endoscopic image of the infant's larynx and trachea

increasing respiratory distress. During the examination, pulse oximetry revealed an oxygen saturation of 91% in room air. The clinical assessment indicated intercostal retractions, a barking cough, and stridor (Fig. 53.1).

Questions

1. Which is the most appropriate first examination for the infant described above?
   A. Barium swallow
   B. Flexible fiber-optic laryngoscopy
   C. Neck magnetic resonance imaging (MRI)
   D. X-ray of the neck and chest
   E. Bronchoscopy
2. Which syndrome may be associated with congenital SGS (more than one correct answer possible)?
   A. 22q11 deletion
   B. Turner's syndrome
   C. Down's syndrome
   D. CHARGE syndrome
   E. Williams syndrome
3. Which of the following statements are true about SGS (more than one correct answer possible)?
   A. The congenital form is more common than acquired SGS
   B. The prevalence of stenosis among intubated neonates ranges from 0% to 2%
   C. In cases of congenital SGS, the airway's size typically does not change as the child grows
   D. The extent of subglottic stenosis is evaluated using the Cotton-Myer grading system, with grade I indicating up to 10% constriction
   E. Stenosis of the subglottis is defined as a diameter of 4 mm or less in full-term infants (normal diameter is 4.5–5.5 mm)
4. Which of the following are risk factors for adult-acquired SGS (more than one answer is possible)?
   A. Traumatic intubation
   B. Granulomatosis with polyangiitis
   C. Prolonged duration of intubation
   D. Laryngopharyngeal reflux
   E. All of the above
5. Following bronchoscopy, evidence of SGS grade II with normal glottis was identified. Which of the following treatments could be employed as a final treatment for the patient described above (more than one answer is possible)?
   A. CO_2 laser use
   B. Antibiotics
   C. Balloon dilation
   D. Partial cricotracheal resection
   E. Tracheostomy

Answers

1. **B**

   Awake flexible fiber-optic laryngoscopy is a valuable initial test that can be performed on an outpatient basis to rule out conditions from the level of the nose to the vocal cords. However, it offers limited visualization of the area above the vocal cords. Bronchoscopy remains the gold standard diagnostic tool for confirming the presence of SGS [1]. In microlaryngoscopy and bronchoscopy, the larynx undergoes examination through suspension laryngoscopy under general anesthesia with spontaneous breathing. Subsequently, the trachea and bronchi are inspected either using a ventilating bronchoscope or by inserting a plain telescope via the laryngoscope [2]. The abovementioned examinations complement each other. Flexible fiber-optic laryngoscopy assesses dynamic airway collapse, vocal cord mobility, and possible laryngomalacia, while rigid direct laryngoscopy and bronchoscopy investigate upper and lower airway structures [1]. Airway radiographs can facilitate the assessment of the airway's overall structure and enable estimation of the length of stenosis. However, their value is limited and should be used additionally in the patient's assessment. In cases where a vascular lesion is suspected to impact the lower airways, MRI of the neck and chest becomes crucial [2, 3]. Additionally, if a child has a history of swallowing or feeding difficulties, a modified barium swallow remains an essential diagnostic procedure [3].

2. **A, C, D**

   Congenital SGS ranks as the third most prevalent congenital airway anomaly following laryngomalacia and vocal fold paralysis and is frequently associated with syndromic conditions such as trisomy 21, CHARGE, and 22q11 deletion syndromes. Developmental anomalies are uncommon, representing about 5% of individuals with SGS [4]. Failure in the recanalization process of the airway within the cricoid cartilage, originating from the sixth branchial arch, leads to SGS, which can manifest as membranous or more usually cartilaginous constriction [1].

3. **B, E**

   Pediatric SGS may be congenital or acquired. Since the 1970s, cases of congenital stenosis have been surpassed by acquired stenosis, which arises due to prolonged endotracheal intubation, lasting for approximately more than 4 weeks [2, 5]. In neonates who undergo intubation, the reported occurrence of SGS ranges from 0% to 2%. Unlike older individuals, most neonates can endure extended periods of intubation without experiencing subglottic damage. In congenital SGS, as the child grows, the airway generally increases in size over time, often eliminating the necessity for additional surgical procedures after initial management. However, children with severe SGS represent an exception to this typical clinical situation [6]. The subglottis represents the narrowest part of the airway in infants and young children. A subglottic diameter of 4 mm or less is deemed stenotic in a full-term neonate, while a diameter of 3 mm or less is considered stenotic in a preterm neonate. The severity of SGS is assessed using the Cotton-Myer grading system, which categorizes it as follows: grade I (up to 50% stenosis), grade II (51–70% stenosis), grade III (71–99% stenosis), and grade IV (no discernible lumen) [7]. Subtle types of SGS, ranging from grade I to grade II, cause stridor, difficulty breathing during exertion, and recurrent croup. Conversely, more severe forms of SGS, graded III or IV, can result in challenging intubations and an inability to be ventilated using a mask and may necessitate a tracheotomy [8].

4. **E**

   In adults, acquired SGS is primarily due to endotracheal intubation. Contributing factors that elevate the risk encompass various elements: traumatic intubation, prolonged intubation duration, repeated extubations and reintubations, inappropriate size of the laryngeal tube, and movement of either the patient or the endotracheal tube. Endotracheal tubes can harm subglottic tissues, causing erosion, disrupted cilia, a higher risk of infection, and scar formation [9]. Other causes include autoimmune conditions such as granulomatosis with polyangiitis and cases categorized as idiopathic, while infections are less common contributors [10, 11]. Specific factors contributing to SGS development relate to chronic inflammation, such as laryngopharyngeal reflux. Patients with diabetes are at an increased risk for SGS, as diabetes changes the inflammatory profile and affects a patient's capacity to recover following an injury [12].

5. **A, C**

   The standard therapy for children with grade I or II typically involves expanding the airway, often carried out using a CO_2 laser to make radial incisions in the stenosis and/or employing pressure-regulated balloons for dilation [3, 13]. Balloons present several benefits by applying a purely radial force around the stenosis, reducing the risk of airway rupture or mucosal injury, and decreasing the necessity for open airway surgery by up to 80% [14]. However, in cases of congenital cartilaginous SGS, the use of laser and dilation may worsen the stenosis; thus, open procedures are preferred [15]. Conversely, individuals with more severe SGS (grades II, III, and IV) or multiple narrowings in the airway, or those for whom successful outcomes are not attained via endoscopic methods, are more inclined to necessitate open reconstruction procedures, such as laryngotracheal reconstruction (LTR) or partial cricotracheal resection (PCTR) [3, 6, 8]. LTR can be conducted to widen the airway either in the forward, backward, or both directions simultaneously [8]. The operation could be conducted in a single stage or double stage. Single stage is recommended for patients with a localized issue, absence of tracheostomy, or minimal ailment at the tracheostomy area, alongside minimal pulmonary, cardiac, or other accompanying health conditions, while double stage is recommended for patients with notable concurrent health conditions, remaining lung problems, airway problems in multiple areas, or structural irregularities causing challenges during intubation [8, 16]. In case of complete stenosis, such as severe grade III SGS or grade IV SGS, PCTR is usually used. PCTR is a resection method where the scarred portion is excised, and the healthy trachea is elevated to substitute the absent cricoid. The trachea is stitched in place to fill the removed cricoid section [7]. In severe conditions, patients may need tracheostomy placement. Tracheostomy can be avoided by performing the anterior cricoid split after at least two extubation failures in premature or young infants [17, 18]. For patients with either isolated anterior or isolated posterior SGS, options include an anterior cricoid split with cartilage graft or a posterior cricoid split with cartilage graft, respectively [1].

References

1. Marston AP, White DR. Subglottic stenosis. Clin Perinatol. 2018;45(4):787–804.
2. Bailey M, Hoeve H, Monnier P. Paediatric laryngotracheal stenosis: a consensus paper from three European centres. Eur Arch Otorrinolaringol. 2003;260(3):118–23.
3. Cotton RT. Management of subglottic stenosis. Otolaryngol Clin N Am. 2000;33(1):111–30.
4. Bottero S, Peradotto F, Roma R, Tucci F. Laryngotracheal reconstruction in glottic-subglottic stenosis associated with DiGeorge syndrome in a four and a half-month-old infant. Acta Otorhinolaryngol Ital. 2015;35(1):53–7.
5. Cakir E, Atabek AA, Calim OF, Uzuner S, AlShadfan L, Yazan H, Ozturan O, Cakir FB. Post-intubation subglottic stenosis in children: analysis of clinical features and risk factors. Pediatr Int. 2020;62(3):386–9.
6. Jefferson ND, Cohen AP, Rutter MJ. Subglottic stenosis. Semin Pediatr Surg. 2016;25(3):138–43.
7. Myer CM 3rd, O'Connor DM, Cotton RT. Proposed grading system for subglottic stenosis based on endotracheal tube sizes. Ann Otol Rhinol Laryngol. 1994;103(4 Pt 1):319–23.
8. Hanlon K, Boesch RP, Jacobs I. Subglottic stenosis. Curr Probl Pediatr Adolesc Health Care. 2018;48(4):129–35.
9. Hawkins DB. Pathogenesis of subglottic stenosis from endotracheal intubation. Ann Otol Rhinol Laryngol. 1987;96(1 Pt 1):116–7.
10. Pasick LJ, Anis MM, Rosow DE. An updated review of subglottic stenosis: etiology, evaluation, and management. Curr Pulmonol Rep. 2022;11(2):29–38.
11. Axtell AL, Mathisen DJ. Idiopathic subglottic stenosis: techniques and results. Ann Cardiothorac Surg. 2018;7(2):299–305.
12. Nicolli EA, Carey RM, Farquhar D, Haft S, Alfonso KP, Mirza N. Risk factors for adult acquired subglottic stenosis. J Laryngol Otol. 2017;131(3):264–7.
13. Eskander A, de Almeida JR, Irish JC. Acute upper airway obstruction. N Engl J Med. 2019;381(20):1940–9.
14. Hautefort C, Teissier N, Viala P, et al. Balloon dilatation laryngoplasty for subglottic stenosis in children. Arch Otolaryngol Head Neck Surg. 2012;138:235–40.
15. Monnier P, George M, Monod ML, Lang F. The role of the CO2 laser in the management of laryngotracheal stenosis: a survey of 100 cases. Eur Arch Otorrinolaringol. 2005;262(8):602–8.
16. Smith LP, Zur KB, Jacobs IN. Single- vs double-stage laryngotracheal reconstruction. Arch Otolaryngol Head Neck Surg. 2010;136(1):60–5.
17. Silver FM, Myer CM 3rd, Cotton RT. Anterior cricoid split. Update 1991. Am J Otolaryngol. 1991;12(6):343–6.
18. Walner DL, Cotton RT. Acquired anomalies of the larynx and trachea. In: Cotton RT, Myer III CM, editors. Practical pediatric otolaryngology. Philadelphia/New York, NY: Lippincott Raven; 1999. p. 524.

Foreign Body Aspiration in Children

54

Vaios Kaminiotis and Marios Stavrakas

Abstract

Foreign body aspiration (FBA) is a common pediatric emergency, especially in children younger than 3 years old (Na'ara et al., Ear Nose Throat J, 99:47–51, 2020). The clinical presentation varies from asymptomatic state to acute respiratory failure, which could lead to death if not urgently treated. The most common symptoms include persistent cough, localized decreased breath sounds, localized wheezing, dyspnea, and fever. Out-of-hospital reported mortality rate is about 36.4%, whereas in-hospital mortality ranges between 0.26% and 13.6% due to complications mainly of hypoxia. In the USA, FBA causes around 5% of all accidental deaths in children (Rizk and Rassi, Eur Ann Otorhinolaryngol Head Neck Dis. 128:169–174, 2011). The most commonly found aspirated object is food due to a choking episode, which cannot be easily identified in a chest X-ray (Upreti and Gupta, Indian Pediatr, 52:659–60, 2015). A study showed that half of the aspiration accidents occurred under adult supervision. This shows that educating the public against choking hazards is imperative (Nichols et al., Int J Pediatr Otorhinolaryngol. 76:169–173, 2012). In most cases, the foreign body is located in the right bronchial tree due to wider lumen than left and having a more acute angle with the trachea.

V. Kaminiotis (✉)
Harefield Hospital, Guy's and St Thomas' NHS Foundation Trust, London, UK

M. Stavrakas
ENT Head and Neck Surgery Department, University Hospitals Plymouth NHS Trust, Plymouth, UK

Case Presentation

You are on call, and a 2-year-old child presents himself with his parents in A&E. His parents are worried because their son has been coughing for the last 1 week. The chest physician referred the child to you because he could not detect anything in physical examination, and his chest X-ray was clear. On a more detailed medical history that you take, you find out that the cough started soon after his grandparents went him for a walk and fed him nuts. You also notice localized decreased breathing sound in his right lower lobe. The child had at least one choking crisis over the past week and started to suffer from low-grade fever the last 24 h.

Questions

1. Which is the clinical presentation of foreign body aspiration in children?
   A. Pneumonia
   B. Atelectasis

N. Tsetsos et al. (eds.), *Otolaryngology Study Guide*, https://doi.org/10.1007/978-3-031-77374-7_54

C. Asphyxia
D. Bronchiectasis
E. All of the above

2. Which are the main reasons of in-hospital mortality due to foreign body aspiration in children?
   A. Severe laryngeal edema
   B. Hypoxic brain damage
   C. Cardiac arrest
   D. Tracheal/bronchial laceration
   E. All of the above
3. Which is the most common object of aspiration in children that may cause death?
   A. Seeds
   B. Chicken and fish bones
   C. Nonfood substances
   D. Gums
   E. Peanuts
4. What additional radiographic features on chest X-ray can assist diagnosis if the foreign body is not opaque?
   A. Pleural effusion
   B. Hyperinflation
   C. Kerley B lines
   D. Hilar lymphadenopathy
   E. None of the above
5. In the case presented, what would be the most suitable course of action?
   A. Rigid/flexible bronchoscopy
   B. Oral antibiotics
   C. Do nothing
   D. New chest X-ray in 1 week
   E. Antihistamine medications

Answers

1. **E**

   Aspiration of foreign body in children could remain undiagnosed for a long period. The symptoms vary and could include atelectasis, bronchiectasis, pneumonia, and asphyxia depending on the size of the bronchi obstructed [1, 2].
2. **E**

   Studies report children's deaths due to complications during rigid/flexible bronchoscopy (hypoxic arrest, bronchial rupture) or soon after (cardiac arrest, respiratory arrest) [3, 4].
3. **C**

   Data from CDC in the USA showed that 160 children <14 years old died from aspiration of a foreign object in 2001 (41% from food and 59% from nonfood). But regarding nonfatal choking-related episodes, food was responsible in 59.5% of the cases [5, 6]. As already mentioned, most FBAs occur in children <3 years old. Generally speaking, under the age of 3, the foreign body is usually organic; over the age of 5, it is inorganic.
4. **B**

   Indirect radiographic signs that can direct our diagnosis are atelectasis, hyperinflation, mediastinal shift, pneumonia, and pneumothorax. The classic appearance is unilateral hyperinflation due to ball-valve effect. The clinician should keep in mind that the X-ray can be normal in 11–26% of cases and the X-rays are only an aid to airway endoscopy. If there is strong clinical suspicion, endoscopy should be planned [7, 8].
5. **A**

   If FBA in a child is suspected (history of sudden choking, persistent cough, localized decreased breathing sounds), then flexible or rigid bronchoscopy should be performed without delay [9]. If the child is stable, the procedure can be carried out the following morning, especially if pediatric ENT expertise is necessary. Exceptions to this include unstable symptoms, organic material that can release oil (e.g., peanut) and granulation formation or could swell, and batteries [8].

References

1. Na'ara S, Vainer I, Amit M, Gordin A. Foreign body aspiration in infants and older children: a comparative study. Ear Nose Throat J. 2020;99(1):47–51.
2. Karakoç F, Karadağ B, Akbenlioğlu C, Ersu R, Yıldızeli B, Yüksel M, Dağlı E. Foreign body aspiration: what is the outcome? Pediatr Pulmonol. 2002;34(1):30–6.
3. Upreti L, Gupta N. Imaging for diagnosis of foreign body aspiration in children. Indian Pediatr. 2015;52(8):659–60.

4. Fidkowski CW, Zheng H, Firth PG. The anesthetic considerations of tracheobronchial foreign bodies in children: a literature review of 12,979 cases. Anesth Analg. 2010;111(4):1016–25. https://doi.org/10.1213/ANE.0b013e3181ef3e9c.
5. Rizk H, Rassi S. Foreign body inhalation in the pediatric population: lessons learned from 106 cases. Eur Ann Otorhinolaryngol Head Neck Dis. 2011;128:169–74.
6. Centers for Disease Control and Prevention. Nonfatal choking-related episodes among children—United States. MMWR Morb Mortal Wkly Rep. 2001;51(42):945–8.
7. Nichols BG, Visotcky A, Aberger M, Braun NM, Shah R, Tarima S, Brown DJ. Pediatric exposure to choking hazards is associated with parental knowledge of choking hazards. Int J Pediatr Otorhinolaryngol. 2012;76:169–73.
8. England RJ, Shamil E, editors. Scott-brown's essential otorhinolaryngology, head & neck surgery. CRC Press; 2022.
9. Midulla F, Guidi R, Barbato A, Capocaccia P, Forenza N, Marseglia G, et al. Foreign body aspiration in children. Pediatr Int. 2005;47(6):663–8.

Part VI

Head and Neck/Laryngology

55 Benign Vocal Fold Lesions

Paraskevi Karamitsou and Alexandros Poutoglidis

Abstract

Benign vocal fold lesions are frequently associated with harsh or excessive vocal usage. The likelihood of developing these nonmalignant lesions can be heightened by factors such as tobacco use, allergies, infections, laryngopharyngeal reflux, and alcohol intake. Approximately half of the patients who consult an ENT clinic due to voice alterations are diagnosed with a benign vocal fold lesion. The membranous vocal fold's structure, from the interior to the exterior, comprises the squamous epithelium, Reinke's potential space, vocal ligament, and thyroarytenoid muscle, also known as the vocal muscle. A comprehensive analysis of the patient's medical history and a meticulous larynx examination are vital for prompt diagnosis and treatment. The type of vocal fold lesions discovered during the physical examination will determine whether conservative or surgical treatment is required. The primary reasons for choosing surgery include cancer suspicion and persistent hoarseness in a benign lesion unresponsive to conservative treatment. Given that these lesions are often due to voice overuse, abuse, or misuse, voice therapy sessions conducted by a certified speech pathologist could help eradicate detrimental behaviors and instruct patients on appropriate voice care.

P. Karamitsou
ENT Head and Neck Surgery Department,
"G. Papanikolaou" General Hospital of Thessaloniki,
Thessaloniki, Greece

A. Poutoglidis (✉)
ENT Department, Lister Hospital, East and North
Hertfordshire NHS Trust, Stevenage, UK

N. Tsetsos et al. (eds.), *Otolaryngology Study Guide*, https://doi.org/10.1007/978-3-031-77374-7_55

Case Presentation

A 57-year-old man visited the ENT clinic with a complaint of a voice change that had been persisting for a month. He did not report any other symptoms. His medical history included hypertension and dyslipidemia. He was a smoker, with a habit of 15 cigarettes per day for the past 35 years. He did not consume alcohol. The patient also mentioned that he worked in a noisy environment and often had to raise his voice or use it aggressively. During a rigid laryngoscopy, a small polyp was found, originating from the middle of the left vocal fold. This polyp did not result in any insufficiency of the glottis gap (Fig. 55.1). A surgery was planned, and the polyp was successfully excised using direct microlaryngoscopy under general anesthesia. The histology report confirmed the benign nature of the lesion. The patient was discharged the day after the surgery. Considering the link between unilateral hemorrhagic vocal fold polyps and voice use, a brief

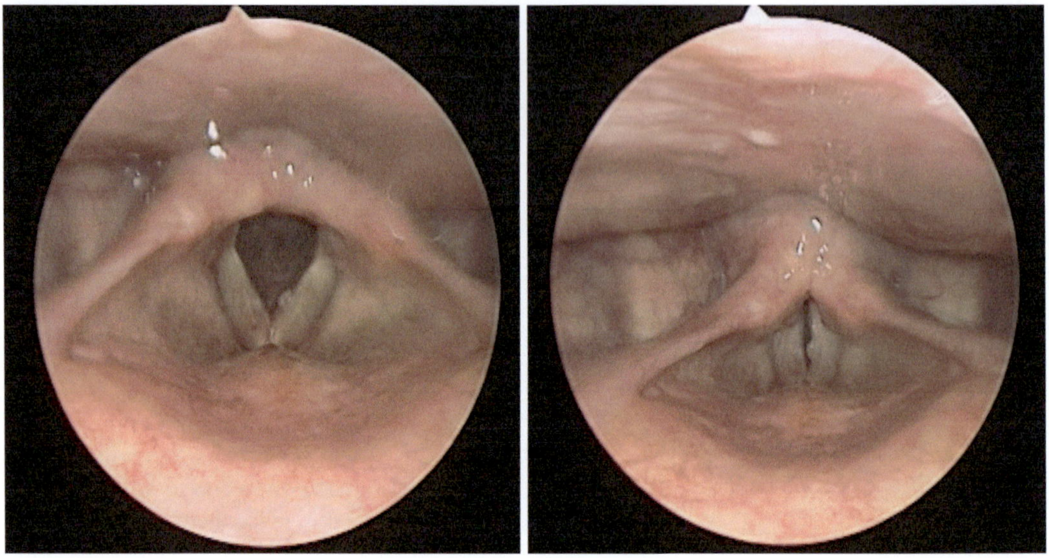

Fig. 55.1 A small polyp originating from the middle of the left vocal fold

course of voice therapy was suggested. The patient was also advised to quit smoking.

Questions

1. Unilateral hemorrhagic vocal fold polyp etiologies include:
   A. Chronic infections of the upper airway
   B. Voice overuse, abuse, or misuse
   C. Cigarette smoking
   D. Allergies
   E. Laryngopharyngeal reflux
2. The most appropriate therapeutic intervention for a vocal fold polyp includes:
   A. Medication
   B. Behavioral treatment
   C. Transoral surgical excision
   D. Transoral laser microsurgery
   E. Watchful waiting
3. Treatment of bilateral Reinke's edema includes:
   A. Smoking cessation and voice therapy
   B. Transoral laser microsurgery (carbon dioxide laser, blue laser, KTP laser)
   C. Cordectomy
   D. Proton pump inhibitors
   E. Watchful waiting
4. Which of the following sentences is true for recurrent laryngeal respiratory papillomatosis?
   A. HPV-6 and HPV-11 are the responsible pathogens.
   B. It is strongly related to malignant transformation.
   C. Surgery is the gold standard treatment.
   D. It is more aggressive in adults.
   E. Recurrences are not often after surgical excision.
5. Laryngeal granulomas:
   A. Are mostly located in the anterior part of the vocal folds.
   B. Gastroesophageal reflux is not associated with their pathogenesis.
   C. Are often related to intubation.
   D. May be transformed into malignant lesions.
   E. Patients should discontinue the anti-reflux treatment after a successful surgical procedure.

Answers

1. **A, B, C, D, E**

   Unilateral hemorrhagic vocal fold polyps can be caused by a variety of factors including trauma; overuse, abuse, or misuse of the voice; cigarette smoking; allergies; laryngopharyngeal reflux; alcohol consumption; and chronic infections of the upper respiratory tract [1]. Extreme vocal exertion can lead to the rupture of capillaries within the mucosa due to shearing forces. This can result in blood seeping from a deep capillary, causing an accumulation that changes the contour of the margin and hardens the mucosa. The process of wound healing and remodeling can lead to the formation of a hemorrhagic vocal fold polyp.

2. **C, D**

   Voice therapy sessions conducted by a certified speech pathologist can help eliminate harmful behaviors and educate patients on proper voice care. A small hemorrhagic polyp may disappear within a few months with conservative treatment, but surgery is usually necessary to restore the normal appearance of the vocal fold and voice capabilities. In cases where laryngopharyngeal reflux is present, acid reflux can lead to hyperemia. Unlike vocal nodules, hemorrhagic vocal fold polyps are unlikely to resolve with voice therapy alone [2, 3]. Surgical removal is often required [2, 4], and transoral laser microsurgery is a suitable treatment option [5]. The laser dissection targets the thrombosed contents of the polyp, sparing much of the stretched overlying mucosa. The prognosis for vocal rehabilitation following precision surgery is excellent [5].

3. **A, B, D**

   Reinke's edema is defined by the buildup of fluid in the Reinke's potential space of the vocal folds, resulting from vascular congestion in the superficial lamina propria. This chronic inflammatory disorder initially leads to hoarseness and, if not treated, can progress to airway obstruction. Factors such as smoking, gastroesophageal reflux, and voice overuse are closely associated with the onset of this condition. As such, the initial steps in managing Reinke's edema involve smoking cessation, use of proton pump inhibitors, and voice therapy. If the condition progresses due to noncompliance with these measures, surgical intervention may become necessary to prevent potential airway collapse. The surgical approach is guided by the principle of removing the excess edematous superficial lamina propria while preserving the remaining epithelium to ensure satisfactory voice quality. The accuracy of this procedure can be improved with the use of contemporary laser technology [6, 7].

4. **A**

   Recurrent laryngeal respiratory papillomatosis is a chronic viral condition. It is strongly associated with human papillomavirus (HPV) types 6 and 11 in its pathogenesis. Conversely, HPV oropharyngeal cancer is linked to HPV-16 and HPV-18. While HPV-6 and HPV-11 are not typically associated with cancer development, they do cause the continuous and recurrent growth of papillomas throughout the respiratory tract. The juvenile form of recurrent respiratory papillomatosis is considered more aggressive. Hoarseness is the most prevalent symptom among patients, and in severe cases with multiple lesions, airway collapse is a possibility. Surgical intervention does not cure the condition but helps alleviate the symptoms. Often, multiple procedures are required to restore voice function or prevent airway collapse in advanced cases. Surgery should be conservative, preserving the vocal fold epithelium to avoid scar formation. The need for multiple surgeries has led to the development of office-based procedures to circumvent the risks and costs of general anesthesia. Modern treatments like the monoclonal antibody bevacizumab and the antiviral drug cidofovir appear to be valid options for disease management. Lastly, vaccination against the HPV strains responsible can provide immunization and should be considered to achieve herd immunity [8–11].

5. **C**

Laryngeal granulomas are primarily linked to extended periods of intubation or multiple instances of intubation. They usually form in the posterior section of the vocal fold, just in front of the arytenoid cartilage. Another contributing factor that frequently results in granuloma formation is gastroesophageal reflux. Proton pump inhibitors are the initial treatment of choice, with surgery being considered for persistent cases or those presenting with hoarseness. However, even after successful removal, patients should maintain their treatment due to the potential risk of recurrence [12, 13].

References

1. Garcia RH, Defaveri J, Domingues MA, de Albuquerque e Silva R. Vocal polyps: clinical, morphological, and immunohistochemical aspects. J Voice. 2011;25(1):98–106.
2. Johns MM. Update on the etiology, diagnosis, and treatment of vocal fold nodules, polyps, and cysts. Curr Opin Otolaryngol Head Neck Surg. 2003;11(6):456–61.
3. Pinto D, Cohn JE, Panossian H, Sataloff RT. Secondary features of hemorrhagic true vocal fold polyps. Ear Nose Throat J. 2020;99(3):NP29–30.
4. Spiegel JR, Sataloff RT, Hawkshaw M, Rosen DC. Vocal fold hemorrhage. Ear Nose Throat J. 1996;75(12):784–9.
5. Byeon HK, Han JH, Choi BI, Hwang HJ, Kim JH, Choi HS. Treatment of hemorrhagic vocal polyps by pulsed dye laser-assisted laryngomicrosurgery. Biomed Res Int. 2015;2015:820654.
6. Dewan K, Chhetri DK, Hoffman H. Reinke's edema management and voice outcomes. Laryngoscope Investig Otolaryngol. 2022;7(4):1042–50.
7. Hess MM, Fleischer S, Ernstberger M. New 445 nm blue laser for laryngeal surgery combines photoangiolytic and cutting properties. Eur Arch Otorrinolaringol. 2018;275(6):1557–67.
8. Derkay CS, Bluher AE. Update on recurrent respiratory papillomatosis. Otolaryngol Clin N Am. 2019;52(4):669–79.
9. Yiu Y, Fayson S, Smith H, Matrka L. Implementation of routine HPV vaccination in the management of recurrent respiratory papillomatosis. Ann Otol Rhinol Laryngol. 2019;128(4):309–15.
10. Fortes HR, von Ranke FM, Escuissato DL, Araujo Neto CA, Zanetti G, Hochhegger B, Souza CA, Marchiori E. Recurrent respiratory papillomatosis: a state-of-the-art review. Respir Med. 2017;126:116–21.
11. Shoffel-Havakuk H, Halperin D, Yosef L, Feldberg E, Lahav Y. Lesions of the posterior glottis: clinical and pathologic considerations and treatment outcome. J Voice. 2014;28(2):263e1–8.
12. Ma L, Xiao Y, Ye J, Yang Q, Wang J. Analysis of therapeutic methods for treating vocal process granulomas. Acta Otolaryngol. 2015;135(3):277–82.
13. Martins RHG, Dias NH, Soares CSP, Gramuglia ACJ. Treatment of laryngeal granulomas. Int Arch Otorhinolaryngol. 2019;23(3):322–4.

Laryngopharyngeal Reflux

56

Konstantinos Garefis

Abstract

Laryngopharyngeal reflux (LPR) is an inflammatory condition affecting the tissues of the upper aerodigestive tract due to the reflux of gastric or duodenal contents, leading to morphological changes. This condition is relatively common, affecting about 8–20% of the general population. LPR significantly impacts patient's quality of life, presenting with recurrent symptoms such as the sensation of a foreign body in the throat, throat clearing, hoarseness, and excessive throat mucus. Assessment includes the use of specific clinical scores and clinical examination. LPR clinical signs, such as posterior commissure hypertrophy, interarytenoid/laryngeal erythema, and thick adhesive laryngeal mucus, are relatively nonspecific and can be seen in other disorders. Diagnosis is not standardized and may be based on objective examinations, empirical treatment, and biochemical tests. Differential diagnoses include esophageal and gastric pathologies and upper airway pathologies, among others. Treatment involves lifestyle and dietary modifications, anti-reflux medications according to individual patient characteristics, and surgery in some resistant cases.

K. Garefis (✉)
2nd Academic ORL, Head and Neck Surgery Department, Aristotle University of Thessaloniki, Papageorgiou Hospital, Thessaloniki, Greece

Case Presentation

A 45-year-old female presents with chronic throat discomfort, including hoarseness, throat clearing, and globus sensation. She reports an increase in symptoms after the consumption of high-fat foods and occasional heartburn. Laryngoscopy reveals posterior commissure hypertrophy, interarytenoid erythema and edema, endolaryngeal sticky secretions, and nodularity of the posterior pharyngeal wall (Fig. 56.1). The rest of the ENT examination is unremarkable.

Questions

1. Which of the following statements are true about LPR (more than one correct answer possible)?
   A. LPR symptoms are found in 43% of outpatients visiting ear, nose, and throat departments
   B. Pepsin leads to inflammatory reaction and dry (sticky) mucus hypersecretion
   C. Consumption of chocolate, feta cheese, and chips can induce LPR
   D. Young subjects feel acid reflux less strongly than elderly
   E. Women show dysphonia more often than men

N. Tsetsos et al. (eds.), *Otolaryngology Study Guide*, https://doi.org/10.1007/978-3-031-77374-7_56

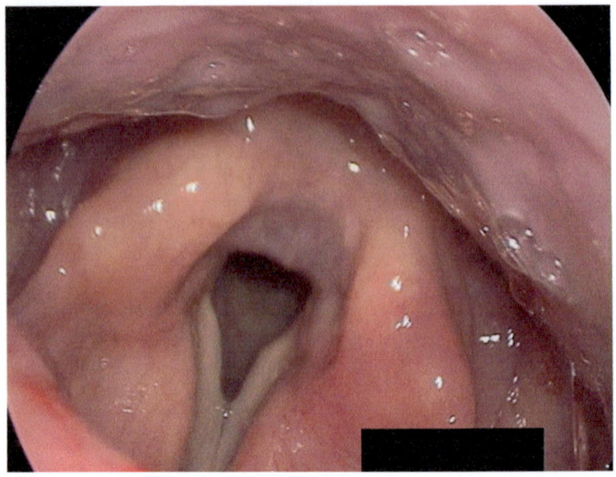

Fig. 56.1 Endoscopic image of patient's larynx

2. Which of the following are frequent LRP's symptoms and signs (more than one correct answer possible)?
   A. Globus sensation, posterior commissure hypertrophy
   B. Throat clearing, vocal fold atrophy
   C. Hoarseness, endolaryngeal mucus
   D. Heartburn, laryngeal/arytenoid inflammation
   E. Dysphagia, subglottic edema
3. The diagnostic workup for LPR may include (more than one correct answer possible):
   A. Multichannel intraluminal impedance-pH metry
   B. Barium swallow test
   C. Empirical therapeutic trial
   D. Pepsin detection
   E. Magnetic resonance imaging (MRI)
4. Differential diagnosis of LPR includes (more than one correct answer possible):
   A. Eosinophilic esophagitis
   B. Chronic rhinosinusitis
   C. Chronic obstructive pulmonary disease
   D. None of the above
   E. All of the above
5. Which of the following treatments should you use for the patient described above (more than one correct answer possible)?
   A. Diet and lifestyle
   B. Alginate
   C. Surgery
   D. Pantoprazole
   E. All of the above

Answers

1. **B, C, E**

LPR symptoms are present in 10–15% of outpatients in ear, nose, and throat clinics and affect 1% of patients in primary care settings [1]. LPR arises from macroscopic and microscopic changes in the mucosa of the upper aerodigestive tract. Irritation of the mucosa leads to inflammation and excessive production of dry, sticky mucus, as pepsin reduces mucin expression and bicarbonate secretion. The buildup of sticky mucus causes symptoms. Additionally, mucosal chemoreceptors in the distal section of the esophagus, which are stimulated by stomach acid reflux, can also cause mucus hypersecretion and accompanying symptoms [2]. A variety of foods can induce LPR, such as fatty fish, fish oil, fatty chicken, high-fat meats (kidneys, bacon, rib steak, roast, salami, etc.), shallots, spicy foods, chili, onions, garlic, tomatoes, chocolate, ice cream, whole milk, hard cheese, full-fat cheese, strong alcohol, red and rose wines, sparkling beverages (water, soda, beer, etc.), coffee, tea, citrus juices (orange, lemon, grapefruit), butter, spicy sauces (mayonnaise, mustard, ketchup, etc.), and sweets [3]. The prevalence of LPR varies by gender and age. Women are more likely to experience dysphonia due to various anatomical, histological, and functional factors [2, 4]. Consequently, diagnosis is quicker in women because of more noticeable laryngeal findings

[2]. In elderly individuals, age-related sensorineural degeneration results in a reduced perception of acid reflux [2, 4].

2. **A, C**

Globus sensation, hoarseness, excess throat mucus, throat clearing, and postnasal drip are the most frequent symptoms, occurring in over 70% of patients with LPR [2, 4]. However, these symptoms are nonspecific and also appear in other airway pathologies, complicating clinical diagnosis [4]. GERD-related symptoms, such as heartburn, are less common in LPR, as most episodes involve gaseous reflux rather than liquid; fewer than 50% of patients exhibit acid reflux or pyrosis [2, 4]. Typical clinical signs of LPR include posterior commissure hypertrophy, interarytenoid and laryngeal erythema, and thick, adhesive endolaryngeal mucus [1, 4]. However, like the symptoms, these signs are relatively nonspecific and are also seen in other airway disorders [4]. Additional laryngeal and extralaryngeal findings and symptoms that may be linked to LPR, but are not yet included in current clinical evaluations, include tongue tonsil hypertrophy, coated tongue, pharyngeal granulations, hypo- and oropharyngeal erythema, vocal fold erythema, retrocricoid erythema and edema, tongue burning, throat pain, odynophagia, eructation, nausea, and dyspepsia [1].

3. **A, C, D**

There is no gold standard for diagnosing LPR; however, the two most widely used methods are multichannel intraluminal (MII) impedance-pH metry and, when this is unavailable, positive response to a well-executed empirical treatment trial. Pepsin detection is increasingly utilized as a diagnostic biomarker. Currently, MII impedance-pH metry is considered the most reliable method for diagnosing LPR. However, due to its cost, unavailability, and other limitations, diagnosis is often based solely on empirical therapeutic trials. This empirical approach involves using clinical scores, such as the Reflux Symptom Index (RSI) and the Reflux Finding Score (RFS), at the initial assessment and prescribing proton pump inhibitors (PPIs) for a 3-month period. If there is no improvement, the PPI may be continued for an additional 3 months. A diagnosis of LPR is only made if the patient improves after 3 or 6 months of therapy. For nonresponders, the diagnosis remains uncertain and requires further examination. Clinical diagnosis is challenging because many LPR symptoms are common to other conditions affecting the laryngeal and pharyngeal regions. Therefore, it is crucial to exclude all cofactors or differential diagnoses before confirming LPR through an empirical therapeutic trial. Pepsin or trypsin detection, which can be performed on saliva or pharyngeal/laryngeal biopsies, is a promising diagnostic tool. These analyses can complement MII impedance-pH metry in patients presenting with LPR symptoms. Currently, the combination of symptoms, signs, positive MII impedance-pH metry results, and pepsin or trypsin detection is considered the closest approach to a gold standard for diagnosing LPR [2, 4].

4. **E**

Based on the main LPR symptoms, differential diagnosis includes situation from:

- Esophageal and gastric pathologies (eosinophilic esophagitis, Zenker diverticulum, mycotic esophagitis, esophageal ectopic gastric mucosa, cricopharyngeal muscle spasm, esophageal spasm, inferior esophageal sphincter spasm, achalasia cardia, gastroparesis, neoplasia).
- Upper airway pathologies (infections: chronic rhinosinusitis, mycosis, recurrent angina, tuberculosis, rheumatologic/autoimmune disorders: rheumatic arthritis Sjogren's syndrome, laryngeal sarcoidosis, amyloidosis, granulomatosis with polyangiitis, allergy, laryngeal musculoskeletal disorders: laryngeal function disorders, muscle tension dysphonia, benign or malign tumors, anatomic disorders: size and shape of the epiglottis, tongue, tonsil hypertrophy, uvula hypertrophy, traumatic and other: laryngeal fracture, upper aerodigestive tract injury, cervical osteophytes, aging voice, upper aerodigestive tract neoplasia, thyroid disease).

  - Non-upper airway pathologies (pulmonary pathologies: chronic obstructive pulmonary disease, asthma, neuropsychiatric/psychological pathologies: stress, anxiety, depression, drugs) [3, 4].

5. **A, B, D**

   Management of LPR may involve both behavioral changes and medication. Adjustments to diet and lifestyle have a significant role in treatment. Specifically, avoiding unhealthy lifestyle factors such as stress, late meals, aerophagy, smoking, alcohol, spices, coffee, tea, and fizzy drinks, as well as a low-protein, high-fat diet, is recommended [4]. Treatment for LPR, based on characteristics identified through MII-pH monitoring (such as types of reflux: acid, nonacid, mixed, and the timing and positioning of reflux episodes: upright, recumbent, daytime, nighttime), includes dietary and behavioral modifications, along with the use of PPIs with or without alginate or magaldrate for a minimum of 3 months. Patients with acid and mixed LPR are treated with PPIs and alginate or magaldrate, while those with nonacid LPR are treated with alginate or magaldrate alone. PPIs should be administered twice daily [1, 4]. After the initial 3-month treatment, therapy can be extended for an additional 3 months if needed. About 25–50% of patients may experience a chronic course of the disease. For these patients, maintaining dietary management and lifestyle modifications are essential. Severe recurrences of LPR can be managed with short-term treatment using PPIs and alginate (or magaldrate) based on the patient's specific needs. Physicians should avoid long-term use of PPIs due to their potential side effects [2, 3]. Laparoscopic fundoplication is a viable treatment for reflux that does not respond to medication and dietary changes, although its effectiveness for LPR is debated, with success rates varying from 44% to 94% [4].

References

1. Lechien JR, Bobin F, Muls V, Mouawad F, Dapri G, Dequanter D, Horoi M, Thill MP, Rodriguez Ruiz A, Saussez S. Changes of laryngeal and extralaryngeal symptoms and findings in laryngopharyngeal reflux patients. Laryngoscope. 2021;131(6):1332–42.
2. Lechien JR, Saussez S, Karkos PD. Laryngopharyngeal reflux disease: clinical presentation, diagnosis and therapeutic challenges in 2018. Curr Opin Otolaryngol Head Neck Surg. 2018;26(6):392–402.
3. Lechien JR, Akst LM, Hamdan AL, Schindler A, Karkos PD, Barillari MR, Calvo-Henriquez C, Crevier-Buchman L, Finck C, Eun YG, Saussez S, Vaezi MF. Evaluation and management of laryngopharyngeal reflux disease: state of the art review. Otolaryngol Head Neck Surg. 2019;160(5):762–82.
4. Lechien JR, Mouawad F, Bobin F, Bartaire E, Crevier-Buchman L, Saussez S. Review of management of laryngopharyngeal reflux disease. Eur Ann Otorhinolaryngol Head Neck Dis. 2021;138(4):257–67.

Recurrent Respiratory Papillomatosis

57

Konstantinos Garefis and Iordanis Konstantinidis

Abstract

Recurrent respiratory papillomatosis (RRP) is an uncommon benign tumor of the aerodigestive tract that primarily affects the larynx in both pediatric and adult populations. It derives from localized Human Papillomavirus (HPV) infection and presents with wartlike growths in the airway, which can affect voice and airway patency. RRP is characterized as juvenile onset (before 12 years) or adult onset (after 12 years). Clinical manifestations include various nonspecific symptoms, such as hoarseness, cough, voice change, wheezing, stridor, and airway obstruction leading to respiratory failure. Papillomas manifest as single or multiple exophytic, pedunculated masses. While infrequent, RRP carries the risk of transforming into squamous cell carcinoma. Diagnosis is based on visualization of the lesions through laryngoscopy or bronchoscopy and biopsies. Computed tomography (CT) is a useful imaging tool. Histopathological examination confirms the diagnosis. Currently, there is no absolute cure for RRP; although adjuvant pharmacologic therapies exist, surgery remains the primary treatment approach. HPV vaccines might delay RRP recurrence and decrease its occurrence by preventing HPV transmission to infants.

Case Presentation

An 81-year-old heavy-smoker male presented to the Emergency Department with stridor and dyspnea persisting for 10 days. He reports hoarseness for about 1 year. During the examination, pulse oximetry revealed an oxygen saturation of 84% in room air. Flexible laryngoscopy revealed multiple exophytic lesions obstructing almost the entire laryngeal lumen. The rest of the ENT examination was unremarkable. Due to the laryngeal obstruction, intubation could not be performed. Therefore, the patient underwent tracheostomy under local anesthesia, followed by biopsies taken under general anesthesia. Histopathological examination confirmed the diagnosis of RRP. Helical CT of the lower respiratory system showed no abnormalities. After 15 days, the patient underwent surgery for the surgical removal of papillomas using potassium-titanyl-phosphate (KTP) laser. Unfortunately, the patient did not attend the recommended follow-up at 1 month; on the contrary, he appeared in the clinic 10 months after his operation (Fig. 57.1).

K. Garefis (✉) · I. Konstantinidis
2nd Academic ORL, Head and Neck Surgery Department, Aristotle University of Thessaloniki, Papageorgiou Hospital, Thessaloniki, Greece

N. Tsetsos et al. (eds.), *Otolaryngology Study Guide*, https://doi.org/10.1007/978-3-031-77374-7_57

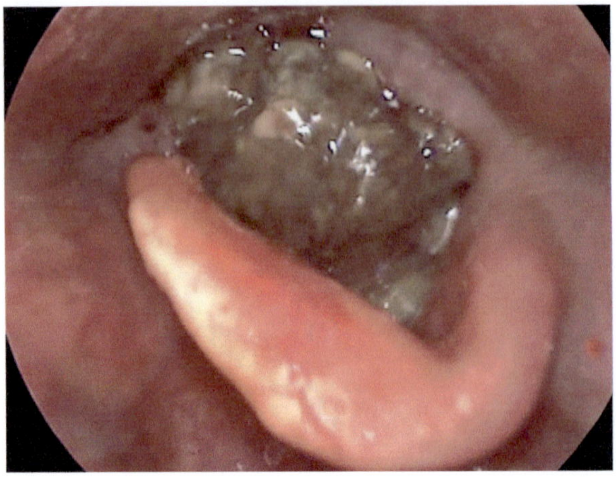

Fig. 57.1 Endoscopic image of the patient's larynx during his last appointment, 10 months postoperatively

Questions

1. Which of the following statements are true about RRP (more than one correct answer possible)?
   A. The disease is more prevalent in children
   B. The most common site for the lesion is the larynx
   C. The adult form develops frequently in women and recurs less frequently than in children
   D. In adults, hoarseness is the most common finding
   E. RRP is usually diagnosed with chest X-ray
2. Which subtypes of HPV are most commonly associated with RRP?
   A. 11 and 16
   B. 6 and 16
   C. 6 and 11
   D. 16 and 18
   E. 6, 11, 16, and 18
3. The most frequent presenting symptoms in children with RRP are (more than one correct answer possible):
   A. Dysphagia and poor weight gain
   B. Dyspnea with exertion
   C. Progressive dysphonia and stridor
   D. Odynophagia
   E. Chronic cough
4. Which of the following variables present a significant risk factor for malignant transformation of RRP in adults (more than one correct answer possible)?
   A. Number of surgical interventions
   B. Age of the patient
   C. Treatment by cidofovir
   D. Absence of HPV DNA on polymerase chain reaction of papilloma specimen
   E. Tobacco use
5. What could be the future treatment options for the patient described above (more than one correct answer possible)?
   A. Surgical removal
   B. Cidofovir local injection
   C. High-dose oral steroid burst
   D. Azathioprine
   E. Radiation therapy

Answers

1. **A, B, D**

   RRP is more frequent in children, with an estimated occurrence of around 4.3 cases per 100,000 compared to 1.8 cases per 100,000 in adults [1, 2]. RRP is also known as laryngeal papillomatosis or glottal papillomatosis. It primarily affects the larynx; however, papillomas can manifest in various sites throughout the respiratory system, with trachea being the most frequent location of extralaryngeal involvement. Other locations include the oropharynx, oral cavity, nasopharynx, nose, and, less commonly, pulmonary parenchyma [1–3]. Involvement of the lower respiratory tract is observed in just 2–5% of cases of laryngeal papillomas, with pulmonary tissue being affected in 1% of occurrences. The juvenile form of RRP tends to be aggressive, characterized by multiple papillomatous lesions and a high likelihood of recurrence. Conversely, the adult form, more prevalent in males, usually shows limited spread and recurs less often. RRP usually presents with general airway symptoms such as chronic cough, hoarseness, stridor, and difficulty breathing, with hoarseness being the most common symptom in adults. Severe cases can result in airway obstruction and respiratory distress. RRP diagnosis can be confirmed by flexible fiber-optic or direct laryngoscopy or bronchoscopy, depending on the site of the lesions [2, 3]. Moreover, narrow-band imaging (NBI) endoscopy is a useful diagnostic method in differentiating benign from malignant laryngeal lesions [4]. Histopathology of biopsied tissue establishes the definitive diagnosis. While chest X-ray findings are seldom used for diagnosing, helical CT is the preferred imaging method, particularly for assessing tracheobronchial and pulmonary lesions [2].

2. **C**

   RRP is a multifaceted condition primarily caused by two strains of HPV: HPV 6 and HPV 11. Notably, subtypes 6 and 11 are responsible for over 90% of RRP cases, with HPV 11 being more frequent [1, 2]. HPV 11 is probably the more virulent strain of the two, and a younger age at presentation is associated with a more severe course of the disease [5, 6]. Additionally, other HPV subtypes such as 16, 18, 31, and 33 have been associated with RRP, although they occur with lower frequency [2].

3. **C**

   Children typically exhibit symptoms between the ages of 2 and 6, with equal distribution between genders. Those affected by HPV 11 typically show signs at notably younger ages compared to those affected by HPV 6 [3]. In children, RRP commonly manifests with a triad of symptoms: progressive dysphonia, stridor, and respiratory distress. This clinical picture often mimics common laryngeal and respiratory conditions like laryngitis, asthma, bronchitis, and croup, which can lead physicians to misdiagnosis [2, 3]. Symptoms often become more severe due to the rapid proliferation of lesions, increasing the risk of airway obstruction [2]. Additional symptoms may involve persistent coughing, recurrent infections of the upper respiratory tract, and hemoptysis [3].

4. **B, E**

   While relatively uncommon, RRP poses the risk of malignant transformation, predominantly towards bronchogenic squamous cell carcinoma, which may emerge decades after the disease onset, especially in patients with prior extension to the tracheobronchial tree. Furthermore, malignant transformation rarely occurs in the laryngeal variant of the disease without affecting the distal airway. Malignant transformation rates range from 3% to 7% in adults and less than 1% in children [2]. Contributing factors encompass infection with high-risk HPV subtypes (16 and 18), tobacco use, previous radiotherapy, cytotoxic medication usage, p53 gene mutation, and heightened activity of 2′-5′-oligoadenylate synthetase [2, 7, 8]. Notably, smoking has been shown to affect the expression of p53, a pivotal characteristic in malignant transformations across various tissues [8]. Although traditionally perceived as low risk, HPV subtypes 6 and 11, particularly subtype 11, also carry the potential for malignant progression. The exact mechanism behind malignant transformation remains uncertain. However, the oncogenic potential of HPV is associated with its disruption of the cellular cycle, consequently altering cellular differentiation control [2].

5. **A, B**

   The treatment of choice for RRP is surgical removal. The primary goals of surgery are to ensure that the airway remains unobstructed and to maintain satisfactory voice quality. Complete elimination is not always the objective, as HPV is thought to persist in laryngeal epithelial cells whether visible papillomas are present or not. The conventional approach to treating RRP typically involves surgically removing the lesions in a hospital operating room while the patient is under general anesthesia. This is usually done using KTP lasers or microdebriders, although some surgeons may also utilize CO_2 lasers or cold steel instruments. However, the introduction of flexible fiber delivery systems has enabled laser procedures to be performed in office, offering potential time and cost savings for healthcare and increased convenience for patients [9]. Tracheostomy might be necessary for advanced disease with a significant risk of laryngeal airway blockage, particularly in cases where numerous interventions have proven ineffective. However, tracheostomy carries the risk of spreading infection to the lower airways [1]. Surgery stands as the main treatment approach for RRP; nevertheless, around 20% of RRP patients necessitate adjuvant therapy since surgery alone is insufficient to manage the disease. Adjuvant therapies include the use of cidofovir, interferon, bevacizumab, celecoxib, and PD-1 inhibitor [9]. Cidofovir is an antiviral commonly used as adjuvant treatment, typically administered intralesionally and has shown good results. It is well tolerated, with limited systemic toxicity [1, 9].

References

1. Carifi M, Napolitano D, Morandi M, Dall'Olio D. Recurrent respiratory papillomatosis: current and future perspectives. Ther Clin Risk Manag. 2015;11:731–8.
2. Fortes HR, von Ranke FM, Escuissato DL, Araujo Neto CA, Zanetti G, Hochhegger B, Souza CA, Marchiori E. Recurrent respiratory papillomatosis: a state-of-the-art review. Respir Med. 2017;126:116–21.
3. Seedat RY. Juvenile-onset recurrent respiratory papillomatosis diagnosis and management—a developing country review. Pediatr Health Med Ther. 2020;11:39–46.
4. Saraniti C, Gallina S, Verro B. NBI and laryngeal papillomatosis: a diagnostic challenge: a systematic review. Int J Environ Res Public Health. 2022;19(14):8716.
5. Derkay CS, Wiatrak B. Recurrent respiratory papillomatosis: a review. Laryngoscope. 2008;118(7):1236–47.
6. Benedict JJ, Derkay CS. Recurrent respiratory papillomatosis: a 2020 perspective. Laryngoscope Investig Otolaryngol. 2021;6(2):340–5.
7. Fusconi M, Grasso M, Greco A, Gallo A, Campo F, Remacle M, Turchetta R, Pagliuca G, De Vincentiis M. Recurrent respiratory papillomatosis by HPV: review of the literature and update on the use of cidofovir. Acta Otorhinolaryngol Ital. 2014;34(6):375–81.
8. Donne AJ, Hampson L, Homer JJ, Hampson IN. The role of HPV type in recurrent respiratory papillomatosis. Int J Pediatr Otorhinolaryngol. 2010;74(1):7–14.
9. Ivancic R, Iqbal H, deSilva B, Pan Q, Matrka L. Current and future management of recurrent respiratory papillomatosis. Laryngoscope Investig Otolaryngol. 2018;3(1):22–34.

58 Laryngeal Cancer

Alexandros Poutoglidis and Evropi Forozidou

Abstract

Laryngeal cancer is the most prevalent form of malignancy in the head and neck region. Squamous cell carcinomas make up the majority of laryngeal tumors, accounting for about 95% of cases, and primarily affect the glottis or supraglottis. The division of the larynx into these specific parts is important due to their distinct embryological development and lymphatic drainage patterns. The main risk factors for laryngeal cancer are smoking and heavy alcohol consumption, and the combination of these factors significantly increases the likelihood of developing the disease. The symptoms experienced by patients depend on the location of the tumor. Glottic cancer typically presents with hoarseness, while supraglottic neoplasms often do not cause early symptoms and may be discovered when a neck lump is noticed. Endoscopy is the preferred clinical assessment method for identifying laryngeal growths. Once a diagnosis is confirmed through histopathological examination, staging is necessary to determine the appropriate treatment approach. Early-stage laryngeal cancer (stages I and II) can often be treated with a single form of therapy, whereas advanced cases (stages III and IV) may require multiple modalities to achieve a curative response. The prognosis for early-stage cancer is generally favorable, but recurrences may necessitate salvage total laryngectomy, which can significantly impact the quality of life.

Case Presentation

A 67-year-old man visited an ear, nose, and throat clinic with a main complaint of worsening hoarseness that had been occurring for the past 5 months. He had a history of heavy smoking for 35 years.

During the physical examination, a glottic tumor was identified using a flexible endoscope. The tumor appeared ulcerated and protruding, but not easily crumbled. It was located in the posterior third of the right vocal fold and did not affect mobility (see Fig. 58.1). Neck palpation did not reveal any abnormalities, and computed tomography scans of the head, neck, and chest did not show any pathological findings.

Under general anesthesia, a panendoscopy was performed to evaluate the upper aerodigestive tract. Biopsies confirmed the presence of a squamous cell carcinoma (SCC) in the glottic region of the right vocal fold. The tumor was classified as stage I cT1aN0M0.

A. Poutoglidis (✉)
ENT Department, Lister Hospital, East and North Hertfordshire NHS Trust, Stevenage, UK

E. Forozidou
ENT Head and Neck Surgery Department, "G. Papanikolaou" General Hospital, Thessaloniki, Greece

N. Tsetsos et al. (eds.), *Otolaryngology Study Guide*, https://doi.org/10.1007/978-3-031-77374-7_58

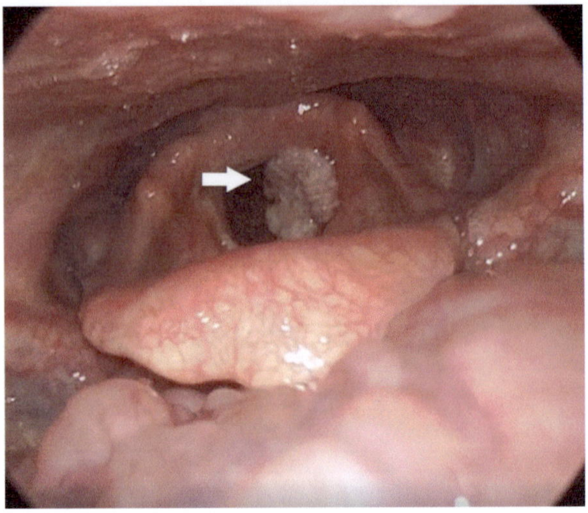

Fig. 58.1 Inflexible endoscopy. An exophytic growth in the posterior third of the left vocal fold (arrow)

The patient was informed about the test results and was presented with the options of radiotherapy or cordectomy as potential treatments. The patient chose to decline surgery and opted for radiotherapy in order to improve voice quality.

Questions

1. An absolute contradiction to conservation laryngeal surgery is:
   A. Paraglottic space invasion
   B. Pre-epiglotic space invasion
   C. T3 glottic cancer
   D. Cricoarytenoid joint invasion
   E. Salvage cases
2. Supraglottic cancer rarely involves:
   A. Infrahyoid epiglottis
   B. Suprahyoid epiglottis
   C. Pre-epiglottic space
   D. Hyoid bone
   E. Arytenoids
3. Supraglottic laryngeal cancer most commonly metastasizes in lymph nodes of level:
   A. I
   B. II
   C. III
   D. IV
   E. VI
4. Early glottic cancer can be better treated by:
   A. Cordectomy
   B. Radiotherapy
   C. Chemotherapy
   D. Cordectomy + adjuvant radiation
   E. Concomitant chemoradiation
5. Local advanced laryngeal cancer (T4aN0M0) should be better treated by:
   A. Conservational laryngeal surgery
   B. Total laryngectomy
   C. Concomitant chemoradiation
   D. Induction chemotherapy + radiotherapy
   E. Total laryngectomy + adjuvant radiation

Answers

1. **D**

   Conservation laryngeal surgery is recommended for both glottic and supraglottic carcinomas as a means of preserving the organ. This includes vertical partial laryngectomy (VPL) and supracricoid partial laryngectomy with cricohyoidoepiglottopexy (SCPL-CHEP) for glottic tumors and supraglottic laryngectomy (SL) with or without cricohyoidopexy (CHP) for supraglottic cancers [1]. Successful oncological and functional outcomes can only be achieved if local control is feasible. The cricoarytenoid joint is the fundamental functional unit of the larynx, and any sacrifice of this joint will result in permanent laryngeal dysfunction [2]. Therefore, conservation laryngeal surgery is not possible in cases where the tumor originates or infiltrates the cricoarytenoid joint. Invasion of the pre-epiglottic and paraepiglottic spaces, however, is not considered a contraindication as SCPL-CHP or VPL can be employed, respectively. Prior radiotherapy presents a challenge for conservation laryngeal surgery as it may impair laryngeal function. However, in, most cases, the operation can still be performed effectively [3].

2. **D**

   The clinical doctor should always consider the detailed anatomy of the larynx. Petiole is the lowest part of the laryngeal surface of the epiglottis and is often mistaken for a cyst or neoplasm. Supraglottic cancer can involve various subsites (ventricle, epiglottis, arytenoids, arytenoepiglottic folds) of the supraglottis [4]. It tends to metastasize early through the extensive lymphatic network and spread locally due to weak anatomical barriers. The fenestrations of the infrahyoid epiglottis are the main reason for tumor extension into the pre-epiglottic space. The complex embryological development of the larynx provides a strong anatomical barrier that resists glottic extension even in advanced cases. Total laryngectomy specimens always include the hyoid bone, although infiltration of the hyoid bone is rare even in advanced supraglottic cancer [5]. Preserving the hyoid bone is important for postoperative swallowing. Additionally, in cases of conservation laryngeal surgery, SC aPL with CHP can be performed even in some transglottic tumors.

3. **B**

   Supraglottis is characterized by a rich lymphatic network. Supraglottic cancer may present with dysphagia, otalgia, or hemoptysis, but these symptoms often appear late. In contrast, hoarseness is an early indicator of glottic cancer, leading to earlier detection. A neck lump in level II of a patient with a long history of smoking should always raise suspicion of metastatic supraglottic cancer. The aggressive nature of supraglottic cancer determines the treatment modalities. In early-stage supraglottic cancer, a single-modality treatment is usually sufficient. The treatment plan should include the neck, except for T1N0M0 tumors. When surgically treating supraglottic cancer >T1, the specimen should include at least bilateral levels II and III of the neck. Occult metastasis in other levels, with clear levels II and III, is very rare [6]. It should also be noted that bilateral or contralateral metastasis is quite common.

4. **A, B**

   Glottic cancer is rarely diagnosed at an advanced stage. Vocal fold involvement leads to early hoarseness and prompt patient presentation. T1 and T2 tumors are rarely associated with neck metastasis due to the limited lymphatic network in the glottis. Therefore, neck treatment can be omitted from the treatment plan. Studies have shown that a single-modality treatment is sufficient for achieving oncological clearance. Patients should be given the option of either radiotherapy or cordectomy, as both have similar oncological outcomes but different side effects [7]. Radiotherapy provides better voice quality but may result in xerostomia, hypothyroidism, local irritation, and an increased risk of a second primary tumor in the treated area. Surgery avoids these limitations but often results in inferior voice quality. Patients should be able to make an unbiased decision based on their preferences. Lastly, it should be noted that radiotherapy cannot be used again in salvage cases.

5. **E**

   T4a tumors are characterized by moderately advanced local disease, with tumor growth involving the thyroid or cricoid cartilage and/or structures beyond the larynx (such as the thyroid gland, trachea, esophagus, tongue muscles, or strap muscles). Trials in the 1990s suggested that T4a tumors could be treated with conservative treatment (a combination of chemotherapy and radiotherapy) to preserve the larynx [8]. This led to significant changes in clinical practice, with a decrease in total laryngectomies. However, the reality showed a significant increase in both recurrences and deaths. Current data supports the use of total laryngectomy and adjuvant radiotherapy as a better treatment approach for locally advanced laryngeal cancer (T4a) [9]. On the other hand, in T3 cancer, surgical options (total laryngectomy or hemilaryngectomy in selected cases) and conservative treatment (concomitant chemoradiation) have similar oncological outcomes, and the patient can make a decision after receiving unbiased information [9].

References

1. Teknos TN, Hogikyan ND, Wolf GT. Conservation laryngeal surgery for malignant tumors of the larynx and pyriform sinus. Hematol Oncol Clin North Am. 2001;15:261–76.
2. Sinha S, Agarwal JP, Mahajan A, et al. Implications of limited exolaryngeal disease and cricoarytenoid joint involvement in organ conservation protocols for laryngopharyngeal cancers: results from a prospective study. Head Neck. 2021;43:1289–99.
3. Chen MM, Holsinger FC, Laccourreye O. Salvage conservation laryngeal surgery after radiation therapy failure. Otolaryngol Clin N Am. 2015;48:667–75.
4. Tsetsos N, Poutoglidis A, Vlachtsis K, Stavrakas M, Nikolaou A, Fyrmpas G. Twenty-year experience with salvage total laryngectomy: lessons learned. J Laryngol Otol. 2021;135:729–36.
5. Timon CI, Gullane PJ, Brown D, et al. Hyoid bone involvement by squamous cell carcinoma: clinical and pathological features. Laryngoscope. 1992;102:515.
6. Xu Y, Zhang Y, Xu Z, et al. Patterns of cervical lymph node metastasis in locally advanced supraglottic squamous cell carcinoma: implications for neck CTV delineation. Front Oncol. 2020;27(10):1596.
7. Demir B, Binnetoglu A, Gurol E, Oysu C. Comparison of voice quality of life in early stage glottic carcinoma treated with endoscopic cordectomy using radiofrequency microdissection electrodes, laser cordectomy, and radiotherapy. J Voice. 2021;35:477–82.
8. Department of Veterans Affairs Laryngeal Cancer Study Group, Wolf GT, Fisher SG, Hong WK, et al. Induction chemotherapy plus radiation compared with surgery plus radiation in patients with advanced laryngeal cancer. N Engl J Med. 1991;324:1685–90.
9. Sanabria A, Chaves ALF, Kowalski LP, et al. Organ preservation with chemoradiation in advanced laryngeal cancer: the problem of generalizing results from randomized controlled trials. Auris Nasus Larynx. 2017;44:18–25.

Oropharyngeal Cancer

59

Alexandros Poutoglidis and Paraskevi Karamitsou

Abstract

The oropharynx is a common location for malignant tumors, with squamous cell carcinomas accounting for over 90% of cases. The incidence of oropharyngeal cancer has significantly increased in the past decade, primarily due to the transmission of human papillomavirus (HPV). Non-HPV-related oropharyngeal cancer is associated with smoking and alcohol consumption, similar to most head and neck cancers. HPV-related oropharyngeal cancer predominantly affects younger individuals with no history of heavy smoking or alcohol use and often presents with early neck metastasis. Its pathogenesis is linked to the overexpression of the p16 protein. Currently, HPV-16 and HPV-18 are the only viruses clearly associated with the development of head and neck cancer, making p16 immunohistochemistry essential in every oropharyngeal tumor biopsy. Fortunately, HPV-related oropharyngeal cancer shows a better response to treatment and is associated with a more favorable prognosis. A unique staging system has been developed for managing these patients with early-stage cancer often treated with a single modality and advanced stages requiring multimodal approaches. Transoral laser microsurgery and robot surgery are innovative techniques that contribute to achieving favorable oncological and functional outcomes. Lastly, lymphomas, salivary gland neoplasms, and mesenchymal tumors are rare malignancies that can occur in the oropharynx.

A. Poutoglidis (✉)
ENT Department, Lister Hospital, East and North Hertfordshire NHS Trust, Stevenage, UK

P. Karamitsou
ENT Head and Neck Surgery Department, "G. Papanikolaou" General Hospital of Thessaloniki, Thessaloniki, Greece

Case Presentation

A 45-year-old woman came to an otolaryngology department with a primary complaint of a lump on the left side of her neck that had been present for 2 months. Her medical history was otherwise unremarkable. Upon physical examination, a small ulcerated mass was found at the top of her left tonsil. The mass was fragile and protruding. A small cystic mass was also detected in the left level II area during neck palpation. A flexible endoscopy showed no other abnormalities. A computed tomography (CT) scan revealed a small mass of less than 1 cm in the left tonsil and a round lymph node with central necrosis on the same side, with the largest dimension being 2 cm (Fig. 59.1). The patient had a biopsy of the tonsil mass under local anesthesia. The biopsy and immunochemistry confirmed the diagnosis of squamous cell carcinoma p16(+). The patient

N. Tsetsos et al. (eds.), *Otolaryngology Study Guide*, https://doi.org/10.1007/978-3-031-77374-7_59

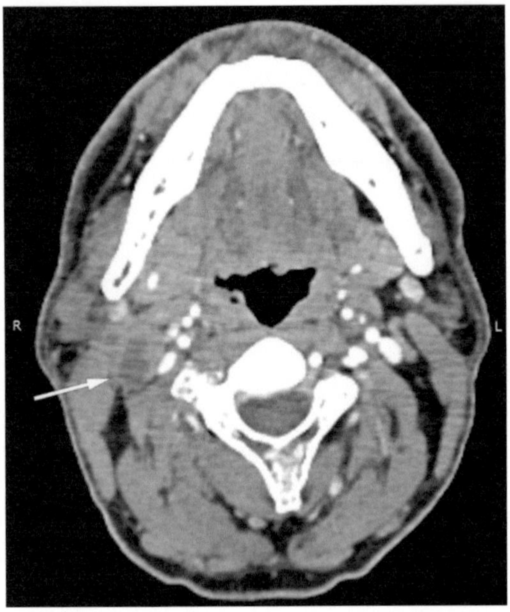

Fig. 59.1 A computed tomography demonstrates the presence of a metastatic lymph node in the right level II (arrow). Central necrosis of the lymph node is characteristic of metastatic disease

was classified as having stage I HPV oropharyngeal cancer with a cT1N1M0 stage and underwent radiotherapy for the oropharynx and neck. The treatment was highly successful, and 5 years later, she remains disease free.

Questions

1. p16 overexpression is responsible for:
   A. Tp53 suppressor gene inactivation
   B. Rb product of retinoblastoma suppressor gene inactivation
   C. E6 and E7 protein overexpression
   D. Oncogenesis in larynx
   E. Poorer prognosis
2. A cT3N2MO HPV oropharyngeal cancer is considered:
   A. Stage I
   B. Stage II
   C. Stage III
   D. Stage IVA
   E. Stage IVB
3. A 47-year-old patient is presented with a proven [after fine needle aspiration (FNA)] metastatic squamous cell carcinoma p16(+) of a lymph node in level II. However, he underwent a thorough investigation with physical examination–endoscopy–CT scans and PET/CT, but a primary tumor has not been identified. This tumor is considered:
   A. Still cancer of unknown primary
   B. T0 nasopharyngeal cancer
   C. T0 salivary gland cancer
   D. T0 oropharyngeal cancer
   E. Metastatic lung cancer
4. Transoral laser microsurgery (TLM) is a novel technique for the treatment of oropharyngeal cancer. Which of the following are relative or strong contradictions?
   A. Trismus
   B. Prior irradiation
   C. p16(+) tumors
   D. Significant inferior extension of the tumor
   E. Lymphomas
5. Factors associated with non-HPV-related squamous cell carcinoma of the oropharynx are:
   A. Non-keratinizing tumors
   B. Older age
   C. Multiple sex partners
   D. Smoking
   E. N0 neck in a tumor >T2

Answers

1. **A, B, C**

   Overexpression of p16 can cause cancer in the oropharyngeal mucosa. However, it has not been linked to other types of head and neck cancers [1]. There are no significant statistical differences in laryngeal cancer between HPV-positive and HPV-negative patients [2]. p16 produces the oncoproteins E6 and E7, with E6 inactivating the tumor suppressor gene tp53 and E7 inactivating Rb, a product of the retinoblastoma tumor suppressor gene. This mutation results in further overexpression of the p16 protein, leading to cancer. Fortunately, the treatment response is better than in traditional non-HPV-related oropharyngeal cancer, and concurrent chemoradiation is effective even in advanced stages [3]. Systematic HPV vaccination could potentially eradicate oropharyngeal cancer [4].

2. **B**

HPV oropharyngeal cancer uses a different staging system from non-HPV-related cancers [5]. Even large tumors with multiple lymph node metastases can be considered early stage and treated with less invasive methods. This benefit improves patient quality of life due to lower toxicity. It is important to note that the neck is almost always included in the treatment plan and should be treated as the primary focus. Therefore, a surgical approach in the oropharynx should usually be accompanied by a selective neck dissection. The specimen will then determine the pathological staging and the need for further adjuvant treatments. Some authors consider sparing level IIb due to its rare involvement [6].

3. **D**

Currently, head and neck cancer of unknown primary is a rare clinical condition. The decrease in its incidence is related to advancements in technology, particularly the use of PET/CT scans [7]. HPV oropharyngeal cancer tends to metastasize early and is often presented with neck metastases at level II. Often, the primary tumor cannot be identified after clinical examination, and even PET/CT may give a false-negative result for the primary tumor [8]. Therefore, clinical staging of p16(+) oropharyngeal cancer includes the category T0, which is characterized by a tumor with no identified primary but with histopathologically proven p16(+)-positive lymph nodes [5]. This biological behavior is explained by the aggressive lymphovascular nature of the p16(+) tumors [9]. In nasopharyngeal cancer, there is a similar category for lymph nodes positive in Epstein-Barr virus (EBV) [5].

4. **A, B, D, E**

Transoral laser microsurgery (TLM) is a new technique with significant advantages for the treatment of oropharyngeal cancer [10]. Avoiding a transmandibular access and a pharyngotomy greatly improves the patient's postoperative course. Like all new medical advancements, TLM was met with great enthusiasm. However, there are several limitations that restrict its use in certain cases. Adequate oral access is necessary for wide exposure. Patients with trismus or reduced transverse mandibular dimension are not suitable candidates for TLM. Additionally, significant lower tumor extension contradicts TLM even in patients with good mouth opening [11]. In these patients, a neck dissection incision can be used to approach the tumor via a pharyngotomy to avoid compromising the integrity of the mandible. Lastly, prior radiation therapy is a contraindication for TLM. Lymphomas, being hematological malignancies, are not treated with surgery.

5. **B, D, E**

Squamous cell carcinoma is the most common tumor of the oropharynx, accounting for 90% of cases [12]. HPV, a sexually transmitted disease that has become widespread in recent decades, is often established in the oropharyngeal mucosa due to multiple sexual partners and oral sex [4]. Patients with p16(−) oropharyngeal cancer are usually over 60 years old and have a long history of smoking and alcohol use. Their tumors are keratinizing neoplasms and do not metastasize early. Even a T3NOMO clinical presentation seems to be common. In contrast, HPV-related tumors tend to be non-keratinizing growths with very early metastasis and affect people aged 40–60 years [12].

References

1. Berdugo J, Rooper LM, Chiosea SI. RB1, p16, and human papillomavirus in oropharyngeal squamous cell carcinoma. Head Neck Pathol. 2021;15:1109–18.
2. Fusconi M, Campo F, Gallo A, et al. Laryngeal cancer, HPV DNA vs E6/E7 mRNA test: a systematic review. J Voice. 2017;31:248.e1–5.
3. Mehanna H, Robinson M, Hartley A, et al., De-ESCALaTE HPV Trial Group. Radiotherapy plus cisplatin or cetuximab in low-risk human papillomavirus-positive oropharyngeal cancer (De-ESCALaTE HPV): an open-label randomised controlled phase 3 trial. Lancet. 2019;393:51–60.

4. Tsentemeidou A, Fyrmpas G, Stavrakas M, et al. Human papillomavirus vaccine to end oropharyngeal cancer: a systematic review and meta-analysis. Sex Transm Dis. 2021;48:700–7.
5. Huang SH, O'Sullivan B. Overview of the 8th edition TNM classification for head and neck cancer. Curr Treat Options Oncol. 2017;18:40.
6. Gross BC, Olsen SM, Lewis JE, et al. Level IIB lymph node metastasis in oropharyngeal squamous cell carcinoma. Laryngoscope. 2013;123:2700–5.
7. Albertson M, Chandra S, Sayed Z, Johnson C. PET/CT evaluation of head and neck cancer of unknown primary. Semin Ultrasound CT MR. 2019;40:414–23.
8. Tsetsos N, Poutoglidis A, Arsos G, et al. ^{18}F-FDG-PET/CT interpretation pitfalls in patients with head and neck cancer. Am J Otolaryngol. 2022;43:103209.
9. Toman J, Von Larson S, Umeno H, Kurita T, Furusaka T, Hasegawa H, Prasad ML, Sasaki CT. HPV-positive oropharyngeal cancer via p16 immunohistochemistry in Japan. Ann Otol Rhinol Laryngol. 2017;126:152–8.
10. Golusiński W, Golusińska-Kardach E. Current role of surgery in the management of oropharyngeal cancer. Front Oncol. 2019;9:388.
11. Hinni ML, Zarka MA, Hoxworth JM. Margin mapping in transoral surgery for head and neck cancer. Laryngoscope. 2013;123:1190–8.
12. Tanaka TI, Alawi F. Human papillomavirus and oropharyngeal cancer. Dent Clin N Am. 2018;62:111–20.

60 Speaking Valves

Evropi Forozidou and Alexandros Poutoglidis

Abstract

Total laryngectomy often results in significant postoperative complications, including loss of voice. To enhance the patient's quality of life, it is crucial to address speech and voice rehabilitation as soon as possible. Three primary techniques have been developed for voice rehabilitation: (1) esophageal speech, (2) speaking valves, and (3) electrolarynx. Esophageal speech often results in a weak voice due to the limited capacity of the stomach and esophagus (60–80 mL), and the electrolarynx produces a mechanical sounding voice, which most patients find undesirable. Conversely, speaking valves are used to maintain an artificially created tracheoesophageal puncture (TEP). These valves prevent esophageal contents from entering the trachea, while allowing lung air to pass through the esophagus, producing a sufficiently loud voice. The large capacity of the lungs results in a much louder voice than that produced by esophageal speech. Valve implantation can be done either during total laryngectomy or several months later. The need for postoperative irradiation is not a contradiction for primary implantation. However, speaking valves are not without complications, and patients must take care of them to prevent TEP failure or local infections. Gastroesophageal reflux is the most common factor predisposing to local complications. Unfortunately, in some cases, the TEP must be closed due to persistent failure.

Case Presentation

A 70-year-old man presented to an otolaryngology clinic for a follow-up appointment 3 months after undergoing a total laryngectomy. The patient was disease free and had not experienced any postoperative complications. His permanent stoma was free of secretions and had a large diameter, and the tracheostomy tube had been removed 2 months after the surgery. The total laryngectomy was performed after radiotherapy failure 3 years ago.

Initially, the patient declined the implantation of a primary speaking valve, choosing instead to develop esophageal speech. Despite his motivation, he was not satisfied with the voice outcome and decided to get a speaking valve. Two weeks later, he underwent a tracheoesophageal puncture (TEP) and voice prosthesis implantation under

E. Forozidou
ENT Head and Neck Surgery Department, "G.Papanikolaou" General Hospital, Thessaloniki, Greece

A. Poutoglidis (✉)
ENT Department, Lister Hospital, East and North Hertfordshire NHS Trust, Stevenage, UK

N. Tsetsos et al. (eds.), *Otolaryngology Study Guide*, https://doi.org/10.1007/978-3-031-77374-7_60

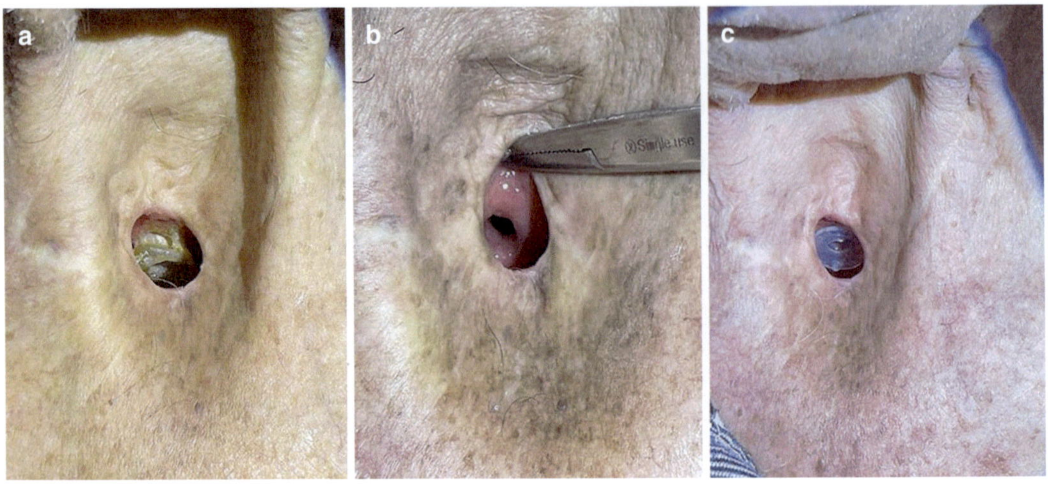

Fig. 60.1 Illustration of a speaking valve replacement. (**a**) Old speaking valve (12 months), (**b**) tracheoesophageal puncture after the removal of the old speaking valve, (**c**) new speaking valve moments after implantation

general anesthesia. The patient developed an excellent voice and was able to deliver a public speech after a year (Fig. 60.1). He was advised that taking care of the valve is crucial, as fungal colonization could cause irreversible failure.

Questions

1. Adjustments and precautions in total laryngectomy technique to achieve a better field for a primary voice prosthesis insertion include:
   A. Delay in the postoperative radiation treatment
   B. Myotomy of upper esophageal sphincter
   C. Section of the sternocleidomastoid muscle attachments in sternum
   D. Pharyngeal closure in an as possible horizontal fashion
   E. Delay of oral feeding
2. Secondary voice prosthesis insertion success is achieved through:
   A. Antibiotic prophylaxis
   B. Preoperative hypertonicity of esophagus solution
   C. Delay in oral feeding postoperatively
   D. Nasogastric tube placement for 10 days
   E. An about 8 mm length of TEP
3. Speaking valve replacement indications are:
   A. A span of 6 months
   B. A good speaking valve should never be replaced
   C. Tracheoesophageal leak
   D. Shortening of the TEP tract
   E. Tumor recurrence
4. Predisposing factors for voice prosthesis failure are:
   A. Gastroesophageal reflux
   B. Distant metastasis
   C. Radiation therapy
   D. Gender
   E. Alcohol consumption
5. What measures should be followed when speaking valve replacement does not suffice for periprosthetic leakage solution?
   A. Closure of the TEP
   B. Shrinkage
   C. Augmentation
   D. Shrinkage with suture
   E. Washer silicon

Answers

1. **B, C, D**

   Primary implantation of a voice prosthesis is favored by the most tertiary institutes. Even cases that will need a postoperative radiation or cases where a laryngectomy is performed after failure of conservative treatment (salvage laryngectomy) are indicated for primary voice prosthesis insertion. Delay on postoperative radiation may cause a devastating oncologic outcome with a local peristomatic recurrence. Valve mechanism prevents aspiration, and oral feeding is not associated with the success of the prosthesis [1]. Myotomy of the upper esophageal sphincter will reduce the hypertonicity of esophagus and improve the overall outcome. Sternocleidomastoid sternal attachment section will prevent a very deep stoma, and thus, TEP will be more functional. Finally, horizontal closure of the neopharynx reduces the tension, prevents a pharyngocutaneous fistula formation, and increases the overall speech outcome [2].

2. **A, B, E**

   Nowadays, secondary voice prosthesis insertion is indicated for patients who are unsatisfied with esophageal speech. Patients mostly desire a louder voice to communicate via telephone. It should be noted that the failure to develop esophageal speech may be the hypertonicity of esophagus that it has not been addressed properly during total laryngectomy. In these cases, it is wise to first perform a chemodenervation of the pharyngoesophageal segment with botulin toxin and then proceed to the implantation [3]. Postoperatively, oral feeding may start immediately, and nasogastric tube is not needed. Valve prevents aspiration, and so patients are encouraged to start their diet. TEP should be placed high in the trachea and not 12 mm below the mucocartilaginous barrier with an optimal length of 8 mm.

3. **A, C, D**

   Speaking valves typically have a lifespan of 4–6 months [4]. Their replacement is a straightforward in-office anterograde process that can be performed without complications. The primary reason for an early replacement is a transprosthetic or periprosthetic leakage [5]. Aspiration of leakage can lead to complications such as pneumonia, making replacement essential. Biofilm growth (bacteria and fungi) is often found on a speaking valve and can cause failure [6]. Clinical evidence has not demonstrated the effectiveness of antifungal agents or antibiotics, so replacement is recommended in all cases of leakage. Before replacement, the length of the TEP should be checked by gently moving the valve in an anteroposterior direction. A highly mobile valve indicates that the length of the TEP has changed, necessitating a reduction in valve number. It is worth noting that the length and thickness of the TEP change naturally, not just due to pathologies. Postoperative reduction of surgical edema and tissue inflammation can decrease the TEP track, potentially rendering the valve unsuitable.

4. **A, C, E**

   Radiation therapy does not contraindicate speaking valve implantation. However, patients who have undergone radiation therapy before or after speaking valve insertion have higher rates of TEP failure [7]. Gastroesophageal reflux is a common issue in patients with laryngeal cancer. Their history of smoking and alcohol consumption is strongly associated with reflux, which can damage the integrity of the neopharynx mucosa. These changes may lead to the development of pathogens and biofilms that interfere with the normal function of a speaking valve or cause enlargement of the TEP [8]. Proton pump inhibitor treatment can help reduce the morbidity of reflux and its local complications on the TEP. Any change in the voice of a speaking valve patient indicates valve dysfunction. Early intervention and valve replacement are associated with better TEP sustainability.

5. **A, B, C, D, E**

   Periprosthetic leakage of a speaking valve does not always necessitate valve replacement. Before surgical closure—and possibly a new attempt at implantation—certain steps should be taken to preserve the TEP. Shrinkage, a natural process that is rarely used these days, involves removing the speaking valve for a few days to allow the TEP to shrink. A nasogastric tube is essential to prevent aspiration. A silicone washer can be used to prevent leakage. It should be placed behind the tracheal flange, just anterior to the problematic mucosa [9]. Another option is a submucosal suture to shrink the TEP. After the suture is placed, a new valve can be inserted. Lastly, augmentation with autologous fat or other bioplastic products like hydroxyapatite may help the TEP avoid permanent failure [10].

References

1. Timmermans AJ, Lansaat L, Kroon GV, et al. Early oral intake after total laryngectomy does not increase pharyngocutaneous fistulization. Eur Arch Otorhinolaryngol. 2014;271:353–8.
2. Deschler DG, Bunting GW, Lin DT, et al. Evaluation of voice prosthesis placement at the time of primary tracheoesophageal puncture with total laryngectomy. Laryngoscope. 2009;119:1353–7.
3. Bartolomei L, Zambito Marsala S, et al. Botulinum toxin type A: an effective treatment to restore phonation in laryngectomized patients unable to voice. Neurol Sci. 2011;32:443–7.
4. O'Connor LR, Morris NR, Paratz J. Physiological and clinical outcomes associated with use of one-way speaking valves on tracheostomised patients: a systematic review. Heart Lung. 2019;48:356–64.
5. Li J, Perez A, Schehl J, Albers A, Husain IA. The association between upper airway patency and speaking valve trial tolerance for patients with tracheostomy: a clinical retrospective study and an in vitro study. Am J Speech Lang Pathol. 2021;14(30):1728–36.
6. Nowak M, Kurnatowski P. Tworzenie biofilmu candida na protezach głosowych Provox 2 oraz Provox Acti Valve [Candida biofilm formation on Provox 2 and Provox Acti Valve voice prosthesis]. Otolaryngol Pol. 2010;64:358–64.
7. Massaro N, Verro B, Greco G, Chianetta E, D'Ecclesia A, Saraniti C. Quality of life with voice prosthesis after total laryngectomy. Iran J Otorhinolaryngol. 2021;33:301–9.
8. Jira D, Pickhard A, Mair L, Zhu Z, Wollenberg B, Buchberger AMS. GERD und adjuvante Radiochemotherapie prädisponieren für rezidivierende Stimmprotheseninsuffizienz [GERD and adjuvant radio-chemotherapy predespose to recurrent voice prosthesis leakage]. Laryngorhinootologie. 2020;99:788–94. German.
9. Hilgers FJ, Soolsma J, Ackerstaff AH, Balm FJ, Tan IB, van den Brekel MW. A thin tracheal silicone washer to solve periprosthetic leakage in laryngectomies: direct results and long-term clinical effects. Laryngoscope. 2008;118(4):640–5.
10. Kasbekar AV, Sherman IW. Closure of minor tracheoesophageal fistulae with calcium hydroxylapatite. Auris Nasus Larynx. 2013;40:491–2.

61 Tracheotomy

Evropi Forozidou and Alexandros Poutoglidis

Abstract

Open surgical tracheotomy is a procedure used to create an opening in the front wall of the trachea. Over the years, percutaneous tracheotomy techniques have been developed, allowing for the placement of the tube at the bedside. Surgical tracheotomy may be necessary in emergency situations or performed electively to assist with mechanical ventilation. The typical procedure begins with positioning the patient in a way that optimizes neck extension. During this time, the surgeon should feel for the neck landmarks to locate the midline and laryngeal cartilages. Usually, a transverse incision is made between the sternal notch and the cricoid cartilage (approximately two fingers above the sternal notch). The next step involves dissecting the subcutaneous tissues and fasciae and moving the strap muscles to the sides. This action exposes the thyroid isthmus, which is then divided and tied off. The trachea is now exposed with only visible, with only the thin pretracheal fascia remaining intact. A window is created in the trachea, at least 0.5 cm below the cricoid cartilage. The final step is removing the endotracheal tube, performing suction if necessary, and inserting the desired tracheostomy tube. The tube is connected to the ventilator, and proper ventilation and end-tidal CO_2 levels are used to confirm correct placement.

E. Forozidou
ENT Head and Neck Surgery Department, "G. Papanikolaou" General Hospital, Thessaloniki, Greece

A. Poutoglidis (✉)
ENT Department, Lister Hospital, East and North Hertfordshire NHS Trust, Stevenage, UK

Case Presentation

A 54-year-old man came to the emergency otolaryngology department with a 2-day history of increasing difficulty swallowing and wheezing. The patient was experiencing stridor even at rest, and a physical examination revealed a rapid heart rate (120 beats/min) and a fever of 38.5 °C. His respiratory rate was 35 breaths/min, and his oxygen saturation was at 54% while on 10 L of oxygen. Upon palpation, a painful swelling was detected on the left side of his neck. The stridor slightly improved after administering adrenaline nebulizers. A flexible fiber-optic endoscopy showed submucosal edema and redness of the larynx along with secretions (Fig. 61.1). Anesthesiologists were unable to intubate the patient, leading to an urgent transfer to the operating suite for an emergency tracheostomy. After stabilizing the patient's airway and breathing, a

N. Tsetsos et al. (eds.), *Otolaryngology Study Guide*, https://doi.org/10.1007/978-3-031-77374-7_61

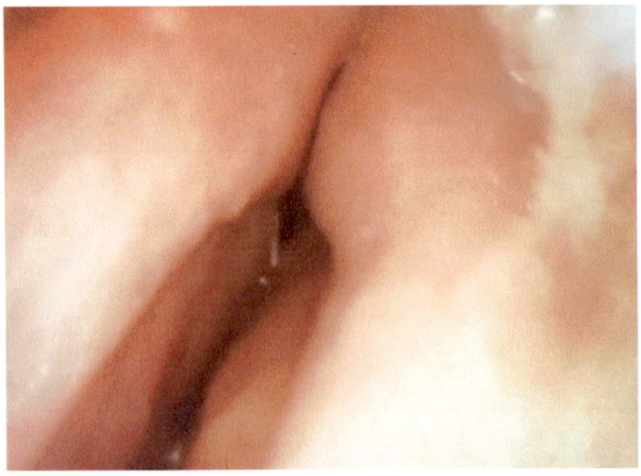

Fig. 61.1 Flexible endoscopy demonstrates the insufficient airway in the level of larynx and the necessity for an immediate intervention

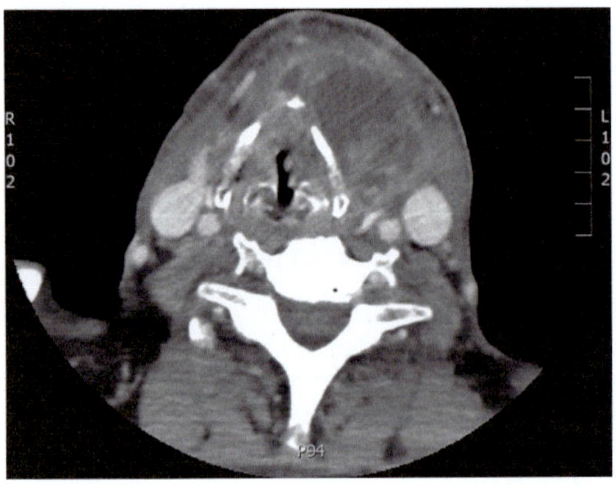

Fig. 61.2 Computed tomography well depicts the formation of an abscess on the left side of the neck. This axial scan is exactly in the level of glottis

neck CT scan revealed a large neck abscess, which was subsequently drained (Fig. 61.2).

Questions

1. Which of the following are indications for an emergency tracheotomy?
   A. Prolonged endotracheal intubation
   B. Upper airway obstruction and failure of endotracheal intubation
   C. Management of major head and neck trauma
   D. Obstructive sleep apnea
   E. Post-cricothyrotomy
2. Which of the following anatomic structures may be used as anatomic landmarks for a safe tracheotomy?
   A. Thyroid notch
   B. Cricoid cartilage
   C. Cricothyroid membrane
   D. Hyoid bone
   E. Sternal notch
3. Which of the following statements are true about tracheotomy?
   A. The thyroid notch is a palpable landmark to identify the superior aspect of the larynx for tracheotomy in infants
   B. Tracheal incision should be performed between the second and third tracheal rings
   C. There are no absolute contradictions to perform tracheotomy
   D. Tracheotomy should generally be performed 30 days after endotracheal intubation
   E. Tracheotomy cuff may be deflated after mechanical ventilation is not needed, and swallowing is normal
4. Which of the following belong to the early complications of tracheotomy?
   A. Tube dislodgement
   B. Tracheoesophageal fistula
   C. Subcutaneous emphysema
   D. Tracheal stenosis
   E. Hemorrhage
5. Which of the following statements are correct regarding pediatric tracheostomy?
   A. The creation of a window with removal of a part of the anterior tracheal wall is mandatory
   B. Cricoid cartilage is lower compared to adults
   C. A chest radiograph is suggested after tube placement
   D. Treacher Collins syndrome, Nager syndrome, and other syndromes that affect the formation of the skeleton often require a tracheotomy to secure the airway
   E. A vertical incision should be preferred in all cases

Answers

1. **B, C, E**

   Emergency tracheostomy is required in cases of acute upper airway obstruction where endotracheal intubation cannot be performed (due to foreign body, angioedema, infections like Ludwig's angina, anaphylaxis, etc.), following a cricothyrotomy (if a cricothyrotomy has been performed, it should be promptly converted into a tracheotomy once the airway is secured), and in the event of penetrating laryngeal trauma or other major head and neck traumas that destabilize the patient [1, 2]. Conversely, elective tracheostomy is indicated for extended intubation, prophylactic tracheostomy before head and neck cancer treatment, obstructive sleep apnea that is resistant to other treatments, chronic aspiration (pulmonary toilet), neuromuscular disease, and subglottic stenosis [3, 4].

2. **A, B, C, E**

   The trachea structure consists of 15–20 incomplete cartilaginous rings. The cricoid cartilage, which is the only complete ring, connects the trachea to the larynx. The trachea's posterior wall is fused with the esophagus's anterior wall. The trachea is located deep to the sternohyoid and sternothyroid muscles, with the thyroid gland isthmus typically overlaying from the second to the fourth tracheal rings. The recurrent laryngeal nerves lie immediately lateral to the cervical trachea. Therefore, thyroid gland dissection should be done carefully to avoid damaging the nerves. Anatomic landmarks include the thyroid notch, cricothyroid membrane (palpable depression between cricoid and thyroid cartilages), cricoid cartilage, and sternal notch. The skin incision is usually made 1–2 cm below the cricoid cartilage [1, 2, 5].

3. **B, C, E**

   Infants have a shortened thyrohyoid membrane, so the hyoid bone is located anterior to the thyroid notch, obscuring the thyroid notch as a landmark for tracheotomy.

   Ideally, tracheotomy should be performed 10–14 days after intubation, but the optimal timing should be individualized based on the risk of continued intubation (i.e., subglottic stenosis) versus the likelihood of extubation [6–11]. A tracheostomy tube can be safely removed when it has been successfully capped for 24–72 h, adequate pulmonary hygiene has been established, there is no need for ventilation, satisfactory absorption capacity is adequate, and there is no evidence of tracheal granulation tissue [12].

4. **A, C, E**

   Tracheostomy complications can be categorized into intraoperative, early postoperative, and late postoperative. The most common intraoperative complication is bleeding, and the platelet count should be at least 50,000 before proceeding with any airway surgery, except in extremely urgent situations [13]. Approximately 5% of patients will have a thyroid innominate artery, which runs along the anterior surface of the trachea, necessitating careful technique in the ligation of the thyroid isthmus [14]. Severe operative complications include pneumothorax, pneumomediastinum, and subcutaneous emphysema, which can occur after inadvertently creating a false passage by placing the tracheotomy tube anterior to the trachea wall or by violating the thorax [15]. Early complications rarely include infections, which can be treated with local wound care, while deeper infections or abscesses may require antibiotics. Acute obstruction of the tracheostomy tube may be caused by blood, mucus, or tube dislodgement. The most feared late complication is tracheal stenosis, which is caused by the pressure due to overinflation of the cuff. High pressure in the trachea might lead to necrosis of the wall due to ischemia. Tracheostomy cuff pressure should ideally be measured at a maximum of 20 cm H_2O. In addition, the high placement of the incision in the immediate subcricoid position is associated with fracture of the cricoid cartilage and subsequent subglottic stenosis. Persistent tracheocutaneous and tracheoesophageal fistulae are other late complications that should always be considered [16].

5. **C, D**

Pediatric tracheostomy is a frequently performed procedure that often leads to significant morbidity. The structure of the larynx and trachea in children differs from adults, necessitating modifications when performing tracheotomies in pediatric cases. The larynx in children is positioned higher, and the framework is softer. As a result, the landmarks for a safe approach are typically higher. Moreover, the soft tracheal framework makes the respiratory tract susceptible to collapse during negative-pressure ventilation [17]. Literature suggests that 3–9% of pediatric patients experience air leak post-tracheostomy tube placement, resulting in conditions like pneumothorax, subcutaneous emphysema, and pneumomediastinum. Consequently, a chest radiograph can be beneficial in ruling out these major complications [18]. Lastly, to prevent unsatisfactory aesthetic outcomes, tracheostomy should be performed using a horizontal incision in a natural skin crease.

References

1. Cheung NH, Napolitano LM. Tracheostomy: epidemiology, indications, timing, technique, and outcomes. Respir Care. 2014;59:895–915.
2. DeLeyn P, Bedert L, Delcroix M, et al. Tracheotomy: clinical review and guidelines. Eur J Cardiothorac Surg. 2007;32:412–21.
3. Rana S, Pendem S, Pogodzinski MS, Hubmayr RD, Gajic O. Tracheostomy in critically ill patients. Mayo Clin Proc. 2005;80:1632–8.
4. Fang CH, Friedman R, White PE, Mady LJ, Kalyoussef E. Emergency awake tracheostomy—the five-year experience at an urban tertiary care center. Laryngoscope. 2015;125:2476–9.
5. Tarazis K, Garefis K, Nikolaidis V, et al. Tracheostomy in the COVID-19 era: a modified approach. Ear Nose Throat J. 2021; https://doi.org/10.1177/01455613211045522.
6. Watters KF. Tracheostomy in infants and children. Respir Care. 2017;62:799–825.
7. Kluge S, Baumann HJ, Maier C, et al. Tracheostomy in the intensive care unit: a nationwide survey. Anesth Analg. 2008;107:1639–43.
8. Huang H, Li Y, Ariani F, Chen X, et al. Timing of tracheotomy in critically ill patients: a meta-analysis. PLoS One. 2014;9:92981.
9. Holevar M, Dunham JC, Brautigan R, et al. Practice management guidelines for timing of tracheostomy: the EAST Practice Management Guidelines Work Group. J Trauma. 2009;67:870–4.
10. Adly A, Youssef TA, El-Begermy MM, Younis HM. Timing of tracheostomy in patients with prolonged endotracheal intubation: a systematic review. Eur Arch Otorhinolaryngol. 2018;275:679–90.
11. Quinnell TG, Pilsworth S, Shneerson JM, et al. Prolonged invasive ventilation following acute ventilatory failure in COPD: weaning results, survival, and the role of noninvasive ventilation. Chest. 2006;129:133–9.
12. Christopher KL. Tracheostomy decannulation. Respir Care. 2005;50:538–41.
13. Kluge S, Meyer A, Kühnelt P, Baumann HJ, Kreymann G. Percutaneous tracheostomy is safe in patients with severe thrombocytopenia. Chest. 2004;126:547–51.
14. Toni R, Della Casa C, Mosca S, Malaguti A, Castorina S, Roti E. Anthropological variations in the anatomy of the human thyroid arteries. Thyroid. 2003;13:183–92.
15. Fernandez-Bussy S, Mahajan B, Folch E, Caviedes I, Guerrero J, Majid A. Tracheostomy tube placement: early and late complications. J Bronchol Interv Pulmonol. 2015;22:357–64.
16. Epstein SK. Late complications of tracheostomy. Respir Care. 2005;50:542–9.
17. König AM. Tracheotomie bei Kindern [Pediatric tracheotomy]. HNO. 2012;60(7):581–9. German.
18. Abode KA, Drake AF, Zdanski CJ, Retsch-Bogart GZ, Gee AB, Noah TL. A multidisciplinary children's airway center: impact on the care of patients with tracheostomy. Pediatrics. 2016;137(2):e20150455.

Sialolithiasis

62

Konstantinos Geronatsios

Abstract

Sialolithiasis is a disease that primarily affects the submandibular salivary glands (approximately 85%). The main symptoms of sialolithiasis are pain and swelling after meals. In cases of prolonged obstruction, infection (sialadenitis) and sometimes abscess formation can occur. It may be related to reduced fluid intake, dehydration, and medication that reduces saliva production. Radiotherapy also causes xerostomia and, as a result, may increase the risk of sialolithiasis. Sjogren's syndrome, an autoimmune multisystemic disorder with main symptoms of dry eyes and xerostomia, can be related to sialolithiasis of the salivary glands. There are also many categories of medication that cause xerostomia. A neck CT scan is an excellent choice for diagnosing sialolithiasis and visualizing sialoliths inside the gland and the duct. MRI is also of high diagnostic value for salivary gland diseases. Sialography is useful because it can also be therapeutic but is not indicated in cases of sialolithiasis. Many clinicians and radiologists believe that ultrasound is the indicated diagnostic investigation for sialolithiasis and sialadenitis. Sialendoscopy is an evolving diagnostic and therapeutic technique for the management of salivary gland disorders.

K. Geronatsios (✉)
ENT Head and Neck Surgery Department,
424 General Military Hospital, Thessaloniki, Greece

Case Presentation

A 32-year-old male presented with a 10-day history of left submandibular swelling that worsened after meals. He has experienced multiple recurrent episodes of swelling over the past 2 years. He is nonfebrile, and there is no trismus. There is also swelling on the floor of the mouth in the area of the left submandibular duct gland. His past medical history is unremarkable, and the rest of the clinical examination is normal. There is no cervical lymphadenopathy, and he has not undergone any recent dental work. A neck CT scan is requested, and the findings are shown in Fig. 62.1. The patient underwent left submandibular gland excision under general anesthesia, revealing a large sialolith obstructing the proximal part of Wharton's duct (Fig. 62.2).

Questions

1. Which salivary glands are most commonly affected by sialolithiasis?
   A. Parotid glands
   B. Sublingual glands
   C. Submandibular glands
   D. Minor salivary glands
   E. All major salivary glands are equally affected

N. Tsetsos et al. (eds.), *Otolaryngology Study Guide*, https://doi.org/10.1007/978-3-031-77374-7_62

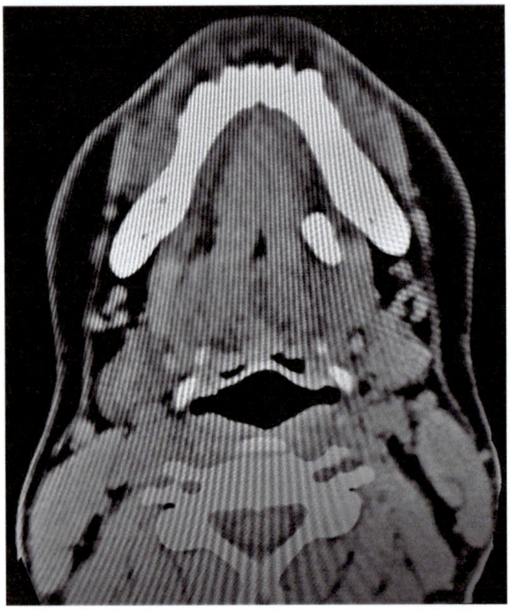

Fig. 62.1 CT neck with contrast. Large sialolith obstructing the proximal part of the Wharton's duct on the left side

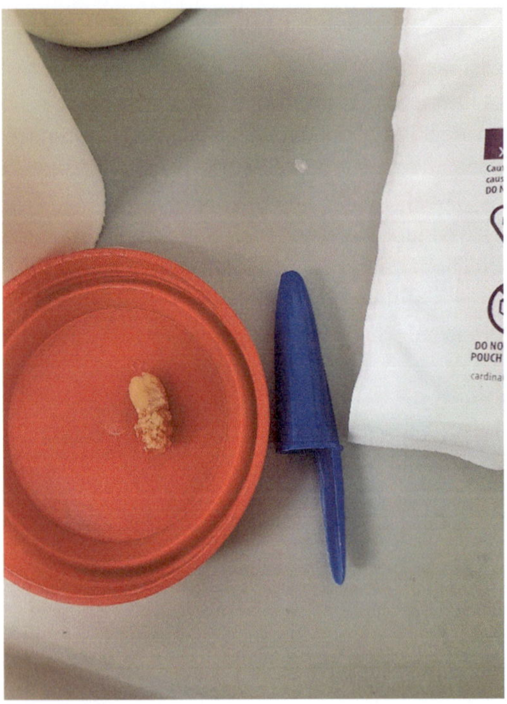

Fig. 62.2 Large Wharton's duct sialolith, measuring 2.11 cm × 0.75 cm. Photo was taken after left submandibular gland excision under general anesthesia

2. Which of the following are causes of sialolithiasis (more than one correct answer possible)?
   A. Dehydration
   B. Clozapine
   C. Sjogren's syndrome
   D. Radiation therapy of the mouth
   E. Parkinson's disease
3. Which of the following imaging test would you prefer for the assessment of a possible sialolithiasis with sialadenitis?
   A. Sialography
   B. Neck CT scan
   C. Plain radiograph
   D. Neck ultrasound
   E. Technetium 99m scan
4. Which of the following are possible complications of submandibular gland excision (more than one correct answer possible)?
   A. Lingual nerve injury
   B. Spinal accessory nerve injury
   C. Hypoglossal nerve palsy
   D. Superior laryngeal nerve palsy
   E. Marginal branch of the facial nerve palsy
5. Which of the following cases of sialolithiasis could be treated with sialendoscopy?
   A. The previous case
   B. Wharton's duct (submandibular gland) stones <5 mm in diameter
   C. All Stensen's duct (parotid gland) stones
   D. All Wharton's duct stones
   E. Intraparenchymal stones >1 cm

Answers

1. **C**

Sialolithiasis is a disease that mostly affects the submandibular salivary glands (approximately 85%) [1–3]. This is due to the alkaline pH and mucus nature of saliva produced by the submandibular glands [1, 2]. Additionally, the flow of saliva through Wharton's duct is against gravity. The saliva produced by the parotid glands is more serous, and less than 15% of sialolithiasis cases affect the parotid glands. Lithiasis of the sublingual and minor salivary glands is quite uncommon

[3]. The main symptoms of sialolithiasis are pain and swelling after meals. Prolonged obstruction can lead to infection (sialadenitis) and sometimes abscess formation.

2. **A, C, D**

   Sialolithiasis may be related to reduced fluid intake, dehydration, and medication that reduces saliva production [3]. Radiotherapy also causes xerostomia, increasing the risk of lithiasis [4, 5]. Sjogren's syndrome, an autoimmune multisystemic disorder with main symptoms of dry eyes and xerostomia, can be related to sialolithiasis of the salivary glands [5, 6]. Clozapine is a medication that causes sialorrhea, which is also a common symptom of Parkinson's disease [7]. There are many categories of medication that cause xerostomia, including antihistamines (H1 receptor blockers), chemotherapy agents, and certain categories of antidepressants, antipsychotics, and analgesics.

3. **B**

   A neck CT scan is a great choice for diagnosing sialolithiasis and visualizing sialoliths inside the gland and the duct. Some disadvantages include the need for thin cuts (1 mm or less) to visualize small stones, the high radiation exposure, and sometimes the lack of exact localization of the sialolith [2, 8]. MRI is also highly diagnostic for salivary gland diseases. Sialography can be performed for both diagnosis and treatment, but is not indicated for cases of sialolithiasis [9]. Many clinicians and radiologists believe that ultrasound is the diagnostic method of choice for sialolithiasis and sialadenitis. However, it is operator dependent, the surgeon cannot have preoperative images, and it can be uncomfortable for the patient in cases of sialadenitis [8, 10]. High-frequency intraoral probes are considered more precise for the diagnosis of sialolithiasis [11]. Plain radiographs lack diagnostic accuracy as some stones are not radiopaque and small stones are not easily visualized [9]. Technetium 99m scan has no indication for these cases.

4. **A, C, E**

   Possible complications of submandibular gland excision are hematoma, wound infection, injury of the mandibular branch of the facial nerve, and lingual or hypoglossal nerve injury [5, 12, 13]. Spinal accessory nerve injury or superior laryngeal nerve palsy could not be related to this operation.

5. **B**

   Sialendoscopy is an evolving diagnostic and therapeutic technique, for the management of salivary gland disorders. Unfortunately, it is impossible to remove all salivary duct and parenchymal stones with this method [14, 15]. It can be done under local or general anesthesia, as a day case, and it is considered as a minimal invasive process. The size and the location of the stones are prognostic factors of the success. Small stones, especially <5 mm in diameter, can be removed easily with sialendoscopy. Larger and parenchymal stones may be difficult to be removed. Combined approaches are also becoming popular. Some clinicians combine lithotripsy before endoscopic removal of a salivary stone.

References

1. Adhikari R, Soni A. Submandibular sialadenitis and sialadenosis [updated 2022 Aug 8]. In: StatPearls. Treasure Island, FL: StatPearls Publishing; 2022.
2. Hammett JT, Walker C. Sialolithiasis [updated 2022 Sep 26]. In: StatPearls. Treasure Island, FL: StatPearls Publishing; 2022.
3. Arifa SP, Christopher PJ, Kumar S, Kengasubbiah S, Shenoy V. Sialolithiasis of the submandibular gland: report of cases. Cureus. 2019;11(3):e4180.
4. Cheng SC, Wu VW, Kwong DL, Ying MT. Assessment of post-radiotherapy salivary glands. Br J Radiol. 2011;84(1001):393–402.
5. Seifert JG. Diseases of salivary glands. Berlin: Springer; 2000.
6. Konstantinidis I, Paschaloudi S, Triaridis S, Fyrmpas G, Sechlidis S, Constantinidis J. Bilateral multiple sialolithiasis of the parotid gland in a patient with Sjögren's syndrome. Acta Otorhinolaryngol Ital. 2007;27:41.

7. Isaacson J, Patel S, Torres-Yaghi Y, Pagán F. Sialorrhea in Parkinson's disease. Toxins (Basel). 2020;12(11):691.
8. Marchal F, Dulguerov P. Sialolithiasis management: the state of the art. Arch Otolaryngol Head Neck Surg. 2003;129(9):951–6.
9. Rzymska-Grala I, Stopa Z, Grala B, Gołębiowski M, Wanyura H, Zuchowska A, Sawicka M, Zmorzyński M. Salivary gland calculi—contemporary methods of imaging. Pol J Radiol. 2010;75:25.
10. Terraz S, Poletti PA, Dulguerov P, Dfouni N, Becker CD, Marchal F, Becker M. How reliable is sonography in the assessment of sialolithiasis? AJR Am J Roentgenol. 2013;201(1):W104–9.
11. Sengupta A, Brown J, Rudralingam M. The use of intraoral ultrasound in the characterization of minor salivary gland malignancy: report of two cases. Dentomaxillofac Radiol. 2016;45(4):20150354.
12. Cumpston E, Chen P. Submandibular excision [updated 2022 Jun 11]. In: StatPearls. Treasure Island, FL: StatPearls Publishing; 2022.
13. Nahlieli O. Complications of traditional and modern therapeutic salivary approaches. Acta Otorhinolaryngol Ital. 2017;37(2):142–7.
14. Zenk J, Koch M, Klintworth N, König B, Konz K, Gillespie MB, Iro H. Sialendoscopy in the diagnosis and treatment of sialolithiasis: a study on more than 1000 patients. Otolaryngol Head Neck Surg. 2012;147(5):858–63.
15. Singh PP, Gupta V. Sialendoscopy: introduction, indications and technique. Indian J Otolaryngol Head Neck Surg. 2014;66(1):74–8.

Parotid Gland Tumor

63

Konstantinos Garefis

Abstract

Tumors of the salivary glands are uncommon, accounting for approximately 3% of head and neck tumors. Around 70–80% of salivary gland tumors occur in the parotid gland, most often in the superficial lobe, and 80% of parotid gland tumors are benign. Common benign parotid gland tumors include pleomorphic adenoma, Warthin's tumor, basal cell adenoma, and oncocytoma, with pleomorphic adenoma being the most frequent and Warthin's tumor the second most common. The most frequent malignant parotid gland tumor is mucoepidermoid carcinoma, followed by adenoid cystic carcinoma, acinic cell carcinoma, carcinoma ex. pleomorphic adenoma etc. A history, clinical exam, imaging tests, and fine needle aspiration cytology or core needle biopsy are nearly essential to diagnose a parotid gland tumor. Pain in the parotid mass, facial nerve weakness, rapid enlargement of the tumor, and numbness of the ear or facial skin—alone or with neck lymphadenopathy—likely indicate malignancy. Surgery is the only treatment for parotid gland tumors. However, the type of surgery (extracapsular dissection, partial superficial parotidectomy, superficial parotidectomy, total parotidectomy with or without neck dissection) depends on the tumor's type and anatomical location.

K. Garefis (✉)
2nd Academic ORL, Head and Neck Surgery Department, Aristotle University of Thessaloniki, Papageorgiou Hospital, Thessaloniki, Greece

Case Presentation

A 62-year-old male smoker was reffered to your Ear, Nose, and Throat (ENT) Department with a 3-year history of a slowly enlarging mass on the left side of his parotid gland region. The mass was painless and movable. Examination of his neck was normal. However, palpation of the opposite parotid gland revealed a small lump. Magnetic resonance imaging (MRI) confirmed the clinical examination findings showing one tumor in the superficial lobe of each parotid gland. A left-side superficial parotidectomy was performed initially, according to fine needle aspiration cytology findings (Figs. 63.1, 63.2, and 63.3).

Questions

1. Which of the following statements are true about Warthin's tumor (more than one correct answer possible)?
   A. It is the second most frequent tumor of the submandibular gland
   B. It can present in both parotid glands
   C. Malignant transformation can occur

N. Tsetsos et al. (eds.), *Otolaryngology Study Guide*, https://doi.org/10.1007/978-3-031-77374-7_63

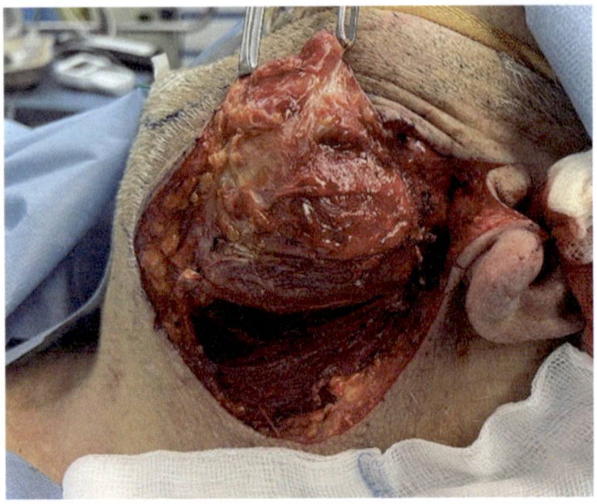

Fig. 63.1 Left superficial parotidectomy. The tumor in the superficial lobe is visible

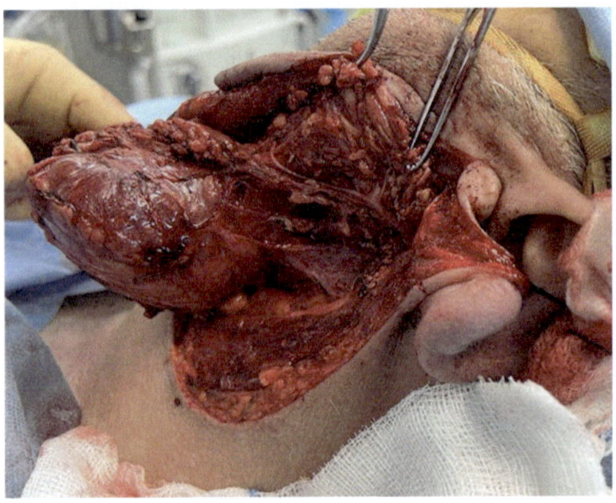

Fig. 63.2 Left superficial parotidectomy. The tumor and the facial nerve are visible

   D. It often occurs in the deep lobe of parotid gland
   E. It can be multiple and ipsilateral
2. Which of the following is the most common tumor of parotid gland?
   A. Pleomorphic adenoma
   B. Warthin's tumor
   C. Mucoepidermoid carcinoma
   D. Adenoid cystic carcinoma
   E. Lipoma
3. In the presence of a parotid mass, which of the following is the most appropriate diagnostic tool to determine its treatment?
   A. Physical examination
   B. Magnetic resonance imaging
   C. Fine needle aspiration cytology
   D. Open biopsy
   E. Ultrasonography
4. Which of the following treatments is the most proper for a fast-growing papillary cystadenoma lymphomatosum tumor?
   A. Radiation
   B. Chemotherapy
   C. Total parotidectomy + radiation
   D. Superficial parotidectomy
   E. Enucleation
5. Which of the following is not a landmark for identifying the facial nerve during parotidectomy (one or more than one correct answer possible)?
   A. The zygomatic process

Fig. 63.3 Excised parotid gland tumor

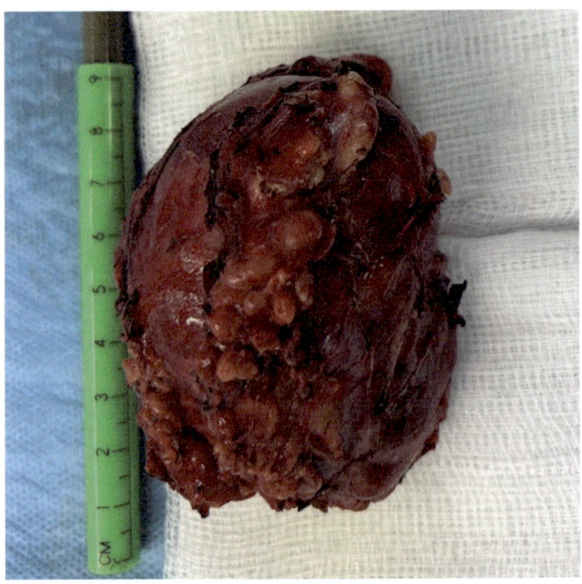

B. The stylomastoid foramen
C. The petrotympanic fissure
D. Digastric muscle
E. Tragal pointer

Answers

1. **B, C, E**

   The Warthin's tumor or papillary cystadenoma lymphomatosum or lymphomatous adenoma or adenolymphoma is a benign tumor of the parotid gland. It is the second most common parotid gland tumor (PGT), after pleomorphic adenoma, comprising approximately about 15% of all PGTs [1]. Moreover, it is more frequent in Caucasians between the sixth and seventh decades of life and in heavy smokers [1]. These tumors can occur bilaterally and/or multiple ipsilaterally with an incidence of about 12% [2]. Generally, PGTs are located in the superficial lobe, which accounts for about 80% of the parotid parenchyma [3]. In addition, Warthin's tumors tend to appear in the parotid tail, with slow growth [4]. Malignant transformation is rare; however, it can occur at a rate of less than 0.1% [1].

2. **A**

   Tumors of the salivary glands account for approximately 3–10% of all head and neck neoplasms. Tumors arise more often in the parotid gland at about 70–80% and in a similar percentage are benign [3–5]. Benign PGTs have a ratio of 3:1 or 4:1 in comparison to malignant PGTs [6]. Pleomorphic adenoma is the most common PGT, representing 35% of all PGTs and 60–70% of all benign PGTs, followed by Warthin's tumor [1, 5, 6]. Malignancies of salivary glands represent about 5–6% of all head and neck cancers [7]. They usually occur in the parotid gland at about 70% [8]. Mucoepidermoid carcinoma is the most frequent type of malignant PGT, comprising approximately 10–15% of all salivary gland neoplasms and 30% of all malignant salivary tumors [4, 8]. Adenoid cystic carcinoma usually occurs in the minor salivary glands, while lipoma is rarely found in the parotid gland [2, 8].

3. **C**

   The fundamental challenge in the management and treatment of parotid masses is differentiating between malignant and benign tumors. This determines the treatment approach. The final diagnosis is usually confirmed after surgery by histological examination. However, fine needle aspiration (FNA) cytology is a quick, safe, simple, inexpensive, complication-free, and accurate diagnostic method when performed by a skilled practitioner, with a sensitivity and specificity of 78% and 87.7%, respectively [9, 10], that can determine the type of PGT preoperatively. Another diagnostic technique with high sensitivity, specificity, and low risk of complications is core needle biopsy [11]. The diagnostic accuracy of FNA cytology and core needle biopsy can be improved with ultrasound guidance [9, 11]. Open biopsy of a PGT is not recommended due to the risk of seeding in the case of malignancy [9]. MRI, computed tomography, and ultrasonography are additional diagnostic tools to assess patients with parotid gland tumors, define the location of the neoplasm, and create the surgery plan. Finally, the history and physical examination are always useful revealing information about the parotid gland mass and the neck [10].

4. **D**

   Papillary cystadenoma lymphomatosum tumor (Warthin's tumor) is situated almost exclusively in the parotid gland. Moreover, it is usually located at the inferior pole of the parotid gland (level II according to the European Salivary Gland Classification). The most common therapy is superficial or partial superficial parotidectomy [12]. Superficial parotidectomy can be performed for every benign tumor of the superficial part of the parotid gland (levels I–III), while partial superficial parotidectomy in cases of large (>4 cm) and medium (3–4 cm) sized tumors of the caudal (level II) and the cranial (level I) part of the parotid gland, respectively [13]. However, extracapsular dissection is an alternative surgical approach for benign PGTs having a similar recurrence rate with superficial parotidectomy and fewer postoperative complications [14]. It can be used "ideally" in small (≤2 cm), well-palpable, and mobile tumors in the periphery of the parotid gland, having no contact to the facial nerve [13]. Total parotidectomy is mainly required in the cases of multiple Warthin's tumors and/or involving the deep lobe [12]. Enucleation is an inadequate surgical approach for parotid gland tumors, due to the increased risk of facial nerve injury and the increased risk of recurrence [13]. Radiation and chemotherapy are additional treatments in some malignant PGTs.

5. **A, C**

   Identifying the facial nerve trunk is essential during parotidectomy because nerve injury may result in inability of muscles on half of the face. There are two approaches to identify the facial nerve trunk: the anterograde and retrograde dissection. Anatomical landmarks have been used to identify the facial nerve early during surgery [15, 16]. The most commonly used landmarks are the stylomastoid foramen, tympanomastoid suture, posterior belly of digastric muscle, tragal pointer, mastoid process, and peripheral branches of the facial nerve [16].

References

1. Fisher R, Ronen O. Cytologic diagnosis of parotid gland Warthin tumor: systematic review and meta-analysis. Head Neck. 2022;44(10):2277–87.
2. Ord RA, Carlson ER. Tumors of the parotid gland. In: Ord RA, Carlson ER, editors. Salivary gland pathology: diagnosis and management. Hoboken, NJ: John Wiley & Sons; 2015. p. 252.
3. Foresta E, Torroni A, Di Nardo F, de Waure C, Poscia A, Gasparini G, Marianetti TM, Pelo S. Pleomorphic adenoma and benign parotid tumors: extracapsular dissection vs superficial parotidectomy-review of literature and meta-analysis. Oral Surg Oral Med Oral Pathol. 2014;117(6):663–76.
4. Gandolfi MM, Slattery W 3rd. Parotid gland tumors and the facial nerve. Otolaryngol Clin N Am. 2016;49(2):425–34.
5. Mashrah MA, Al-Sharani HM, Al-Aroomi MA, Abdelrehem A, Aldhohrah T, Wang L. Surgical interventions for management of benign parotid tumors: systematic review and network meta-analysis. Head Neck. 2021;43(11):3631–45.
6. El Fol HA, Beheiri MJ, Zaqri WA. Comparison of the effect of total conservative parotidectomy versus superficial parotidectomy in management of benign parotid gland tumor: a systematic review. J Craniomaxillofac Surg. 2015. pii: S1010-5182(15)00012-8; https://doi.org/10.1016/j.jcms.2015.01.002.
7. Yan F, Lao WP, Nguyen SA, Sharma AK, Day TA. Elective neck dissection in salivary gland malignancies: systematic review and meta-analysis. Head Neck. 2022;44(2):505–17.
8. Lewis AG, Tong T, Maghami E. Diagnosis and management of malignant salivary gland tumors of the parotid gland. Otolaryngol Clin N Am. 2016;49(2):343–80.
9. Liu CC, Jethwa AR, Khariwala SS, Johnson J, Shin JJ. Sensitivity, specificity, and posttest probability of parotid fine-needle aspiration: a systematic review and meta-analysis. Otolaryngol Head Neck Surg. 2016;154(1):9–23.
10. Carlson ER, Webb DE. The diagnosis and management of parotid disease. Oral Maxillofac Surg Clin North Am. 2013;25(1):31–48. v
11. Witt BL, Schmidt RL. Ultrasound-guided core needle biopsy of salivary gland lesions: a systematic review and meta-analysis. Laryngoscope. 2014;124(3):695–700.
12. Quer M, Hernandez-Prera JC, Silver CE, Casasayas M, Simo R, Vander Poorten V, Guntinas-Lichius O, Bradley PJ, Tong-Ng W, Rodrigo JP, Mäkitie AA, Rinaldo A, Kowalski LP, Sanabria A, de Bree R, Takes RP, López F, Olsen KD, Shaha AR, Ferlito A. Current trends and controversies in the management of Warthin tumor of the parotid gland. Diagnostics (Basel). 2021;11(8):1467.
13. Psychogios G, Bohr C, Constantinidis J, Canis M, Vander Poorten V, Plzak J, Knopf A, Betz C, Guntinas-Lichius O, Zenk J. Review of surgical techniques and guide for decision making in the treatment of benign parotid tumors. Eur Arch Otorhinolaryngol. 2021;278(1):15–29.
14. Albergotti WG, Nguyen SA, Zenk J, Gillespie MB. Extracapsular dissection for benign parotid tumors: a meta-analysis. Laryngoscope. 2012;122(9):1954–60.
15. Poutoglidis A, Paraskevas GK, Lazaridis N, Georgalas C, Vlachtsis K, Markou K, Gougousis S, Fyrmpas G, Keramari S, Tsentemeidou A, Vardaxi X, Garefis K, Poutoglidou F, Tsetsos N. Extratemporal facial nerve branching patterns: systematic review of 1497 cases. J Laryngol Otol. 2022;136(12):1170–6.
16. Righini CA. Facial nerve identification during parotidectomy. Eur Ann Otorhinolaryngol Head Neck Dis. 2012;129(4):214–9.

Parathyroid Disease

64

Nikolaos I. Sakellaris, Eleni I. Sakellari, and Marios Stavrakas

Abstract

Primary hyperparathyroidism is a condition caused by abnormal parathyroid glands producing an excessive amount of parathyroid hormone, resulting in consistently elevated total serum calcium levels. Primary hyperparathyroidism (pHPT) and familial hypocalciuric hypercalcemia (FHH) are both conditions characterized by high calcium levels, but their management and treatment approaches are completely different. pHPT typically requires surgical intervention, while FHH, a genetic condition, is typically managed conservatively because it is benign and does not lead to the complications seen in pHPT. This condition can be diagnosed based on clinical criteria and laboratory studies. Localization of the affected glands can be achieved with imaging studies mainly including ultrasound scan and technetium Tc 99m sestamibi. The most effective treatment for pHPT is parathyroidectomy.

Case Presentation

A 40-year-old lady was referred to the head and neck clinic, with a diagnosis of primary hyperparathyroidism. Her highest corrected calcium was 2.72, with a PTH of 17.9. She was generally well until recently when she has been feeling tired all the time with aches and pains all over, stomach ache, and reduced sleep. She is thirsty and polyureic. There is no history of pancreatitis, and basically she feels 10 years older than she actually is. The imaging on ultrasound and sestamibi (Figs. 64.1 and 64.2) has revealed localization of a 10 mm left-sided parathyroid probable adenoma. Familial hypocalciuric hypercalcemia was already excluded. The patient was consented for a parathyroid exploration.

Questions

1. Which laboratory test is necessary to distinguish primary hyperparathyroidism (pHPT) from familial hypocalciuric hypercalcemia?
   A. Serum total calcium level
   B. Serum parathyroid hormone (PTH) level
   C. Serum creatinine level

N. I. Sakellaris
Department of Otolaryngology, "G. Gennimatas" General Hospital of Athens, Athens, Greece

E. I. Sakellari
Faculty of Health Sciences, Aristotle University of Thessaloniki, AHEPA University Hospital, Thessaloniki, Greece

M. Stavrakas (✉)
ENT Head and Neck Surgery Department, University Hospitals Plymouth NHS Trust, Plymouth, UK

N. Tsetsos et al. (eds.), *Otolaryngology Study Guide*, https://doi.org/10.1007/978-3-031-77374-7_64

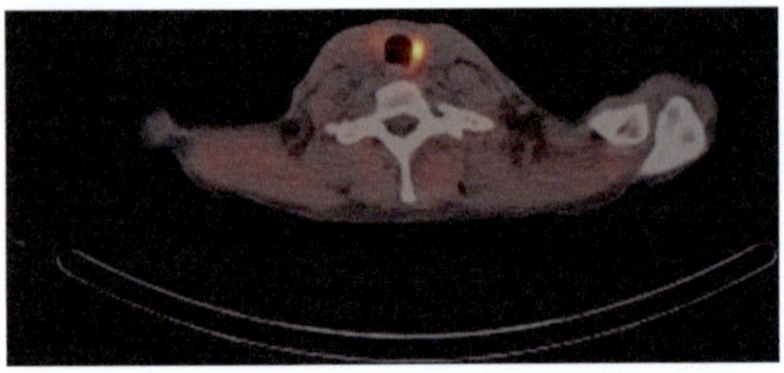

Fig. 64.1 Sestamibi scan demonstrating a focus of retained tracer uptake just behind the left lobe of the thyroid gland

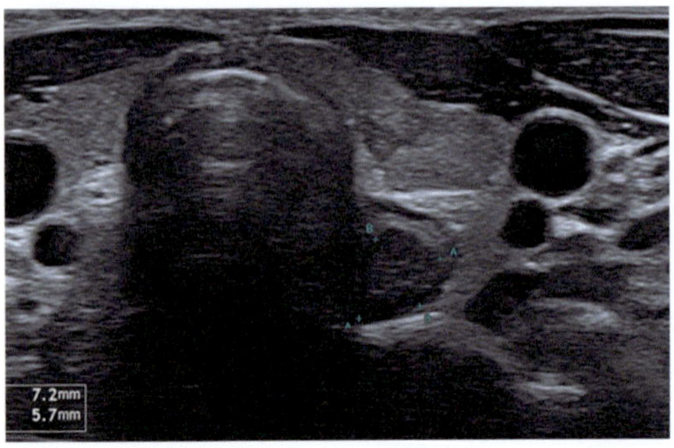

Fig. 64.2 US neck, showing a solid lesion positioned posteromedially to the left thyroid lobe

   D. 24-h urine measurement of calcium and creatinine
   E. Bone mineral density measurement using dual-energy X-ray absorptiometry (DXA)
2. When is parathyroidectomy indicated for patients with pHPT?
   A. For all patients with symptomatic pHPT
   B. For patients with significantly elevated serum calcium levels
   C. For patients with symptoms such as fractures
   D. For patients with evidence of renal involvement
   E. All of the above
3. In patients with pHPT who present with hypercalcemic crisis (rapid-onset, albumin-corrected serum calcium level greater than 14 mg/dL), what is the recommended management approach?
   A. Immediate parathyroidectomy
   B. Intravenous fluid monitoring
   C. Dietary restriction of calcium
   D. Intravenous fluid resuscitation and medical management, followed by parathyroidectomy
   E. High-dose vitamin D supplementation
4. Which of the following statements are true (more than one correct answer possible)?
   A. Imaging results can be used to confirm or exclude the diagnosis of pHPT
   B. Preoperative management should include both sonography and a functional imaging technique
   C. Patients with negative imaging results are not eligible for parathyroidectomy
   D. Preoperative parathyroid fine needle aspiration biopsy is recommended only in specific cases of pHPT
   E. Ultrasonography is accurate in excluding a multiglandular parathyroid disease
5. Which of the following statements are true (more than one correct answer possible)?
   A. Minimally invasive parathyroidectomy is recommended for multiglandular disease (MGD)
   B. Minimally invasive parathyroidectomy is recommended for single parathyroid adenoma
   C. A careful capsular removal with no need of adherent tissue extraction is the preferable option for cases of parathyroid carcinoma
   D. Bilateral exploration is the preferred approach in cases highly suspicious of MGD
   E. Adjuvant external beam radiotherapy should be routinely performed after surgical resection of parathyroid carcinoma

Answers

1. **D**

Primary hyperparathyroidism is a prevalent condition caused by abnormal parathyroid glands producing an excessive amount of parathyroid hormone, resulting in consistently elevated total serum calcium levels [1]. Primary hyperparathyroidism (pHPT) and familial hypocalciuric hypercalcemia (FHH) are both conditions characterized by high calcium levels, but their management and treatment approaches are very different [2]. pHPT typically requires surgical intervention, while FHH, a genetic condition, is typically managed conservatively because it is benign and does not lead to the complications seen in pHPT [2]. FHH can mimic the presentation of pHPT, but it is characterized by low urinary calcium excretion, which can be assessed through a 24-h urine collection test [1]. Patients with FHH typically have urinary calcium levels less than 100 mg/24 h and calcium-to-creatinine clearance ratio less than 0.01 [1]. On the other hand, patients with pHPT will often have higher levels of calcium in their urine due to the overactivity of their parathyroid glands [1].

2. **E**

   The most effective treatment for pHPT is parathyroidectomy [1]. Parathyroidectomy is indicated for all patients displaying symptoms of hypercalcemia such as persistent polydipsia, polyuria, and constipation. It is also recommended for those with end-organ failure, notably nephrolithiasis, nephrocalcinosis, fragility fractures, especially vertebral compression fractures, or established osteoporosis [1, 3, 4]. In general, patients with symptoms impacting their health-related quality of life, such as neurocognitive, psychiatric, and cardiovascular symptoms, are also potential candidates for surgery [1, 3]. Moreover, notable elevation in serum calcium levels by more than 1 mg/dL above normal or an albumin-adjusted serum calcium level of 2.85 mmol/L or above, regardless of symptoms, serves as another indication for surgery [1, 4]. Successful parathyroidectomy not only reduces the risk of kidney stones and may contribute to stabilizing kidney function but also improves bone mineral density and decreases fracture rates. This benefit holds true even for patients with normal or osteopenic bone [1].

3. **D**

   A hypercalcemic crisis is an urgent medical condition characterized by a rapid rise in serum calcium levels above 14 mg/dL, accompanied by manifestations of multiorgan dysfunction [1, 3]. Noteworthy symptoms include acute kidney failure nausea, pancreatitis, and possibility of cardiac arrest [1, 3]. Given its life-threatening nature, immediate intervention is imperative [1, 3]. Prompt management involves intravenous fluid resuscitation and pharmacologic measures tailored to individual symptoms, aiming to stabilize the patient's condition prior to an expedited parathyroidectomy [1, 3].

4. **B, D**

   The main goal of using imaging techniques for pHPT is to achieve precise localization of the affected parathyroid gland and to determine the patients that are suitable for minimal invasive surgery [1, 5]. While the diagnosis of pHPT relies on clinical presentation, laboratory tests, and other diagnostic criteria, imaging results do not serve as diagnostic determinants [1]. The most cost-effective imaging strategy involves a combination of a cervical ultrasonography and a functional imaging technique such as technetium Tc 99m sestamibi [1, 3, 4]. However, both imaging techniques exhibit limited sensitivity in identifying a multiglandular parathyroid disease [1]. Parathyroid fine needle aspiration biopsy is infrequently necessary and not recommended for all cases of pHPT [1]. It can be used in carcinoma suspicious cases [1]. Patients with negative imaging results can still be candidates for parathyroidectomy [1].

5. **B, D**

   The most frequently used surgical approach for primary hyperparathyroidism is minimally invasive parathyroidectomy (MIP), which is recommended for cases with a single parathyroid adenoma [1]. Due to the high percentage of patients with a single adenoma and the advantages of focused surgery, such as lower hypocalcemia rates and cosmetic benefits, MIP is the preferable option [1, 4]. However, considering the 5% chance of persistent or recurrent disease even in patients with a single adenoma, a four-gland exploration should also be considered as an option [4]. In patients with negative imaging results or a high suspicion of multiglandular disease (MGD), bilateral exploration (four-gland) is the preferred operative strategy [1, 4]. In cases of parathyroid carcinoma, a complete resection avoiding capsular disruption and, if necessary, en bloc resection of adherent tissues should be preferred. Postoperative adjuvant external beam radiotherapy can be performed as a palliative option [1]. Successful parathyroidectomy can be assessed intraoperatively by frozen section histological confirmation and PTH level monitoring. A drop in PTH of 50% or more within 10 min of tumor resection indicates a successful parathyroidectomy [6].

References

1. Wilhelm SM, Wang TS, Ruan DT, et al. The American Association of Endocrine Surgeons guidelines for definitive management of primary hyperparathyroidism. JAMA Surg. 2016;151(10):959–68. https://doi.org/10.1001/jamasurg.2016.2310.
2. Shinall MC Jr, Dahir KM, Broome JT. Differentiating familial hypocalciuric hypercalcemia from primary hyperparathyroidism. Endocr Pract. 2013;19(4):697–702. https://doi.org/10.4158/EP12284.RA.
3. Weber T, Dotzenrath C, Dralle H, et al. Management of primary and renal hyperparathyroidism: guidelines from the German Association of Endocrine Surgeons (CAEK). Langenbecks Arch Surg. 2021;406(3):571–85. https://doi.org/10.1007/s00423-021-02173-1.
4. Hyperparathyroidism (primary): diagnosis, assessment and initial management. NICE Guideline, No. 132. London: National Institute for Health and Care Excellence (NICE); 2019. https://www.ncbi.nlm.nih.gov/books/NBK542087/.
5. Piciucchi S, Barone D, Gavelli G, Dubini A, Oboldi D, Matteuci F. Primary hyperparathyroidism: imaging to pathology. J Clin Imaging Sci. 2012;2:59. https://doi.org/10.4103/2156-7514.102053.
6. Smith N, Magnuson JS, Vidrine DM, Kulbersh B, Peters GE. Minimally invasive parathyroidectomy: use of intraoperative parathyroid hormone assays after 2 preoperative localization studies. Arch Otolaryngol Head Neck Surg. 2009;135(11):1108–11.

MIX
Papier aus verantwortungsvollen Quellen
Paper from responsible sources
FSC® C105338

If you have any concerns about our products,
you can contact us on
ProductSafety@springernature.com

In case Publisher is established outside the EU,
the EU authorized representative is:
Springer Nature Customer Service Center GmbH
Europaplatz 3, 69115 Heidelberg, Germany

Printed by Libri Plureos GmbH
in Hamburg, Germany